"As a yoga therapist and parent of two older children with complex needs, I only wish that I had access to Shawnee Thornton Hardy's wise counsel many years ago. Her book, *Yoga Therapy for Children and Teens with Complex Needs*, isn't just a compilation of tools. It is a beacon of hope for those of us struggling to connect with our children. And, best of all, it offers our kids a pathway back home to themselves. With clear examples, practices and scientific evidence, Hardy shows us there is a path forward, even when we feel lost and confused. She explains: 'The practice of yoga is a practice of coming home to ourselves. The intuitive, curious, joyful and present nature of who we truly are beyond our experiences in life. A coming home to our innate wholeness, wellness and interconnectedness with the world.' Thank you, Shawnee, for shining a light in the dark and helping us all find our way home."

—*Jivana Heyman, author of* Accessible Yoga
*and* Yoga Revolution

"Shawnee Thornton Hardy offers her wisdom and expertise with heart and clarity in this much-needed and important resource to support children and teens. This book will provide the reader an accessible and comprehensive guide for assessment and program development strategies, informed by yoga philosophy and practices, integrated with neurophysiology and psychology frameworks."

—*Marlysa Sullivan, DPT, C-IAYT, E-RYT, author of*
Understanding Yoga Therapy

T0385366

*by the same author*

**Asanas for Autism and Special Needs**
Yoga to Help Children with Their Emotions, Self-Regulation and Body Awareness
*Shawnee Thornton Hardy*
ISBN 978 1 84905 988 6
eISBN 978 1 78450 059 7


*of related interest*

**Teen Yoga For Yoga Therapists**
A Guide to Development, Mental Health and Working with Common Teen Issues
*Charlotta Martinus*
*Foreword by Sir Anthony Seldon*
ISBN 978 1 84819 399 4
eISBN 978 0 85701 355 2


**Yoga for Children and Young People with Autism**
Yoga Games and Activities to Engage Everyone Across the Spectrum
*Michael Chissick*
*Illustrated by Sarah Peacock*
ISBN 978 1 78592 679 2
eISBN 978 1 78592 863 5


**Zensations**
*Frank J. Sileo and Christopher Willard*
*Illustrated by Lily Fossett*
ISBN 978 1 83997 679 7
eISBN 978 1 83997 680 3

# Yoga Therapy

## for Children and Teens
## with Complex Needs

### A Somatosensory Approach
### to Mental, Emotional and
### Physical Wellbeing

**Shawnee Thornton Hardy**

Foreword by Amy Wheeler

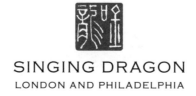

SINGING DRAGON

LONDON AND PHILADELPHIA

First published in Great Britain in 2023 by Singing Dragon,
an imprint of Jessica Kingsley Publishers
Part of John Murray Press

I

Front cover image source: Photography by Tim Hardy. The cover image is
for illustrative purposes only, and any person featuring is a model.

Models featured in the photographs are: Ella Timpe-Calsyn, Kaian Marley White Menezes,
Makena Marilia White Menezes, Lania Star White Menezes, Naiya Paz White Menezes,
Liam Mulcaire-Jones, Aavni Muir Bajaj, Naya Mae Bajaj, Aria Fine, Noam Krentzman.

Body outline, sensations images, breathing, emotions and
animal drawings illustrated by Jesse Hotchkiss.
Figures 6.1–6.4 illustrated by Lior Zackaria Hikrey.
Photographs (excluding Chapter 6) by Tim Hardy shotbyhardy.com.

A CIP catalogue record for this title is available from the
British Library and the Library of Congress

ISBN 978 1 78775 225 2
eISBN 978 1 78775 226 9

Printed and bound in Great Britain by TJ Books Limited

Jessica Kingsley Publishers' policy is to use papers that are natural, renewable and recyclable
products and made from wood grown in sustainable forests. The logging and manufacturing
processes are expected to conform to the environmental regulations of the country of origin.

Jessica Kingsley Publishers
Carmelite House
50 Victoria Embankment
London EC4Y 0DZ

www.singingdragon.com

John Murray Press
Part of Hodder & Stoughton Limited
An Hachette UK Company

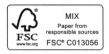

MIX
Paper from
responsible sources
FSC® C013056

# Dedications

I would like to dedicate this book to the children and youth I've worked with throughout the years who are perfectly whole and beautiful, and who have taught me about patience, compassion, perseverance and the importance of being authentic in my work and in my life. To the parents who dedicate their hearts to their children and are *always* doing their best. To the many angels out in the world: parents, teachers, caregivers, therapists, social workers, mental health practitioners and medical professionals, who dedicate their lives to supporting children and helping them to live happier, healthier and more peaceful lives. To my mother, who has embodied strength, resilience and unconditional love, and has taught me what it is to be an empowered woman, tender like a lamb but brave like a lion. To my brothers, whom I admire and love dearly, and to whom I will be forever connected through our shared grief and joys in life. To Willa, Samuel, Ben, Nathaniel and Alexios, my niece and nephews who fill my heart with joy and remind me of the beauty of childhood and the importance of play. To my willful, curious and empathic daughter who is my breath, my heartbeat and my reason for healing, and to my loving husband who is my greatest support, my life partner, my best friend, my safe person and the talented photographer for my book.

I also want to dedicate this book in memory of my beloved uncle who gave me my birth name, Shawnee. Named after a beautiful white horse he once knew. White horses are thought to symbolize strength, freedom and wisdom. Several days after my uncle's passing, a white butterfly landed on my shoulder and rested there for what seemed like an eternity. White butterflies symbolize healing and spiritual transformation, and it is thought that if you see a white butterfly, an angel is looking over you. There are no coincidences in life, only synchronicities. The white horse and butterfly are a reminder to me of both the strength and fragility of life and the importance of embracing each one as we move through the world. May our hearts hold our own strength and fragility with reverence and care. May I embody strength, wisdom and freedom, and may I continue to move towards transformation and healing in myself, so I can best facilitate transformation and healing in others. May I be the horse and the butterfly.

# Contents

# Acknowledgments

I first want to acknowledge my many teachers and mentors who have shared their knowledge and wisdom so graciously. It is in their willingness to share their hearts' work that I have been able to share mine. To my publisher, Singing Dragon, whose patience and understanding allowed me the time and space to heal in order to have the capacity to finish this book. I am grateful for their grace and their belief in the importance of this work. To Peter Levine for developing Somatic Experiencing, to which I attribute a deeper understanding of myself and our body's innate wisdom and ability to heal from prolonged stress and trauma. To my dear friends, whose work I respect and admire, Rachel Krentzman and Ann Magnuson Davis. Thank you for your willingness to contribute your wisdom to this book. To Mallika Varadarajan Iyer, who has been part of my faculty for years, for contributing her pediatric PT expertise. To Mother Earth: it is only with your continued offering of your beautiful animals, trees, lakes, oceans, mountains, sky and earth in which I've taken respite that I am here today. You have been my greatest resource, my inspiration, my co-regulator, my solace in times of despair. May we as human beings honor and care for you. May we not take more than we need. May we recognize that we are not separate from you but part of you.

# Disclaimers

The suggestions for practices in this book are not intended to diagnose or replace medical advice. Each child or teen will present with their own unique physical, sensory, cognitive, social and emotional needs. It is up to the adult to know their scope of practice or limitations when working with a child with complex needs. If you are new to these practices and want to share them with children and teens, it is recommended that you attend educational trainings and receive mentorship from skilled teachers and practitioners in order to learn these tools in an embodied way and apply them safely based on the individual needs of each child or teen. Ahimsa—non-harm—should always be at the forefront of these teachings. As you continue to learn, practice the activities in your own body and apply these tools when working with children and teens; you will begin to develop greater intuition that can only come from practice and experience.

# Foreword

This book has the potential to change the perspective of generations of neuro-divergent kids who are experiencing mental health challenges and the effects of unprocessed trauma. The book is for their parents, educators, mental health professionals, yoga therapists, occupational therapists and physical therapists, and anyone else who works with children and teens. As adults, our goal is to support our youth in allowing the best of humanity to emerge and grow. We want to encourage the special gifts that these kids and teens express so naturally. The question is: "What is the world going to need in the next 30 years?" I believe that we are going to need creative and compassionate humans who think outside the box. Shawnee's book is the perfect resource for helping youth build capacity to navigate the challenges of life and be the embodied, present, reflective, grounded and empowered community members we need for the future.

The main concepts outlined in this book are a perfect marriage between modern neuroscience and the ancient teachings of yoga, aimed to support children and teens to function well in their minds, bodies and lives. The book includes a guide for how yoga and somatic practices can be used in the modern context with children and teens to promote more self-awareness and the ability to manage emotions, be more socially aware, build better relationships and make decisions that support their wellbeing. This book sets the tone for an embodied, *whole-child approach* to health and healing for kids. Shawnee shares time-tested and kid-tested strategies that she has found to be successful in her decades of work with youth.

Her book takes us on a deep journey reviewing the latest neuroscience around kids' brains and how their nervous systems function when under stressful stimuli compared to when they are feeling calm and at ease. Shawnee brings in medical language and research about how to create a regulated and balanced autonomic nervous system. She offers a lens into how trauma impacts brain development and how, without proper support, trauma can lead to overactive nervous system functioning, or even generalized feelings of lack of safety. Shawnee emphasizes the importance of connection and co-regulation between the child and adult, and how this facilitates a felt sense of trust and safety. The experiential tools in the book will not only support youth but also support adults in regulating their own nervous systems. Many caretakers are unaware of the high levels of allostatic load they are carrying around, and it is no wonder that they are not able to regulate themselves, much less co-regulate with the children and teens. If we could get parents, educators and the adults in the room to do these practices alongside the children they live and work with, huge changes would happen at a personal level and also at the systemic and structural levels of education, parenting and healthcare.

Shawnee's reflection on her own childhood, filled with dysfunction, addiction and loss in her family of origin, reminds us of our humanity, our capacity to endure challenges and our ability to find meaning and purpose in the ups and downs of life. Throughout the book, she offers moments to pause and reflect on our own childhood experiences, find compassion for our younger selves and tend to our inner children with understanding and care. Shawnee was a highly sensitive being who spontaneously found that nature could help her to co-regulate so that she could move from survival to resilience, and finally a state of thriving in adulthood. It was these early experiences that set the stage for Shawnee to find her dharma, or life purpose. Her purpose is to help other highly sensitive, neuro-diverse, anxious, depressed or traumatized children and teens understand how to regulate themselves from the inside out. She offers tools to educators, parents, therapists and healthcare providers to support kids in building self-awareness, self-agency and emotional stability in order to move through the world with more confidence, curiosity and connection. Isn't that what we all want for our kids and for the future of humanity? I can empathically say "YES!" I wish my parents and I had been able to read this book as we navigated my personal trials in middle school and high school. These were some of the most traumatic times of my life, which I am still working through the negative impacts of to this day. For we must not forget, the seeds we plant today are the flowers of tomorrow. Immerse yourself in Shawnee's book and use the information to plant positive, balanced and nourishing seeds that will set the stage for the collective future of humanity.

With gratitude for Shawnee and her second book,

*Amy Wheeler, PhD., C-IAYT*
*Founder of Optimal State Yoga Therapy School and Yoga Nidra School, Former*
*President of the Board of the International Association of Yoga Therapists (2018–2020)*

# Preface

Before reading this book, I invite you to picture your younger self.

Your younger self may show up as an infant, toddler, adolescent or teen. As you picture your younger self, notice any characteristics or qualities that come to mind. Notice if your younger self is in a certain place. Notice what your younger self is doing. Notice the expression on the face of your younger self. Notice the posture. Notice the energy. Tell your younger self, "I am here with you."

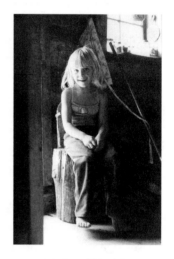

If emotions begin to arise, acknowledge them, allow them, and let your younger self know that you are here, now, to be a compassionate witness to any sadness, grief, anger or pain that may show up. Imagine your adult self holding the hand of your younger self tenderly, with unconditional love and compassion. Place your hands on your heart and repeat these words to your younger self: "I see you, I hear you, I love you, I value you."

So much of our work with children comes from our capacity to connect with our own inner child, to hold our younger parts with compassion and to continue to do our own inner-child healing work so we are able to show up for the children we serve from a place of love and healthy connection.

When I picture myself as a young child, I see a little girl with raggedy blonde hair and gapped teeth, climbing trees, building forts with sticks and riding her dirt bike in the mountains of Montana. She's sensitive, curious, inquisitive and a girlish tomboy. She has an insatiable love for reading and wants to be a teacher someday. She loves to write—words are her escape. She is tender and kind, and she loves animals. She has a sensitive heart that can love deeply but be hurt easily. She spends her days sitting beneath the aspen trees, daydreaming of traveling to far-off places. She loves to draw. She is timid and shy, with an inner strength and resilience she doesn't yet know she has. Someday she wants to make a difference in the world.

This little girl is how I found my heart's work and how I came to write this book.

I grew up in the mountains of Montana in a tiny round log house with my mom, my dad and my two brothers. We didn't have electricity or running water. We had little money, but we were rich in the abundance of trees, mountains, creeks, waterfalls and nature that surrounded us. I speak of this because I believe nature "saved" me, and it has continued to be my greatest resource.

Life was a struggle at times. My dad was an alcoholic, critical, unpredictable and sometimes abusive. He angered easily, and much of my childhood I remember fearing him. I wasn't allowed to show emotion around him or in response to his behavior. If I showed sadness, I was "whiny," if I showed anger, I was "bitchy," so I learned to stuff my emotions down and believed that they weren't important. My mom is a loving and caring person, and is now my best friend and greatest support, but in those early years of my life, she wasn't able to be the emotionally present parent I needed. She herself was in a state of survival, and much of her energy went toward my dad and her co-dependent relationship with his addiction. I spent much of my early childhood feeling alone and without the emotional and physical protection from those who were responsible for protecting me. Many times in my growing up, my boundaries were crossed. In fact, at the time I didn't really have a sense of what a boundary was, let alone that I could have boundaries. On many occasions throughout my childhood and teenage years, I received unsolicited attention from adult men that felt shameful. Shame that would eventually become part of my perception of myself. I absorbed the shame of others as part of who I was.

When I turned 13, I moved into town with my brother, cousin and an "adult chaperone" in order to attend high school. We saw our parents when they came to town from the mountains, but we were essentially on our own. We had a lot of freedom, but there was a deep-rooted need in my survival being to always "be in control." I had a passion for running and placed a lot of my energy into competing in cross country. I was on the varsity team as a freshman. I was driven, a perfectionist and fully in control, or so I thought.

In my teenage years, my dad's addiction got increasingly worse. He had developed a considerable amount of back pain and began taking Percocet as a means to alleviate his pain. This began the spiral of addiction to other drugs. He would often come to town to get his fix, perhaps as an escape from life and all of its responsibilities. There was a point where all we saw was this stranger, drugged out and drunk, who sometimes didn't even recognize where he was or who we were. I felt a tremendous amount of anger toward him and also a responsibility to take care of him. This is the role he had given me. To take care of him when my mom wasn't around to do that for him. It was a cycle of co-dependence that I would carry with me into my adult life.

Memory is an interesting thing. I have very little memory of joyful times with my dad, even though I know there were glimpses. The memory that stands out for me is the last words I said to my dad before he died. He had come to town to do what he had always done. He was drunk and I was angry. I was angry that he didn't care enough about us to stop drinking and doing drugs. I was angry about all of the times he hurt me. I wanted him to feel the pain he had caused his family. We got into an argument, and I told him I hated him. He left. I felt guilt and shame for hurting him, so I made up a bed for him on the couch and waited for him to come home, but he never did. The next day, I found out my dad had died of a drug overdose. A lethal injection someone else had given him. These same people took him to the hospital and, rather than bringing him inside, dropped him off outside, leaving him there to die cold and alone. I was 15. The me who had felt so in control began to unravel after my dad's death. When I would drink, though it wasn't often, it was to get drunk. To drown my sorrows and escape from the pain. In the midst of the grief, just six months later, I was raped. I didn't tell anyone. My last years of high school, I lost my sense of self. I felt alone in my grief and shame. I felt broken. I developed bulimia, which I now know was my own attempt to purge the deep emotions that just felt too overwhelming for me to bear. I stopped running and struggled to make it to my classes. I had suicidal ideation and felt such a tremendous feeling of survivor's guilt. I felt as though I should have saved my dad, and that I was a failure because I didn't. This would haunt me for years into my early adulthood, and I would find myself in relationships where I was living out this role as being the "fixer," saving my partners from their addictions, dismissing my own needs for the sake of others.

At age 17, right after my graduation, I moved to Boston. All I wanted to do was escape. Escape the small town where everyone knew my story. Escape the pain and grief. Escape the memories of the past. Escape the anxiety and the feelings of loneliness. Even though the grief and anxiety still remained, it was the best decision I could have made for myself. A new chapter, a new beginning.

It's not a surprise that I ended up working as a nanny and a teaching assistant at a preschool. I was fiercely mature, independent and driven at the age of 17. I had always felt a love for children and had always known that I wanted to be a teacher. I took joy in reading my little brother's bedtime stories. I remember lining up my porcelain dolls in a row, as if they were my pupils and I had important lessons to teach them.

For some it takes a lifetime to realize their Dharma and life's purpose. For me, it was always known. Perhaps it was my own feeling of missing the experience of a carefree childhood or my heart's understanding of the struggles of childhood and adolescence that drew me to this work. Perhaps it was my desire to show up for children in the ways that others weren't able to show up for me. Perhaps it was the deep sense of purpose that working with children brought to me. Perhaps it was the contagious energy of joy and curiosity that children evoke.Perhaps it was my own subconscious way of beginning my journey of healing my inner, wounded child.

In yoga, we speak of gurus, a Sanskrit term for mentor, guide or master. My first guru was a young boy named Austin who was attending the preschool where I was assisting. He was unique, quirky, loveable and brilliant in his own way. He had a fascination with vacuum cleaners and could tell you the names of all the brands and all the parts that made up the whole of a vacuum. He struggled with connecting to the other children and had difficulty managing the uncomfortable emotions that came from the different ways in which his brain and body understood and navigated the world. He had a single mom, Sarah, who was doing her best in raising a child who was not easily understood by others. Perhaps it was his brilliance and his unique way of seeing the world. Perhaps it was my own lived experience of feeling as if no one else understood me. Perhaps it was simply just divine intervention that we were drawn to one another. This was my first insight into the world of autism, and I longed to learn and understand more so I could help Austin and other children who were struggling. He was my teacher, and I was his. He is the one who directed me on my path toward my heart's work. I honor him and the impact he had on my life and am forever grateful for his teachings.

Fast-forward years later and nearly two decades of working with children with diverse needs and backgrounds when my love for working with children and my passion for yoga merged.

It wasn't until my early 30s that I found yoga, or, more accurately, yoga found me. It was a hugely challenging and transitional time in my life. I was going through a divorce, was a single mother, had been diagnosed with Hashimoto's thyroiditis, was experiencing significant back pain, and my lifelong experience of anxiety was elevated to a point that felt overwhelming and paralyzing. When I took my first yoga class, I cried almost the whole way through. I felt a cathartic release of grief and sadness that I had been holding in for so long. As I became dedicated to my practice, I experienced a feeling of strength, embodiment and inner peace that I had never felt before. My yoga practice was a way for me to be in my body, connect to my emotions and attend to myself and my needs. I found, with consistent practice, that I was less anxious, more focused and more present in my life.

It became my mission and passion to share these practices with the children I was working with. All of the children I had worked with over the years had experienced some form of trauma. Many were severely abused as children. Many struggled with sensory integration challenges, learning and communication difficulties. Many children were navigating the world with disability, chronic pain and fatigue. Many struggled with anxiety and depression. Most of the children's nervous systems were dysregulated, which significantly impacted their learning, behavior, communication and social connection with others.

I began to adapt the traditional yoga practices I had learned in my yoga training toward children with diverse needs, and I explored breathing, movement and mindfulness practices as tools to support increased body awareness, focus and attention, self-regulation (including emotional regulation), communication, self-confidence, self-esteem and social connection. Yoga became an integral part of my educational and behavioral programming in the classroom. We took frequent "yoga breaks" throughout the day and integrated yoga into the learning curriculum. The incredible impact I saw these practices have on the children inspired me to write my first book, *Asanas for Autism and Special Needs: Yoga to Help Children with Their Emotions, Self-Regulation and Body Awareness*.

Thus came my desire to share the tools I had developed with other teachers so that these transformational practices could be shared with a greater number of children. It has been my authentic experience that all too many children with diverse needs are left out of opportunities and experiences simply due to the lack of education and training of the adult supports and equal access in the community. The deepest intention of my work is to make the practices of yoga and mindfulness inclusive and accessible to children of all brains, bodies and abilities. It has been my greatest honor and gift to be able to offer trainings to others who have a common passion and desire to share these practices with all children. The people whom I've had the pleasure of meeting in the trainings are from around the world with such diverse backgrounds in their work with children. They have enriched my life in so many ways, and I have learned so much from them. That feeling of loneliness and not being understood by others that I carried with me for so long diminished when I found my heart Sangha. The connection with so many beautiful humans fills me up and inspires me to keep moving forward on this path.

As I merged my two passions and continued on my journey of yoga therapy studies, I had the opportunity to do many private yoga sessions with children of varying ages with varying needs throughout the years. Through these experiences, I grew as a yoga therapist and learned a great deal from the children I worked with. My lifelong experience in working with children and my studies in yoga therapy had merged in such an effortless and synchronous manner. One can only call it *destiny*.

Now as I continue my journey of teaching and learning, I have been called to trauma work. I am grateful to have completed three years of study in Somatic Experiencing developed by Peter Levine, which brought even more clarity to my path and my purpose. I often say studying the Somatic Experiencing training happened at the best time and also the worst time in my life. At the start of the training, I had just been in a significant car accident and was experiencing symptoms of PTSD. Throughout the duration of the three-year trauma training, I had a near-death car accident, witnessed my uncle drown before my eyes and was diagnosed with breast cancer. All of this amidst a global pandemic. There were moments in that period of time that I could sense myself contracting, isolating from others and going into a state of immobilization and freeze. My traumatic experiences from my childhood and recent traumas became over-coupled. My neuroception of the world was that it was a dangerous place, that I was going to lose the people I loved, that I shouldn't trust myself or others; should I allow myself to feel joy, something terrible and tragic would surely happen. Over the duration of those three years, I was also fortunate to have studied developmental trauma and healing applications with Kathy Kain and Stephen Terrell. This gave me a greater understanding of my own attachment style and how important in my own healing it was to have a compassionate witness, a safe base of support. My experience showed me that healing happens *in relationship* with others. Even in the midst all of the trauma, the grief, the desire to contract and hide from the world, I was learning in real time about the nervous system and how trauma impacts the way we move through the world. I was also learning tools to help me navigate moving through those traumas, current and from my childhood. Knowledge is empowering.

The merging of all of my life experiences, my own childhood and recent life traumas, my deep love for and connection with children with complex needs, my devotion to healing my own inner child and adult wounds, my passion for and belief in yoga and somatic practices, my insatiable desire to learn and grow, and my heart's longing to be of good service in the world are what have brought me here, to this moment, writing this book. I truly believe we can turn our pain into purpose. Through our own lived experience, we can serve as a beacon of hope to others.

It is my intention that this book serves as a resource for others to support children and teens in navigating the world with more curiosity, confidence and connection. Our children are our greatest hope for our future. May they feel seen, heard, loved and equally valued. May this book be a conduit to healing in the world.

## INNER CHILD

*There is a voice in your heart*
*Longing to be heard*
*An invisible child*
*Hoping to be seen*
*Tiny hands reaching out*
*Wishing to be held*
*In bearing witness*
*To suffering untold*
*Showing up*
*With love and grace*
*Wounds can mend*
*Hand in hand*
*Your grown-up self*
*Your younger one*
*Together*
*Knowing now*
*You'll never again*
*Feel alone*

Shawnee Thornton Hardy

It is my hope as you move through this book that you tend to your own inner child. It is in our own healing work, showing up for our younger parts, that we can best show up for others. Throughout the book, I offer *inner-child reflections*. I invite you to *pause and reflect* when you arrive at each one. If it calls to you, you may want to have a designated journal to write, draw and explore with compassion and curiosity.

Chapter 1

# What Is Yoga Therapy?

Embodying a Whole-Child Approach

## WHAT IS YOGA THERAPY?

Although all yoga is potentially therapeutic and healing, yoga therapy is the specific application of yogic tools—postures/exercises, breathwork, meditation techniques and more—to address an individual's physical, mental and emotional needs.

IAYT—the International Association of Yoga Therapists—defines yoga therapy as "the process of empowering individuals to progress toward improved health and well-being through the application of the teachings and practices of Yoga" (IAYT, n.d.).

According to IAYT, the application of yoga therapy is from one or more of three perspectives:

1. The application of shakti-krama: The use of yoga to gain a sense of power, i.e., the power of muscular strength, concentration, engaging in challenging postures and experiencing stamina.
2. The application of chikitsâ-krama: The use of yoga to heal specific physical ailments in the body, such as impurities in the organs (doshas) or energy centers (chakras) and channels (nâdîs).
   - Healing from sickness (chikitsâ).
   - The prevention of or protection from sickness (rakshana).
   - If sickness and protection is not needed, the acquiring of knowledge and skill is necessary (shikshana).
3. The application of âdhyâtmika-krama: The use of yoga beyond the physical to a deeper understanding of the limited sense of self. One's true self as unchanging (purusha) and all that is changing (prakriti).

(Miller, n.d.)

Yoga therapists have in-depth training to help them assess the individual and develop a therapeutic protocol uniquely designed to support them in their healing. They work with individuals to address their specific goals while considering any limitations or challenges they might be experiencing. The emphasis in a yoga therapy session is to work in partnership and collaboration with the individual so they build a sense of self-agency and self-empowerment in their own ability to improve their wellbeing. We as yoga therapists are facilitators of healing, but true healing is in the hands of the individual. Of course, children rely on this co-facilitation and consistent support of an adult, but they too can learn to pilot their own planes and build a sense of agency in how they move through the world. The practices a yoga therapist recommends could include:

- movement ranging from gentle to vigorous
- breathing techniques
- meditation or visualization practices
- physical postures that address specific areas of discomfort or musculoskeletal imbalances
- any combination of tools like these.

## THERAPEUTIC YOGA APPLICATIONS

This book emphasizes therapeutic approaches to support children and teens with mental, emotional and physical wellbeing. The therapeutic approaches emphasized include:

- asana, movement and somatic practices
- breathing strategies
- meditation and visualization practices
- chanting and sound
- mantras and mudras
- attunement and co-regulation
- connection with nature
- expressive arts therapy
- other holistic approaches.

According to a recent research summary on yoga therapy for pediatrics, gathered from multiple databases, including 13 randomized controlled trials, yoga shows promising results in terms of its benefits for children and adolescents. The results of the summary showed the following (Evan *et al.*, 2016).

Physical health challenges:

1. **IBS (irritable bowel syndrome)**: Reduction in abdominal pain and gastrointestinal symptoms related to IBS.
2. **PCOS (polycystic ovary syndrome)**: Yoga was found to be more effective than physical exercise for improving glucose metabolism in adolescent girls with PCOS.
3. **Poor physical coordination**: Decreased negative responses in Children's Body Satisfaction test.

Psychosocial wellbeing:

1. Improvements in behavior and attention in children with attention deficit hyperactivity disorder (ADHD).
2. Improved IQ and social adaptation in children with intellectual disabilities.
3. Greater reduction in symptoms and lowered food preoccupation in adolescents with eating disorders.
4. Improvement in self-esteem and self-regulation in children coping with stress.
5. Improvement in scores of voluntary engagement, rumination, intrusive thoughts and emotional arousal in underserved youth.
6. Improvement in anger control and fatigue/inertia outcomes and reduction in mood disturbance, mood anxiety and negative affect in well children.

## EMBODYING A WHOLE-CHILD APPROACH
Yoga therapy for youth and the contents of this book emphasize embodying a whole-child approach when working with children and youth—seeing the child through a lens of compassion and recognizing they are whole and beautiful beings without the need for "fixing" or "making better." The emphasis is on supporting children and youth with building capacity and resilience, and recognizing their strengths and their own inner power and agency to navigate the challenges of life and develop healthy coping skills to support their overall wellbeing and connection to the world around them.

### Meeting Therapeutic Goals Through Yoga
Throughout my years of integrating yoga practices into my work with children, what has stood out to me the most is the many ways yoga can be integrated into multiple therapeutic modalities to support meeting specific therapeutic goals. I've had the opportunity to meet people from around the world with a variety

of pediatric backgrounds such as occupational therapy, physical therapy, speech therapy, behavior therapy, mental health, the medical field and education. It has amazed me how the practices I teach in my trainings can apply to the therapeutic needs of so many children in so many areas of focus. I refer to yoga therapy as "stealth therapy" because it is non-competitive, fun and playful, and doesn't feel like "therapy" even though there are many therapeutic benefits that come from the practices. The opportunities are limitless for ways to integrate yoga into other therapeutic and educational modalities in order to enhance learning, memory, movement, coordination, daily functional skills, communication, self-regulation, executive functioning, mental, emotional and physical wellbeing, and meeting individualized therapeutic goals. Yoga is a perfect adjunct therapy or practice to add to other therapies and can be implemented in creative and seamless ways that are child-oriented and therapy-focused.

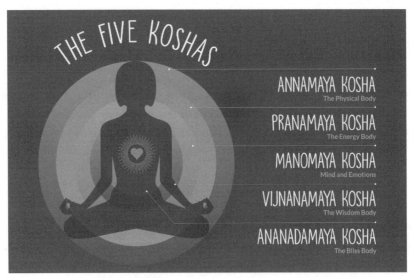

**Figure 1.1** The five koshas
© *Yoga Therapy for Youth (www.yogatherapyforyouth.com)*

### More than the Physical Body

Yoga is a comprehensive, holistic approach to wellbeing. Rather than solely addressing the physical body, yoga acknowledges that there are five bodies, five layers of self or being that must be addressed for optimal health and healing.

These are known as the koshas, layers or sheaths, moving from the physical outer body (gross) to the deeper, more inner layers (subtle) of the core. Think of Russian dolls—each layer or sheath within the outer layers (see Figure 1.1). These layers or sheaths are interconnected and interrelate with one another. What happens with one layer affects all other layers. Therefore, when addressing an overall sense of wellness, we must consider all layers. This in essence is embodying a whole-child approach—considering the whole "being" of the child and how they navigate and interact with the world rather than simply their physical state.

The five koshas are a journey from our physical experience of the world to the very essence of who we are.

### Physical Body (Annamaya Kosha)

The outermost layer is the physical body (organs, bones, muscles, tissues and skin). *Anna* translates to "food" or "physical matter," and *maya* translates to "made of." The annamaya kosha is the layer that most are familiar with when it comes to the practice of yoga. We connect with this layer through the experience of our physical body in yoga asana as well as the physical experience of disease or illness. We also experience the world around us through the physical body in relation to touch and physical connection with others.

Children learn about themselves and the world around them through their physical bodies. Their brains develop and grow through the interaction of their bodies with their environment. As early as infancy, their bodies are the vessels through which children experience the outside world. They are the conduits through which children develop, learn, explore, connect and communicate. Our bodies and brains are in constant communication with one another. The afferent messages—communication from the somatic, body-based sensations to the brain—are the foundation for how we "embody" the world.

The term "embodiment" literally means being "in body." As children become more connected to their bodies, there is a greater connection to the world around them. This deeper, more embodied connection impacts all aspects of their development and relationships in and with their environment. Greater embodiment allows children to navigate their bodies and nervous systems with more confidence and ease, decreases stress and anxiety and supports self-regulation, which directly impacts learning, mood, behavior and social relationships with others. A more "embodied" child is a more present, connected and regulated child.

The emphasis in exploring and balancing the physical body with children and youth is through connection to their bodies and developing healthy ways of taking care of their physical being.

### Focus for Annamaya Kosha

- Asana and movement
- Body awareness activities
- Nutrition
- Proper rest and restoration

## Energy Body (Pranamaya Kosha)

Sheathed by the physical layer, the energetic body is referred to as pranamaya kosha. This layer is composed of the body's subtle life-force energy, *prana*. Prana coordinates all physiological activity in the body, such as the pumping of the heart, lymphatic flow and physiological waste. Imbalances within this energetic body greatly affect the overall functioning of the physical body as well as the mental body. The way in which we breathe governs our physical and mental/emotional state, and our physical and mental/emotional state impacts the way in which we breathe. Unstable or erratic breathing can cause the mind to become agitated and the systems of the body to function irregularly. When we balance our breath, we also bring more balance to the mind and body.

The sign of the first moments of life is when a baby is born and takes its first breath. Our breath not only governs our physical and mental/emotional wellbeing but is also a key factor in our communication and expression of our own unique voice. Our breath is the only autonomic function that we can control. Breathing practices can support children with regulating their nervous system states and emotions, which are directly connected to their physical experience in the world.

The emphasis in exploring and balancing the energetic body with children and youth is through connection to their more subtle being.

### Focus for Pranamaya Kosha

- Pranayama, breathing strategies
- Music and sound
- Chanting
- Chakras

## Mental Body (Manomaya Kosha)

The third body, manomaya kosha, consists of our mind and emotions. This layer governs our thoughts, feelings and sensations. *Manas* is translated as "mind" or "thought process."

Many of us in the modern world often have an overactive or agitated manomaya kosha. Constant anxiety, worried thoughts and an agitated mind greatly impact our nervous system and, in turn, our emotions. This layer also governs our five senses and the way in which we receive and process information from our internal and external environments. Through the practice of yoga and mindfulness, we are able to ease the mind, soothe the nervous system and recover from stress and fatigue. The practices offered in yoga also support us in connecting to our senses, so we are able to be in the world through a more present and embodied experience.

Children often have very active minds and imaginations. They are still developing their ability to self-regulate. Yoga, somatic practices and mindfulness tools can support sensory integration, calming the mind and managing difficult emotions, which impacts their general sense of mental/emotional wellbeing.

The emphasis in exploring and balancing the mental/emotional body with children and youth is through awareness of their thoughts and emotions and developing tools for focus, concentration and self-regulation.

### Focus for Manomaya Kosha

- Mantras and mudras
- Integrating the eight senses
- Meditation and visualization
- The gunas

## Wisdom Body (Vijnanamaya Kosha)

When we begin practicing yoga, we experience the first three layers—physical (asana), energy (pranayama), mental (meditation and mindfulness)—through linking our breath with our physical practice and bringing more awareness to our thoughts and emotions. The fourth layer is more subtle and requires more internal awareness. With continued practice, this layer is cultivated over time.

Beneath our thoughts, sensation and emotions lies an inner knowing, a higher intelligence in our wisdom body. This deeper layer is vijnanamaya kosha, *vijnana* translating to "intellect."

Our intuition, sense of self and ability to self-reflect are all parts of our wisdom body. Here we develop a deeper awareness and insight of who we are and how we relate to the world around us.

The practice of yoga helps quiet the mind (mental body) so we can listen more deeply to our intuition, our inner knowing that goes beyond thought and reason. We begin to pay attention to our sensations, emotions and thought patterns, and become more attuned to the deeper layers of ourselves. Self-awareness precedes self-regulation. As children develop more self-awareness of their body sensations, thoughts and behavior patterns, they become more connected to their intuition. Intuition is the ability to sense or "see" something without the need for conscious reasoning. It is our inner sight that guides us—that "gut feeling" that tells us when something *feels* right or wrong. As children develop this skill, inevitably there is more of a felt sense of confidence, an inner knowing and connection to their inner truth. As children become more connected to their truth, they are more able to set healthy boundaries, assert self-agency and allow their inner wisdom to guide them. Essentially, what we want children and youth to develop is independence, autonomy, healthy relationships and the confidence to be their authentic selves—to take up space in the world and let their inner lights shine!

The emphasis in exploring and balancing the wisdom body with children and youth is through awareness of their internal sensations, connection to their inner knowing and developing tools to support self-awareness, self-confidence and self-agency.

### Focus for Vijnanamaya Kosha

- Meditation and visualization
- Boundaries, self-agency and self-esteem
- Interoception

### Bliss Body (Anandamaya Kosha)

The deepest layer of our being, anandamaya kosha, our bliss body, *ananda* translating to "bliss." In this state, we are connected to our authentic self where we experience joy, unbounded freedom and connection in which time and space does not exist.

This experience of the deepest layer, the bliss body, often occurs when we are in deep and loving connection with another being, when we are so present in doing something we love that we are not aware of time, and moments when we feel most alive and most like ourselves.

Children who come from loving and attuned homes can often naturally connect to their bliss body even more than adults. When children are younger, they are often more able to experience uninhibited joy and connection to the world around them because their minds and nervous systems have not yet been distorted or filled with fear and anxiety from experience in the outside world. Children have a natural curiosity and see the world with awe and wonder. Their imaginations are active, and they are able to see the "magic" all around them. As children grow older, their fearful or unpleasant experiences can begin to override their deeper connection to their wisdom and bliss bodies.

The practice of yoga is a practice of coming home to ourselves. The intuitive, curious, joyful and present nature of who we truly are beyond our experiences in life. A coming home to our innate wholeness, wellness and interconnectedness with the world.

The emphasis in exploring and balancing the bliss body with children and youth is through relationship, curiosity, play and supporting the child in connecting to their authentic self.

Focus of Anandamaya Kosha

- Resourcing
- Expressive arts
- Nature
- Connection and attunement
- Play

## PAUSE AND REFLECT

Imagine a moment in time when you were doing something you love or when you were in a place you felt deeply connected to. As you think back to that experience or place, what were the sensations or emotions you felt in that moment? Were you looking at the clock, checking the time or thinking of your to-do list? Or did you experience a sense of presence and connection where time did not exist? These are moments of *bliss*—what can be referred to as *resources* that remind us of who we are and connect us to our most authentic self. These moments of presence can be experienced through time in nature or places we love, doing activities that bring us joy, spending time with people or animals we love who nurture our souls, moments of connecting to our creative self and through the experience of play.

Invitation to journal in response to this question.

## EMBODYING A WHOLE-CHILD APPROACH IN THERAPEUTIC YOGA

Throughout this book, we will be exploring working therapeutically with children and youth through the lens of the five koshas, exploring each layer and how they interrelate with one another. Every child is a unique and complex human being. Through the exploration of the five koshas and therapeutic tools for wellness, the intention is to support children to connect to their bodies, develop more awareness of their thoughts and emotions, develop more awareness of their internal sensations, learn tools to regulate their nervous systems, build capacity and resilience, build self-confidence and self-esteem, and develop connection to their innate wholeness, wellbeing and interconnectedness with other people, plants, animals and the earth as a whole.

## THE EIGHT LIMBS OF YOGA
### What Are the Yoga Sutras?

*The Yoga Sutras* is a succinct but complete manual of Raja Yoga, meaning royal yoga. Raja Yoga is an ancient yogic science. Patañjali was not the creator of Raja Yoga but the first known to systematize it in a complete text. *The Yoga Sutras* is considered one of the primary books of Raja Yoga and the foundation for most forms of modern yoga today.

The Sanskrit word *sutra* means thread. Each sutra is interconnected, like beads on a thread. Patañjali's manual is made up of 196 sutras in four chapters. The practice as codified by Patañjali is called ashtanga yoga. *Ashta* is the Sanskrit word for eight, and *anga* translates to limb, fold or part. *The Yoga Sutras* describes an eightfold path to help cultivate a life of purpose, meaning and connection, which is where the term "eight limbs of yoga" comes from.

> *Yoga anga anushtanat ashuddhi kshaye jnanadi Apthiraviveka khyatehe.*

> "By the sustained practice of the eight limbs of yoga, the impurities are destroyed and the light of wisdom, discrimination shines forth."

> (Sutra II:28; translation Graphics, 2020)

Sejal Shah references an explanation of Sutra II:28 by Gurudev Sri Sri Ravi Shankar which states:

> Human consciousness is like a seed. A seed has the possibility of a tree, of the leaves, of a branch, of fruits, of flowers, of multiplication; so also the human mind. A seed needs a proper ground, proper conditions, sunlight, water, proper soil for it to sprout and blossom. Similarly human consciousness and human mind. Either the seed can be dormant for years, keeping its possibility within itself, or it starts blossoming, sprouting. The sprouting of the seed of human consciousness is *viveka* – discrimination. Freedom comes with *viveka*, discrimination.

> (Shah, 2020)

What is the importance of cultivating discernment or discrimination in children and teens? Discernment means "the power or faculty of the mind, by which it distinguishes one thing from another, as truth from falsehood, virtue from vice; acuteness of judgment; power of perceiving differences" (Websters Dictionary 1828, n.d.).

To have discernment is the root of our decision-making and problem-solving ability. When we have clear discernment, we see and act in truth and integrity. We recognize what is false and real. We are able to notice our false perception of reality versus what is true reality. We are able to discriminate between right and wrong. We recognize the impact we have on those around us and make the right effort to engage in the world with a sense of care for others. We make decisions based in truth, integrity and consideration for ourselves and all living beings.

## Yamas and Niyamas (the First Two Limbs)

The yamas and niyamas are the foundation of yoga. Yoga is an ancient and sophisticated system that extends beyond just doing physical asanas. Yoga literally is a *way of living*. Yoga is designed to bring more awareness not only to our bodies but also our thoughts, behaviors and the ways in which we relate to the world around us. Yoga offers an experiential journey through the layers of our being in which, through practice, we learn to live in the world with more consciousness and intention.

The yamas and niyamas can be thought of as guidelines and ethical disciplines or restraints and observances. They are the offerings of wisdom that give direction of how to live a more joyful, connected and authentic life.

The eight limbs form a sequence from the outer to the inner and act as a guide in our yoga practice and exploration of ourselves. The teachings of the yamas and niyamas can be woven into your sessions with children and teens in creative and seamless ways. Integrating the eight limbs in your sessions supports children and teens in exploring yoga beyond just physical poses or breathing practices. As they explore the yamas and niyamas, they learn to connect more deeply with themselves and the world around them.

Below is a simple guide to the yamas and niyamas and how to describe them to children and teens.

### Yamas (Restraints)

**Ahimsa:** Practice non-harm with each thought, word and action towards oneself and others. Be kind to yourself, other people and all living things.

**Satya:** Be honest, be truthful, stand in your truth, speak your truth with compassion for yourself and others. Use your voice to speak up for others.

**Asteya:** Do not take from others what does not belong to you. Be generous and giving to others.

**Brahmacharya:** Practice moderation. Use your energy wisely.

**Aparigraha:** Practice gratitude, non-attachment and letting things go.

### Niyamas (Observances)

**Saucha:** Cleanliness of mind and body. Take care of your body through good hygiene and healthy food. Respect your environment and clean up after yourself.

**Santosha:** Be content with what you have. Love yourself for who you are. Practice gratitude.

**Tapas:** Channel your energy in positive ways. Connect with life-force energy, joy and enthusiasm. Continue to strive for personal growth.

**Svadhyaya:** Study and learn about yourself and the world around you. Continue to grow and evolve as a human being.

**Ishvara Pranidhana:** Trust the source in yourself and surrender to the will of the universe or a higher power.

## SEL—SOCIAL EMOTIONAL LEARNING

According to the Collaborative for Academic, Social, and Emotional Learning (CASEL), SEL or Social Emotional Learning is an integral part of education and human development. SEL is the process through which all young people and adults acquire and apply the knowledge, skills and attitudes to develop healthy identities, manage emotions and achieve personal and collective goals, feel and show empathy for others, establish and maintain supportive relationships, and make responsible and caring decisions (CASEL, 2022).

The five core CASEL competencies are:

- **Self-awareness:** The ability to recognize and name personal emotions as well as to understand one's own needs, strengths and limitations.
- **Self-management:** The ability to regulate one's own emotions and behaviors in order to get along with others and achieve desired goals in life.
- **Social awareness:** The ability to understand what others are feeling and be able to see their perspective. A foundation for empathy.
- **Relationship skills:** The ability to form positive social relationships, work together and deal effectively with conflict.
- **Responsible decision making:** Making positive choices around personal and social behavior. Making responsible decisions and recognizing the impact decisions have on oneself and others.

### SEL and the Eight Limbs

When teaching the eight limbs of yoga to children, the emphasis is very much in alignment with the standards or pillars of SEL—in particular, the yamas and niyamas (social awareness). Along with the yamas and niyamas, asana and pranyama help children cultivate a deeper connection to their bodies, emotions, behaviors and sense of self, and provide tools for self-regulation (self-awareness and self-management). The continued practice of meditation, visualization and activities that support focus and concentration help children build a greater capacity to make healthy and responsible decisions (responsible decision making). As they continue to explore their external and internal worlds, build self-regulation skills and develop an awareness of how their behaviors impact themselves and others, they are able to recognize how we are all interconnected (relationships skills), and therefore their thoughts, words and actions will reflect this sense of interconnectedness with other people, animals and the planet.

## CHAKRAS

Chakra or *cakra* (pronounced chuh-kra) is a Sanskrit word meaning "wheel" or "circle."

Chakras are accepted in the practice of energy work and energy medicine, and are considered to be the vital energy centers that exist within each one of us. The chakras are "subtle," meaning they can't be seen by the human eye or touched physically.

The chakras have been visualized and described as spinning wheels, vortexes of energy or rotating spheres or discs of energy.

The chakra energy systems were described in ancient Indic systems both Vedic and Tantric as far back as 1500–500 BC. The teachings from both systems were handed down orally before being recorded in writing, which explains the lack of the exact date of origin (Schneider & Cooper, 2019). The Vedic system of knowledge, upon which the Hindu religion and much of the philosophical teachings of yoga are based, is contained in the *Vedas*, which are sacred texts. The Sanskrit word "veda" means "knowledge." The Tantric system arose within the same time period, drawing from the Vedic teachings.

The chakras can be thought of as types of invisible, energetic organs, each self-contained and having functions that relate to and impact specific parts of the whole human system. They help regulate and generate functions that impact us physically, energetically, emotionally, mentally, sensorially, intuitively and spiritually (Helbert, 2019).

The chakras provide insight into the energetic and more subtle systems of our body. Each chakra is associated with a physical location in the body as well as specific organs and functions. Our chakras reflect our experience with physical sensations, thoughts, emotions and how we interact with ourselves and the world around us.

When we are subjected to stress or trauma, our homeostasis goes out of balance and our chakras can become blocked or imbalanced. Each chakra inter-relates with the others; when one chakra is out of balance, it will impact the other chakras. Our foundational chakras are the root and sacral chakras, which is where we experience a sense of safety and connection.

## Maslow's Hierarchy of Needs and Chakras

We can relate Maslow's hierarchy of needs to the chakras and see the correlation between the two.

Maslow asserts that at the bottom of the pyramid are our **basic needs**:

- physiological—related to food, water, shelter and proper rest
- safety—related to security, a familiar and predictable environment and freedom from illness or harm.

In the middle of the pyramid are our **psychological needs**:

- belonging and love—intimate relationships, friendship, connection with others, feeling valued and included
- esteem—feelings of purpose and accomplishment.

At the top of the pyramid are our **self-fulfillment needs**:

- self-actualization—achieving one's potential, creativity and expression of true self.

The same is true with the chakra system as shown in Figure 1.2.

Self-actualization cannot occur until the preceding needs are met; therefore, we work from the bottom up when working with human growth and healing. This is also the intention in working with a child's nervous system from the old brain to the new brain, or bottom-up approach. We address a child's felt sense of safety and security in their nervous system, then progress to their learning and higher-order thinking.

I have found that children and teens become quite interested and excited learning about their chakras and ways to balance them. Children and youth have an openness about subtle practices that adults may often be suspicious of or hesitant to try because they have to "see it to believe it." Children are much more open to imagination, visualizing and believing in things that they can't necessarily "see." Children are more apt to "believe it to see it." This is the wonder and magic of working with children. We get to open ourselves to the energetic fields and practices that we may have shut out as we moved into adulthood.

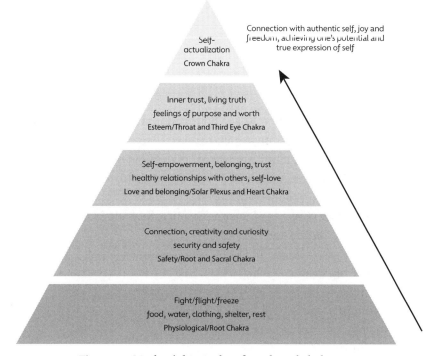

**Figure 1.2** Maslow's hierarchy of needs and chakras

Across the following pages is a simple outline of the chakras, including the translation, color, element, seed sound, vowel sound, musical note, sense, location, association and experience when out of balance and when in balance. Included are suggestions for specific asanas and mantras associated with each chakra. When integrating the chakras into the child's therapeutic protocol, all of these elements can be explored with an intention of balancing their energy systems in order to come back to homeostasis or a felt sense of groundedness, connection, joy, presence, self-agency, self-empowerment and clarity. As you learn more throughout the chapters in this book in regard to sensory processing, anxiety, depression and specific nervous system states, you can refer back to the chakra guide to see how you might implement them in your protocol. There are so many rich and creative ways to integrate the chakras through sound, imagery, body awareness, senses, breath and movement.

## The Seven Chakras
### Root Chakra (Muladhara)

Base of our chakra system.

**Meaning:** *Mula*, root, *adhara*, support or base

**Color:** Red

**Element:** Earth

**Sound:** LAM (Lum)

**Vowel sound:** UH (as in "huh")

**Musical note:** C

**Sense:** Smell

**Location:** Base of the spine, pelvic floor and first three vertebrae

**Associated with:** Grounding, vitality and stability; most instinctual of all chakras; the basis of our survival or "fight/flight/freeze" response

**When out of balance:** Anxiety or depression, fearful, feeling of lethargy or being "stuck," disconnected

**When in balance:** Grounded, secure, resourceful and independent

**Intention:** Grounding and stability

**Asanas and breath:**

- Mountain
- Tree
- Warrior I
- Warrior II
- Airplane
- Low or High Lunge
- Easy Seat
- Monkey Toes
- Spider Legs up the Wall
- Savasana (on back or belly)
- Energy of Breath (downward)
- Elevator Breath

**Mantras:**

- I am grounded
- I am connected to my body
- I am rooted like a tree
- I am loved

- I am okay right now
- I belong
- I make choices that are healthy and good for me
- I am stable
- I am supported by others
- I am here, now

**Daily practices to strengthen root chakra:**

- Spend time in nature
- Look at and listen to images and sounds of nature
- Grounding box (pieces of nature to look, listen, smell, feel)
- Stand barefoot on the earth
- Use the imagery of trees and earth in meditation
- Hug trees!
- Growing plants or gardening
- Roll a ball on the bottoms of feet or massage feet
- Integrate earth images and colors in art
- Create an earth mandala
- Carry a root stone (red carnelian, red jasper, bloodstone)

### Sacral Chakra (Svadhisthana)

**Meaning:** One's own place
**Color:** Orange
**Element:** Water
**Sound:** VAM (Vum)
**Vowel sound:** Oo (as in "you")
**Musical note:** D
**Sense:** Taste
**Location:** Pelvis, hips
**Associated with:** Creativity, pleasure, feeling, emotion, connection
**When out of balance:** Shame, compulsive thoughts and behaviors, anxiety/
   depression, lack of creativity, difficulty experiencing pleasurable
   experiences, disconnection from emotion
**When in balance:** Creative, playful, joyful, passionate, feeling
**Intention:** Creativity and connection

**Asanas and breath:**

- Frog
- Butterfly
- Warrior II
- Triangle
- Tree
- Easy Seat
- Horse
- Giraffe
- River
- Turtle
- Emotions Breaths

**Mantras:**

- I love and enjoy my body
- I take care of myself
- I have healthy boundaries
- I do things I love
- I explore with my senses
- I am passionate
- I am creative
- I feel my feelings
- I am joyful
- I am peace

**Daily practices to strengthen sacral chakra:**

- Make/create something
- Dance and listen to music
- Spend time in nature near water
- Look at images of water and listen to sounds of water
- Do something playful
- Do something or imagine something that sparks joy or brings pleasure
- Carry a sacral stone (citrine, orange carnelian, orange aventurine)

## Solar Plexus Chakra (Manipura)

**Meaning:** Lustrous gem

**Color:** Yellow
**Element:** Fire
**Sound:** RAM (Rum)
**Vowel sound:** Oh (as in "go")
**Musical note:** E
**Sense:** Sight
**Location:** Between the navel and solar plexus
**Associated with:** Self-confidence, self-esteem, willpower, inner power, choice
**When out of balance:** Low self-esteem, anxiety/depression, lack of motivation, difficulty setting healthy boundaries
**When in balance:** Joyful, confident, willing to take chances, sense of self-agency
**Intention:** Confidence, energy and action

**Asanas and breath:**

- Boat
- Plank
- Mountain
- Warrior I
- Warrior II
- Star
- Bicycle
- Frog
- Roller Coaster Twist
- Boxer Breath
- Choo-Choo Breath
- Happy Baby
- Sun Salutations
- Balloon Belly Breath
- Three-Part Breathing

**Mantras:**

- I love and accept myself
- I stand up for myself
- I am strong
- I am courageous
- I am powerful

- I am brave
- I am confident
- I am authentic
- I am the pilot of my own plane
- I have choice
- My inner light is unique and beautiful
- I am a superstar
- I am a warrior

**Daily practices to strengthen solar plexus chakra:**

- Spend time in the sun
- Look at images of the sun
- Gaze at a fire or candle
- Watch the sunrise/sunset or look at images
- Smell yellow flowers
- Drink warm water with lemon
- Draw, color or paint the sun
- Do things that bring laughter
- Carry a solar plexus stone (topaz, yellow tourmaline, citrine, sunstone)

### Heart Chakra (Anahata)

**Meaning:** Unhurt or unstruck
**Color:** Green
**Element:** Air
**Sound:** YAM (Yum)
**Vowel sound:** Ah (as in "la")
**Musical note:** F
**Sense:** Touch
**Location:** Heart, lungs (arms and hands extension)
**Associated with:** Love, warmth, compassion, joy, connection, trust
**When out of balance:** Grief, sadness/depression, disconnection, resentment, closed
**When in balance:** Love, compassion, forgiveness, joy, connection, openness
**Intention:** Love, compassion and trust

**Asanas and breath:**

- Open Book/Close Book

- Bridge
- Camel
- Shark
- Cobra
- Cow
- Star
- Warrior II
- Flamingo
- Self-Hug
- Show Me Ten
- Reach for the Moon
- Wake the Spider
- Mix It Up
- Eagle Arms
- Mountain with Hands at Heart
- "I Am" Breath Mantra
- Heart/Belly Breathing

**Mantras:**

- I receive love
- I love myself
- I love others deeply
- I am grateful
- I am kind
- I receive kindness from others
- I am connected with animals and nature
- I feel love and connection with others
- I am worthy of love and kindness
- I am important
- I am love

**Daily practices to strengthen heart chakra:**

- Visit or look at images of places of beauty
- Look at images that are beautiful to you
- Spend time in nature and take in the many shades of green
- Green look box (green nature items to look at)
- Place pink flowers in home
- Paint with the colors pink and green

- Have plants in the home and spend time watering and bathing them (watering meditation)
- Spend time with people you love (in person or via phone/video)
- Write a list of things you love and use them as resources
- Carry a heart stone (rose quartz, watermelon tourmaline, rubellite)

## Throat Chakra (Visuddha)

**Meaning:** Especially pure
**Color:** Blue/turquoise
**Element:** Ether
**Sound:** HAM (Hum)
**Vowel sound:** EYE (as in "my")
**Musical note:** G
**Sense:** Hearing
**Location:** Neck, throat shoulders (ears and mouth)
**Associated with:** Accepting oneself, authenticity, standing in your truth
**When out of balance:** Self-doubt, negative thinking, anxiety/depression, low self-esteem, not telling the truth
**Intention:** Speaking truth, empowerment

### Asanas and breath:

- Bridge
- Camel
- Snake
- Shark
- Butterfly to Cocoon
- Rabbit
- Butterfly
- Cat/Cow
- Roller Coaster Twist
- Ear Stretch
- Lion's Breath
- Hum Breath/Bee Breath
- Wave Breath
- Emotions Breaths

**Mantras:**

- I speak my truth
- I communicate my feelings with ease
- I can take up space
- My feelings are important
- What I have to say matters
- I have important things to share
- I can express my anger and sadness
- I am a good listener
- I listen to my body
- I stand in my truth
- My words are powerful
- My voice is beautiful

**Daily practices to strengthen throat chakra:**

- Singing and chanting
- Writing in a journal
- Use voice in creative ways (e.g. acting, speaking poetry, spoken word)
- Vocal toning
- Ear stretches and pressure pointing
- Facial massage around the jaw
- Palming of the throat
- Make animal sounds or other empowering vocal sounds
- Practice using voice to set boundaries and speak truth (role-play)
- Listen to soothing music or empowering music
- Draw, color or paint using blue
- Practice listening (sit outside and notice the different sounds you hear)
- Drink plenty of water
- Lie on the ground and look up at the blue sky
- Carry a throat stone (amazonite, turquoise, aquamarine)

## Third Eye Chakra (Ajna)

**Meaning:** To perceive, to command
**Color:** Indigo
**Element:** All elements combined, light
**Sound:** AUM (Om)
**Vowel sound:** Ay (as in "may")

**Musical note:** A

**Sense:** Sight and extrasensory perception

**Location:** In the brain, at the brow, above the base of the nose

**Associated with:** Intuition, imagination

**When out of balance:** Hyperactive mind, disconnection from reality, lack of intuition, brain fog, fear/anxiety, judgment of self and others, black-and-white thinking

**When in balance:** Seeing both inner and outer worlds, connection to all senses, focus, balanced, self-reflective, accepting, intuitive, expansive thought

**Intention:** Focus and clarity

**Asanas and breath:**

- Tree
- Airplane
- Warrior II
- Flamingo
- Triangle
- Eagle
- Open Book/Close Book
- Half Moon
- Child's
- Puppy
- Rag Doll
- Down Dog
- Apple Picking
- Sneaky Peak
- Alternate Nostril Breathing

**Mantras:**

- I listen to my intuition
- I have an inner knowing
- I have an inner wisdom
- I understand myself
- I am wise
- I know myself
- I trust myself
- I love and accept myself

- I am open to learning new things
- I am a source of truth and love
- I listen to my body

**Daily practices to strengthen third eye chakra:**

- Keep a dream journal
- Keep a journal of free-flowing thoughts, intuitions and manifestations
- Meditation practice
- Walking meditation in nature to connect with all of the senses
- Sensory box (items to look, listen, feel, smell, touch and taste)
- Massage from the center of the forehead outward along the top of brows to temples
- Palming
- Limit time on devices
- Eye exercises
- Carry a third eye stone (blue lace agate, amazonite, blue sapphire)

## Crown Chakra (Sahasrara)

**Meaning:** Thousand petal lotus
**Color:** Violet or white
**Element:** Beyond all elements or thought, transcendence of ego
**Sound:** AUM (Om) or silence
**Vowel sound:** EE (as in "me")
**Musical note:** B
**Sense:** Beyond the senses
**Location:** Crown of the head
**Associated with:** Awareness, understanding, serenity, interconnectedness with all, peace, sense of purpose, desire to learn, non-attachment
**When out of balance:** Depression, fearful, distrust, egocentric, attachment
**When in balance:** Gratitude, faith, trust, feeling of one with the universe or divine
**Intention:** Gratitude and connection to all living beings

**Asanas and breath:**

- Balancing poses with weight on top of head
- Tree

- Mountain
- Star
- Flamingo
- Easy Seat
- Butterfly
- Handstand
- Rabbit
- Crocodile
- Monkey
- Inversions with block or chair under head
- Savasana
- Alternate Nostril Breathing
- Three-Part Breathing

**Mantras:**

- I am part of the Divine
- I am source within
- I cherish my heart and soul
- I am joy
- I let go of things that don't serve me
- I offer my pain up to something greater
- I am here, now
- I trust in the universe
- I am present
- I have great worth
- I am important
- I am joyful
- I am whole and beautiful just as I am
- I am grateful
- I am one with nature and all living things

**Daily practices to strengthen crown chakra:**

- Meditation and prayer
- Tapping
- Keep a daily gratitude journal
- Read books that inspire and awaken
- Occipital massage
- Facial Savasana

- Place lavender bunches in your home
- Lavender oil on top of head and occipital ridge
- Do things that spark joy and make you feel most like yourself
- Carry a crown stone (clear quartz, amethyst, moonstone)

Each chakra is connected to specific organs and systems of the body. As you create your protocols, you can integrate the chakras that relate to the child's physical ailments or imbalances.

**Root:** Testes, kidneys, spine
**Sacral:** Bladder, prostate, ovaries, kidneys, gallbladder, bowels, spleen
**Solar Plexus:** Intestines, pancreas, liver, bladder, stomach, upper spine
**Heart:** Heart, lungs
**Throat:** Bronchial tubes, vocal chords, respiratory system, all areas of the mouth, including tongue and esophagus
**Third Eye:** Eyes, pituitary gland, pineal glands, brain
**Crown:** Spinal cord and brainstem

# Chapter 2

# Child Development

## Developmental Milestones: Birth to 17

Child development is a fascinating subject. It involves the biological, psychological and emotional changes that occur from birth to adolescence. There are many factors that influence a child's development, including family structure and history, age, social, physical, psychological, economic, cultural and geographical. In this chapter, we'll explore child development in the areas of physical, social/emotional, cognitive and communication. If we are to work with children and teens effectively, it's important that we have a strong foundation and understanding in child development. When we understand where they are in terms of their own unique development, we can better support their needs and ensure that we are meeting them where they are at.

## PHYSICAL DEVELOPMENT
### Neurodevelopmental Sequence

The neurodevelopmental sequence is the typical movement development in infants that sequentially progresses based upon movement principles. If you observe a baby's movement from birth to approximately age 2, there is a specific sequence of movement they follow as they grow and develop the abilities to roll, crawl, stand, walk and more. It is helpful to know this developmental sequence; not only does it enable us to understand how children develop physically, but it can also help in assessing a child's strength, balance, coordination, energy level, posture, breathing and movement patterns. It can also assist in recognizing gaps in a child's development where they may have missed important movements, which could impact them on many levels. What is important to recognize is that development occurs from the ground up, and movement progresses from proximal to distal. What this means is that the head and trunk develop before the arms and legs, and the arms and legs develop before the fingers and toes. Another example of this is that neck control and head holding develop before trunk control and independent sitting.

When working with children and teens to address movement patterns, one must begin first with lower developmental postures and movements, from the ground up, proximal to distal. Skipping over these foundational movements in working with children who have challenges with movement and coordination will not only impede their progress but could also leave them feeling disoriented and dysregulated. It is also important to consider how a child's sensory system develops. This begins when they are on the ground, exploring, moving, observing and taking in the world around them. They begin to develop both their vestibular and proprioceptive systems when they are closer to the ground. Then, as they become stronger and more stable, they are able to move from the ground to standing because their sensorimotor systems are more developed. Having a child explore movement closer to the ground when they are less coordinated or their sensory system is underdeveloped will give them more of a felt sense of safety and stability. The progression of motor skills goes from simple to complex, from gross motor to fine motor control, and from mass movements to more refined isolated movements. Keep in mind this is an example of typical development, but not all children develop in this way, and not all children are impacted by variations in motor development. It is important to consider the impact that developmental trauma can have on whether or not a baby is given the opportunity, support, safe environment and secure attachment to explore the movements and sensory experiences that are foundational to their physical development. A child's physical development can depend on many factors and can be impacted by brain injury, disability, neglect, abuse, illness and other factors.

According to Harold Blomberg, a Swedish doctor and psychiatrist, there are basic movement patterns that an infant needs to move through sequentially to establish strong foundations and the ability to differentiate in order for movement to become easy, graceful and automatic. These developmental movement patterns are:

- Breathing: The breath is the foundation of all movement patterns that follow. "The breath gives life to movement."
- Mouthing: The mouth is the first to reach, grasp, hold and let go.
- Core-distal connectivity: The connection of all the limbs to the navel or core. Babies must develop a sense of their center before they can reach out and move through the world.
- Head–tail connectivity or Spinal Movement: Differentiation between the front and back of the body. A foundation for developing attention and focus.
- Upper–lower connectivity: Differentiation between the upper and

lower halves of the body. A foundation for experiencing stability and grounding.

- Body-half connectivity: Differentiation between the left and right sides of the body. A foundation for mobility and movement in all directions.
- Cross-lateral connectivity or contralateral movement: The coordinated movement of opposite upper and lower limbs. A foundation for experiencing movement with ease and efficiency.

(Blomberg & Dempsey, 2011, p.40)

What I found to be so fascinating and exciting is that traditional yoga postures mimic the movements and shapes that are part of the neurodevelopmental sequence. Babies are natural yogis! Not only can we use the sequence as an assessment tool, but we can also integrate specific poses that correlate with missing gross motor milestones in the developmental sequence in order to "fill in the gaps." Filling the gaps can assist with bringing the body and nervous system back to balance so a child or teen moves with more ease and flow.

## EXPLORING ASANA AS AN ASSESSMENT OF MOVEMENT PATTERNS AND DEVELOPMENT

As we explore this sequence, we can observe and note areas of imbalance or challenge. The emphasis in using assessment and developing therapeutic protocols is to support nervous system regulation and integration and cohesion of the brain/body systems, rather than "fixing" the structure of the body.

### Neurodevelopmental Sequence Observation and Assessment
Supine (Savasana)

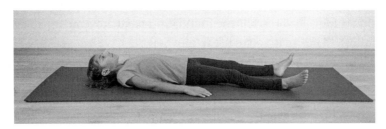

When babies are born, they are placed supine, on their backs, and any initial movement that occurs is often automatic or what is referred to as reflex movement. Their movements are primarily governed by primitive reflexes that interfere with midline activities and dissociation of movement between different parts of the body. They have not yet developed any muscle strength in their necks, so they are not able to raise their heads or initiate any gross volitional/voluntary movement until around 1–2 months of age. They are mostly docile and depend solely on their caregivers to move them about in order to meet their needs.

*What to Observe and Note*

- Breathing patterns

### Happy Baby

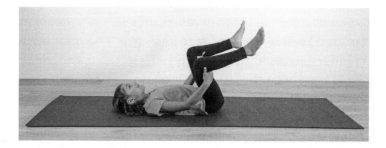

As children start to notice that they have arms, hands, legs and feet, they begin to explore their bodies by grabbing their feet with their hands and even rocking back and forth. This rhythmic movement facilitates not only the beginning of postural and core strength but also sensorimotor development and self-soothing behavior.

*What to Observe and Note*

- Ability to bring hips into flexion
- Ability to rock side to side in a controlled and rhythmic manner

### Cobra

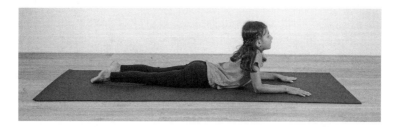

### Roll from Supine to Prone

As the baby gathers more momentum in shifting their weight back and forth on their backs, they are eventually able to roll from their backs onto their bellies, from supine to prone. This is a critical position for development of the muscles in the neck, core and spinal extensors. Babies initially come into the world with only a C-curve or kyphotic curve in their spine. This is considered their primary curve. As they lie prone on their belly and start to lift their head, they begin to develop the first secondary curve at around 3–9 months old, a lordotic curve in their cervical spine. They develop their lumbar and sacral curves between 1 and 3 years of age. Of course, the natural curvature of the spine can be impacted throughout our lifespan by injuries, poor posture and lack of movement.

As babies spend more time on their bellies, they are able to see more in their environment, track moving objects without moving their head and begin to reach for items of interest to them. This not only facilitates increased strength in the neck, trunk and arms, but it also facilitates increased sensorimotor development. As babies reach for items, they are strengthening their hand–eye coordination, and by shifting their weight back and forth, they are continuing to develop their vestibular and proprioceptive systems. This is why tummy time is emphasized so much in child development. There are so many benefits to a child being prone on their bellies!

### What to Observe and Note

- Ability to lift head and shoulders from mat (spinal extension)
- Ability to hold themselves up with their arms
- Ability to shift weight from one side to the other as they reach forward with alternating hands

### Prone to Supine

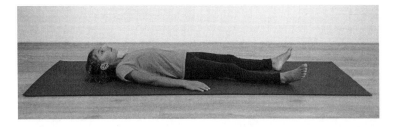

As babies develop more core strength, they are able to roll back and forth from prone to supine and supine to prone, again continuing to develop in areas of postural strength and the sensorimotor system. The motor pattern for rolling also becomes more refined as babies progress from a reflexive log roll (where the whole body turns as one unit) to a segmental roll. With this progression, they are able to dissociate and rotate their upper body followed by their lower body voluntarily in order to roll from prone to supine or supine to prone.

### Seated

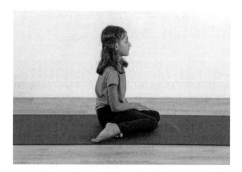 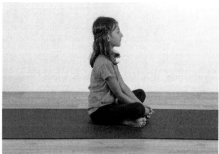

Eventually, babies have enough neck and trunk strength to sit upright. They may initially side sit, which requires less core strength than sitting in a criss-cross position. As they explore their worlds through sitting up, they begin to develop more rotation in their spine as well as their lumbar lordotic curve, which facilitates both the natural curvature of the spine and functional movement. Being in a seated position also allows for movement that crosses the midline, such as reaching one hand across the body to grab a toy. The ability to cross the midline impacts later movement such as crawling and walking as well as reading, writing, attention and regulation. Integration of primitive reflexes also lays the foundation for voluntary dissociation of movement between different body parts, midline and crossing the midline activities.

#### What to Observe and Note

- Ability to sit in a criss-cross position independently
- Is their posture upright or rounded?
- Are their knees in line with their hips?
- Natural curvature of the spine
- Ability to reach hand across body (cross midline)

### Quadruped or Table Pose

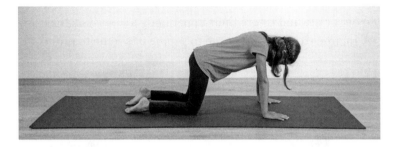

As babies' postural muscles become more developed, and they have developed more strength in their arms and legs, they come onto their hands and knees. In this position, they shift their weight from one side to the other as well as back and forth, helping them continue to develop their balance, strength, reflex and sensory systems.

#### *What to Observe and Note*

- Are they able to hold themselves up against gravity?
- Is there any hypermobility in their elbow joints?
- Is their spine rounded or in extension rather than neutral?
- Is there winging in their shoulders?
- How long can they hold the position without fatiguing?

### Crawl or Animal Walk

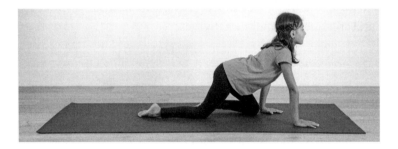

In the photograph above, notice the hyperextension in the child's right elbow when her right upper extremity is in weight bearing.

Crawling is a precursor to walking. When children begin to crawl, it opens up a whole sensory world to them and they begin to develop more of a sense of curiosity, independence and trust in themselves. Crawling to a baby is like a teenager getting their driver's license! They now have the ability to move their bodies where they want them to go and no longer have to rely on their caregiver to take them there. There is so much critical development that happens with crawling, including:

- increased strength and coordination
- increased development of the proprioceptive and vestibular systems
- sensory development
- ability to align one body part over another
- ability to move against gravity
- ability to shift weight from side to side and front and back
- postural control and balance
- midline crossing, which facilitates whole-brain integration
- rhythmic movement that facilitates a more regulated nervous system.

As babies crawl, they are engaging in contralateral movement. Contralateral movement is a diagonal movement of one upper limb with the opposite lower limb. This is a necessary skill in being able to walk with smooth, rhythmic and coordinated movements. When we move in a smooth and rhythmic way, rather than with rigid and uncoordinated movement, we move through the world with more confidence and ease. Our nervous systems love rhythm!

*What to Observe and Note*

- Are they able to demonstrate contralateral movement?
- Are their movements smooth and coordinated?
- Are they showing fatigue from the activity?

### Tall Kneeling or Kneeling Mountain

As babies develop more strength, confidence and coordinated movement, they begin to explore pre-standing movements. They may come up onto their knees in order to make themselves taller and explore the world from a new perspective. Tall kneeling promotes core activation and control.

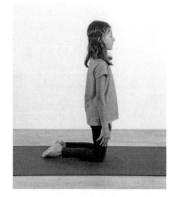

*What to Observe and Note*

- Is their posture rounded or upright?
- Are their joints stacked?
- Do they show a sense of stability in the position?

### Half Kneeling or Low Lunge

Babies may move from tall kneel to half kneel where one knee is on the floor. This facilitates the ability to dissociate flexion movement from extension movement, one hip in extension and one hip in flexion, the same movements that occur in walking. Half kneel also supports hip mobility and balance to prepare for walking.

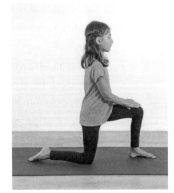

*What to Observe and Note*

- Are they able to shift their body weight to balance on one knee to flex then rotate the opposite hip to bring the foot on that side forward?
- Are they able to balance with minimal effort?
- Are they able to maintain an upright position?
- Are they able to demonstrate the position on both sides?
- Is one side different from the other?

### Standing or Mountain

Now that the baby has developed enough postural strength, and strength in their legs and arms, they begin to explore standing. They may initially explore standing with support by pulling themselves up on a coffee table, couch or other support. This is where you may see them attempting to stand on their own. Falling (when it's in a safe space to do so) actually supports a baby's development of their sensorimotor system. This impacts the integration of the righting reflex, the ability to correct the orientation of their body when it's taken out of its normal upright position.

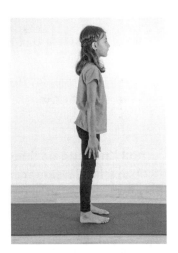

*What to Observe and Note*

- Position of the pelvis (neutral, anterior or posterior tilt)
- Are their joints stacked?
- Is their posture upright or rounded?
- Is there any hyperextension in their knees?

### Squat to Standing or Frog to Mountain

As a baby becomes more confident and stable with standing, you will often observe them moving from a standing to squatting position. This facilitates developing greater strength in the legs and core, as well as balance.

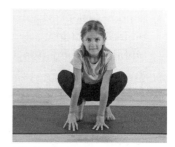

*What to Observe and Note*

- Are they able to move from squat to standing with ease?
- Are they able to stay balanced in the pose?
- Are they able to externally rotate their hips with a normal range of motion?
- Is their posture upright or rounded as they do the pose?

### Walking or Warrior I

Prerequisites for walking with fluidity and ease are the ability to shift weight from one leg to the other in a balanced and coordinated manner.

*What to Observe and Note*

- Are they able to show hip extension of the back hip and hip flexion of the front?
- Are they able to stay balanced in the pose?
- Is their posture upright or rounded as they do the pose?
- Can they demonstrate appropriate shoulder flexion?
- Adequate range of motion in ankles, especially the one in the back to allow dorsiflexion to keep the heel of the back foot on the ground.

### Walking (with support then independently)

The final stage in the neurodevelopmental sequence of movement is walking. At this point, the baby has gone through a significant amount of physical development. Their bodies have literally been moving and growing in order to bring them to their feet and give them the freedom to move about the world with increased independence, strength, endurance and agency. They now have the ability to go from walking to running, jumping, skipping, hopping and so many other movements that continue to facilitate

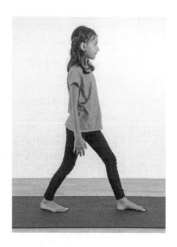

their physical growth and development. Continued exploration of movement supports coordination, balance, well-developed sensorimotor systems, whole-brain integration, attention, learning, social connection, communication and building a foundation for greater mental, emotional and physical wellbeing.

## Additional Movements to Observe

### Transitions

Transition is a change from one neurodevelopmental position to another as the child's sensorimotor system develops and matures. Some examples of motor transitions are moving from quadruped (table pose) to sit, half knee to stand, squat to stand. Assessment of motor transitions is an extremely important part of a thorough assessment. Missing motor patterns or parts of the motor sequence can give important clues to underlying deficits and what to target during the therapeutic session.

When assessing movement transitions, it is also important to look for:

- a variety of motor patterns, which indicates that the child is able to use a variety of muscle groups and combinations to move from one position to another, for example, the child is able to move from table to side sit or from table to heel sit or from table to cross-legged sitting
- adequate core muscle strength, which again lays the crucial foundation for the ability to efficiently transition/move from one developmental pose to another
- ability to control and grade small-range movements
- ability to perform controlled weight shifts
- adequate rotatory movements and control of rotations
- balance to efficiently and successfully complete the transition.

Transitions between different developmental positions can be used not only in assessment but also as part of the treatment in a therapeutic program. Since the developmental positions align so well with the yoga poses, it means that movement transition from one pose to another can be used as an effective tool in both assessment and treatment.

#### Important Transitions

- Moving from supine to prone and prone to supine. Watch for adequate neck flexor–extensor strength as it is the component that initiates this transition.
- Prone to prone movement on forearms. Look for the ability to bring

hands under shoulders to push up onto forearms using neck and upper back extensors, shoulder and elbow extensors.

- Moving into quadruped from prone on forearms, using core muscles and hip flexors to bring knees under hips. Observe whether there is adequate strength in neck, upper back, shoulder and elbow extensors to move into position.
- Quadruped to side sit. Notice ability to rotate and control trunk movement, which is a function of core muscle strength, and dissociate movement of lower extremity as one hip moves into external rotation and the other moves into internal rotation.
- Quadruped to W-sit. A lot of babies will demonstrate this transition during the early phases of their sensorimotor development, as they lack the core strength and the rotatory control needed to perform the quadruped to side sit. As the sensorimotor system matures, they will be able to show more variety by being able to transition into side sit or into squat.
- Moving from prone to plank (resistance, flexing and extending arms). Observe whether there is adequate strength in the core and upper body.
- Moving from Upward Dog to Downward Dog (moving forward and backward).
- Squat to stand. Observe whether there is adequate strength in core, ankle, knee and hip extensor muscles.
- Tall kneel to half kneel. Watch for adequate core strength, weight shift, rotation to bring one foot in front.
- Half kneel to stand transition. Look for active ankle dorsiflexion in the back foot, adequate core strength and balance, knee and hip extensor and ankle plantarflexor muscle strength to push from half kneel to stand.
- Moving through a sequence of poses. Observe motor planning and coordination.

## PAUSE AND REFLECT

Practicing this sequence can be an opportunity for us as adults to experience our own neurodevelopmental repair and explore the resonating effect of the sequence on our own bodies and nervous systems.

I invite you to practice the neurodevelopmental sequence on your own. As you practice, explore each movement slowly and with intention. Imagine yourself as a baby, moving through the sequence with curiosity. With each posture and transition, notice which muscles you feel activating, which muscles you feel stretching, what level of effort is needed in each posture and in each transition from one posture to the next. Look at your hands and feet with awe and wonder. Imagine all the amazing changes that are happening in your body. Orient to your space as if you are taking in your environment for the first time. If you were a baby, what would you reach for? What would you crawl towards? What sounds and expressions might you make as you see the world through fresh eyes? As you are exploring this practice, imagine that your grown-up self is there with you. Watching with excitement and joy. Being witness to your growth and development. Celebrating your every movement. Ever present and available to wipe your tears, should you fall, and offer encouragement, should you become frustrated or in need of support.

Invitation to journal about your experience.

## Important Things to Consider When Assessing Physical Development

### Why Is the Core So Important?

Our core is the foundation for all functional postures and movement. Having good core strength facilitates stability in the spine, upright posture and balance. When children lack appropriate core strength, it impacts their movement, breathing, attention, stamina and ability to learn. Children with weak cores will often present with a collapsed posture, shoulders rounded, forward head posture and eyes moving more towards the ground. Core muscle strength greatly impacts the mechanics of breathing. With the diaphragm being an important part of the core muscle group and the primary muscle of respiration, any weakness in the core (postural) muscles leads to the child using the accessory (movement) muscles to breathe. Thus the child expends more energy for the basic function of breathing. In addition, much of their energy goes towards holding their bodies upright and can take away from the energy they need to attend to other tasks. Think of a child sitting in circle time on the floor, fidgeting, flopping over to the floor, slumping and struggling to focus. Often, a child's inability to sit still and attend to a task at hand can be due to lack of core strength. Because children develop from proximal to distal, weakness in their postural muscles will impact their fine motor skills. We must have well-developed gross motor skills in order to have well-developed fine motor skills. Our core is also the energy center or "sun" of our bodies. When children have weak cores, it can impact their mood, self-esteem and the way they move through the world. It is important to assess a child's core strength when developing a therapeutic protocol. Think of core strength as the foundation of your physical assessment.

### Motor Planning and Bilateral Coordination

Bilateral coordination is the ability to use both sides of the body at the same time in a controlled and organized manner. This can mean using *both sides to do the same thing*, such as catching a ball with both hands, using *alternating movements* such as when crawling or walking, or using *different movements on each side*, such as when tying shoes. Children with vestibular-proprioceptive processing difficulties typically have praxis and bilateral integration difficulties. Asana and movement can be used to both assess bilateral coordination and enhance skills in this area.

Symmetrical movement is when both sides of the body are doing the same thing.

Examples of symmetrical movement in asanas are:

- both arms reaching up in Warrior I
- both arms reaching out to side in Warrior II
- both knees bent and hips externally rotated in Butterfly
- the arms and legs in Table
- tapping body parts with both hands
- Star
- River
- Open Book/Close Book.

Reciprocal movement is when there are alternating movements on each side using rhythmical motion.

Examples of reciprocal movement in asanas are:

- arms alternating during Orange Juice Squeeze
- Marching Yogi (marching in place with alternating bent knees)
- Bicycle
- Reach for the Moon.

Asymmetrical movement is when both sides of the body are performing separate tasks.

Examples of asymmetrical movement in asanas are:

- Warrior poses
- Balancing poses
- Triangle.

Contralateral movement is a diagonal movement of one upper limb with the opposite lower limb. Crawling and walking are examples of contralateral movements.

Examples of contralateral movement in asanas are:

- Hunting Dog, which is done on hands and knees with one arm reaching forward and the opposite leg reaching back
- Shark, which is done on the belly with one arm reaching forward and up while the opposite leg reaches back and up
- Flamingo, which is done standing with one knee bent and lifted while reaching the opposite arm up.

Midline crossing movement is movement in which an arm or leg crosses over to the other side of the body, crossing the midline or "center" of the body.

Examples of midline crossing movement in asanas are:

- Apple Picking
- Eagle
- Roller Coaster Twist
- Bicycle.

### Understanding Social, Emotional and Cognitive Development

It is relatively easy to understand physical growth and development as it is obvious to see; however, social and emotional development often go unnoticed, such as when the child begins to understand sharing, taking turns or making friends. The social and emotional aspects of development relate to the child becoming able to understand and control their emotions while balancing the elements of socializing and interacting with other people around them. Understanding where a child is in their social-emotional development is necessary when developing yoga lesson plans and teaching yoga to children.

Healthy and typical social and emotional development will allow the child to:

- develop healthy relationships
- develop the ability to discover, play, create and learn
- expand attention span
- self-regulate their behavior
- develop a range of appropriate emotions.

Social development helps to shape the child to learn important skills such as proper reactions to matters of emotion. Emotional development is the process of learning how to understand and control emotions (self-monitoring and self-regulation). It's also important to have an understanding of cognitive and communication development. Cognitive development involves information processing, perceptual skills, language and learning. It is helpful to understand these stages of development when teaching the practices of yoga to children and teens. First, we have an understanding of where they are in terms of physical development so we can best support their social/emotional and learning needs; then we can help children build these skills by integrating yoga practice that helps strengthen their areas of development.

Table 2.1 Developmental milestones ages 2–17

| Age (years) | Social | Cognitive | Communication |
|---|---|---|---|
| 2 | • Begin to develop self-awareness<br>• Learn through imitation<br>• Connect with other children but mostly engage in parallel play<br>• Notice cause/effect | • Understand simple concepts (now, later)<br>• Follow simple one-direction requests<br>• Begin pretend play<br>• Begin to recognize and sort objects by shape/color | • Use at least 50 words<br>• Put two words together<br>• Name some body parts or familiar objects (toy, dog)<br>• Speak with mix of made-up and real words<br>• Repeat words |
| 3–4 | • Begin to cooperate with others, take turns and show problem-solving skills<br>• Show wide range of emotions<br>• Imagination is very active at this age | • Identify colors<br>• Understand same and different<br>• Follow three-part commands<br>• Remember parts of stories<br>• Identify common objects/pictures | • Speak 250–500 words<br>• Say name/age<br>• Answer simple questions<br>• Speak in sentences of 5–6 words at age 4<br>• Tell stories |
| 5–7 | • Begin to see others' perspectives and how their actions affect others<br>• Begin to develop sense of self-confidence and mastery of learning | • Begin learning to read and write<br>• Understand concepts of space, time and dimension<br>• Perform simple addition and subtraction<br>• Enjoy planning and building | • Develop oral language skills, acquiring new vocabulary and sentence structures<br>• Begin to reason and argue |
| 8–12 | • Increased perspective taking<br>• Value peer relationships<br>• More sophisticated and complex emotions and interactions<br>• Clear sense of self-identify | • Begin to think hypothetically and logically<br>• Become more goal oriented<br>• Can interpret context of a paragraph and write stories<br>• Can tell time | • Become more confident speakers<br>• May use cursing or slang to fit in with peers<br>• May begin to communicate more with peers than adults as they reach age 12 |

*cont.*

| Age (years) | Social | Cognitive | Communication |
|---|---|---|---|
| 13–17 | • Become very focused on peer relationships with same and opposite sex<br>• Can be very focused on opinions of peers and make choices around peer pressure | • Attain the ability to make decisions based on knowledge of others and their consequences<br>• Build skills to become more self-sufficient | • Teens essentially communicate as adults and want their opinions, thoughts and ideas to be heard and valued<br>• May use more "slang" language with peers |

## TYPICAL DEVELOPMENT VS DELAYED

Children with cognitive delays, physical challenges and social/emotional challenges may present as typical in some developmental areas but not others (e.g. show typical physical development, age-appropriate fine/gross motor skills but delay in social/emotional growth and development). It's important to look at the child as a whole in order to identify their cognitive, physical, communicative and social/emotional needs.

### Early Childhood (Birth to 8 Years)

At around age 1, emotional attachment formation occurs (Vinney, 2019). Attachment theory suggests that the attachment and bonds of love and trust that are formed with caregivers at this age can shape the child later in life. The way the child is cuddled, held, shown affection and played with early in life will set the basis for future adult relationships. Through years 3 to 5, skills in this category include forming relationships with peers, making choices, turn-taking and beginning to develop independence. In this stage of development, the child acquires the ability to imagine, to play well and cooperate with others, and to lead as well as follow (mirroring). The ability to see the perspective of another individual is difficult at this age. During the ages 1–4, children tend to be more impulsive and have less ability to sustain attention for longer periods of time.

Between the ages of 5 and 8, the child enters into a broader peer context in a learning environment and is able to develop close friendships. This is also a time when the child will begin to think about the future and understand more about their place in the world. If the child lacks a secure and trusting early childhood, they are more likely to experience fear, have difficulty forming strong friendships and continue to depend solely on caregivers. At this stage, the child displays empathy for others, has strong likes and dislikes, and responds well to structure and knowing what to expect.

## Middle Childhood (8–12 Years)

Between the ages of 8 and 12, the child can start to form stronger, more complex friendships and peer relationships. It becomes more emotionally important to have friends and develop peer connections. The child will begin to experience more peer pressure and will want to be liked and accepted by friends. As puberty approaches, the child will become more aware of their body. This pre-teen phase is a critical age to ensure self-love and acceptance as body image issues and eating problems are frequently seen at this stage as the child begins to compare themself to others. This stage is also a time when the child will face more academic challenges at school and will develop an increased attention span. The child will also become more independent from the family and more able to see the perspective of others.

## Adolescence (12–18 Years)

The rapid and sudden physical changes and the new intense experiences that adolescents go through make adolescence an important time in emotional development. This is a very self-conscious, sensitive and worrisome time for the individual as they make comparisons about themselves with their peers. Because physical changes may not occur on a smooth, regular schedule, many adolescents go through awkward stages, both with their appearance and physical coordination. Mood swings are common in adolescence and can be attributed to hormones and social, physical and cognitive changes facing the individual. As adolescents begin to separate from their parents and search for identity, they are confronted with the challenge of matching who they want to become with what is socially acceptable. With that said, the adolescent may exhibit unpredictable or contradictory behaviors. Their peer group may become a safe haven in which the adolescent can test new ideas.

In early adolescence, the peer group usually consists of non-romantic friendships, often including cliques, gangs or clubs. Members of the peer group often try to act alike, dress alike, have secret codes or rituals, and participate in the same activities.

In mid- to late adolescence, young people often feel the need to establish their sexual identity by becoming comfortable with their body and sexual feelings. This is a time when adolescents will have a strong focus on forming romantic relationships and dating. Adolescence also marks an important time for cognitive development, as the teen begins to change the way they think and reason about problems and ideas. As they develop more complex cognitive skills, adolescents gain the ability to solve more abstract and hypothetical problems, and they develop a stronger sense of right and wrong.

### Understanding the Adolescent Brain

Adolescence is a stage of great importance in terms of brain development.

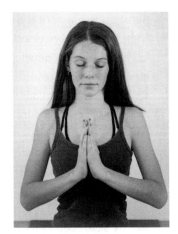

This stage is a period of transition between childhood and adulthood, and is defined approximately as ages 13–17; however, recent research shows that the growth and remodeling of the brain continues into the early to mid-20s (Johnson, Blum & Giedd, 2009).

Two very big things are happening in the brain during this stage of development.

**Synaptic pruning** is the process in which the brain eliminates extra synapses that aren't being used. Synapses are brain structures that allow neurons to transmit an electrical or chemical signal to another neuron. Synaptic pruning is the brain's way of removing connections in the brain that are no longer needed (Cafasso, 2018).

This is where the term "use it or lose it" applies. Synapses that are more active are strengthened, and synapses that are less active are weakened and ultimately pruned. The process of removing the irrelevant synapses is a whittling-down and shaping process like pruning and shaping a tree.

Early synaptic pruning is linked to our genes and later synaptic pruning is linked to our experiences. In essence, this means that children's brains are shaped by their experiences. When a child has a richness of experiences, frequent and ongoing, their synapses are more likely to become permanent compared to a child who receives little stimulation. This second group of children tend to keep fewer brain connections. Between the embryonic stage and age 2, new neurons and synapses are formed at an extremely high rate. In fact, at birth a baby's brain contains 100 billion neurons. As the neurons mature, new synapses are formed. By age 2–3, there are approximately 15,000 synapses per neuron (Graham, 2021).

What is occurring in these early stages of life is the laying of the foundation for the future construction of the building structure. The essential element in laying a firm and stable foundation is healthy attunement from a primary caregiver and rich experience through movement, play, sensory exploration and frequent exposure to new learning experiences, as well as opportunity to practice learned experiences. These are the building blocks for developing healthy connections in the brain.

Between ages 2 and 10, the number of synapses drops dramatically. This is when pruning is taking place more rapidly. During adolescence, there is less synaptic pruning occurring; however, the synapses that are present become more "stabilized" according to the adolescent's experiences and preferences.

**Myelin formation** is the "laying down" of myelin sheaths connecting the remaining linked neurons.

> Myelin enables the remaining and connected neurons to communicate with each other with more coordination and speed. Myelin permits the action potential—the ions flowing in and out of the membrane creating a flow of charge down the long axonal length—to move one hundred times faster. And the resting time between firings, the refractory period, is thirty times quicker. That means neural firing becomes three thousand times quicker with myelination. Practice lays down myelin to enable a skill.

> (Siegel, 2014)

What is interesting about what happens in the brain during adolescent development is that there is a significant decline in the gray matter in the prefrontal cortex (Mills *et al.*, 2016) and there is more activity seen in the limbic system. During adolescence, myelination and synaptic pruning increase in the prefrontal cortex. The decline in gray matter is thought to be correlated to the energy that is going towards synaptic pruning and the fine-tuning of connections between brain cells (Mills *et al.*, 2016).

The prefrontal cortex or frontal lobe is the area of the brain that is responsible for:

- decision making
- problem solving
- communication
- impulse and self-control
- self-reflection.

The limbic system is composed of four main parts: the hypothalamus, amygdala, thalamus and hippocampus. The limbic system is the emotional center of the brain and also the reward center of the brain.

This reduction in gray matter in the prefrontal cortex and increase in activity in the limbic system explains what we see in the emotional behavior of adolescents.

Siegel refers to this as a time when the adolescent brain is "under construction." He describes it this way: "turning off the plumbing and electricity for remodeling" the brain may be a bit messy and disheveled for a period of time until the construction is complete.

Naturally a remodeling zone will not be as functional during the re-constructive process as it will be later on: at times we need to shut-down the electricity or the plumbing during the process. But in the long run, the adolescent brain will result in more refined capacities, more emotional balance, more insight and wisdom, all processes resulting from integrative capacities to create internal well-being and interpersonal health.

(Siegel, 2014)

Behavior we may observe during adolescence includes:

- moodiness
- emotional unpredictability
- risk-taking behaviors
- self-consciousness
- impulsivity
- desire to break away from parental figures
- sometimes illogical/irrational thinking
- challenges with perspective taking.

During adolescence we might see:

- **A greater sensitivity to social evaluation and social judgment:** This is a time when adolescents are hyperfocused on the opinions of their peers, are self-conscious, self-critical and socially awkward, and have an intense desire and need to fit in and feel as though they belong among their peers.
- **Increased sensation-/reward seeking behavior:** During adolescence, there can be increased activities in adrenaline-inducing behaviors and/ or increased addictive tendencies towards drugs, alcohol, pornography, social media, video games, etc.
- **Exploration of identity:** This is often a time when adolescents are exploring their own identities and how they fit into the world around them.
- **Increased interest in sex and sexuality:** This is a time when adolescents begin to explore their sexuality and sexual relationships with others.

Because the adolescent brain has increased activation in the limbic system, their brains can be particularly sensitive to stressors.

Types of stressors include:

- **Biological:** Changes in hormone levels affect development of neurobiological circuits.
- **Population**: Mass events, war and disaster, and community/ socioeconomic issues such as violence, gangs, drugs, poverty can have longer-lasting impacts.
- **Social:** Adolescents need a supportive environment to develop their social identity and connection to peers.
- **Emotional:** Any life stressors such as school pressures, peer issues, family and home life.

Why can this stage of development be a positive opportunity for growth? At this stage in their brain development, adolescents are broadening experiences of social networks and increasing the acquisition of new skills. The time of puberty initiates intense learning and brain development, which leads to structural remodeling and neural reconfiguration of key brain systems. This is a crucial time for the formation of social networks that will have lasting impacts for the rest of their lives (Backes & Bonnie, 2019).

Through the exploration of mindfulness practices such as yoga, expressive and creative arts, music, sound and other experiences, there is linkage of different parts of the brain to one another and integration occurs. Integration is the path to harmony and homeostasis. Siegel notes:

> When linkage and differentiation are not present, chaos and rigidity can emerge. Integration creates the possibility of regulation—of attention, mood, emotion, thought, social interactions, and behavior. And much recent research supports this notion that impaired integration in the brain is at the root of many psychiatric disturbances.
>
> (Siegel, 2014)

The pruning and myelination that is occurring during adolescence is what links those differentiated regions to support integration. What better time to introduce yoga, mindfulness and self-regulation tools? Because these practices come from a more bottom-up approach, they are more accessible to the adolescent brain. The key is educating adolescents on the importance of repetition in their regulation practices so they can become fully integrated into their neural pathways and nervous systems, and they can carry those tools for resilience and regulation into adulthood. We want to educate and empower adolescents to understand how their brains work and what they can do to manage the ups and downs of adolescence.

## DEVELOPING AGE-APPROPRIATE SEQUENCES AND PROTOCOLS

Developing sequences and therapeutic protocols for children must take into consideration their age and stage of development (physical, cognitive, communication and social/emotional).

Below is a general guideline for developing one-on-one sessions and group sessions based on age.

### Ages 2–3

Toddlers are able to mirror and copy others' movements but are still developing their attention, coordination and self-regulation skills. Using simple directional cues such as reach, twist, touch, move, sit, stand, turn, jump will support them in processing information more efficiently. At this stage, they are learning through play, imitation and experience. Integrating a lot of movement, music, rhythm and repetition is recommended. At this stage, children are learning about their bodies, developing spatial awareness and discovering new ways to move their bodies. They are open and curious, and love to explore what their bodies can do! This is a time when children are still very egocentric and view the world mostly from their own perspective; however, it's a great time to begin to introduce awareness of their emotions and feelings as well as those of others.

### Ages 4–6

Children at this stage are full of imagination and can have very active and curious minds. They are continually asking questions and wanting to learn and understand the world around them. They begin to develop the capacity to pay attention for longer and are building more capacity with managing their emotions. They become much more aware of others' perspectives and, as they mature, become more engaged in connected and interactive play, negotiation and exploration with other children their age. This is a time to emphasize building empathy, self-awareness and awareness of others.

This is also a good time to teach the importance of movement and create a love for yoga. This time is the foundation for their future years!

Integrating stories, themes and playful games and activities as well as activities that focus on social/emotional learning and self-regulation is recommended. Children at this stage love to make up their own poses and stories. Give them ample opportunity to explore their bodies, to come up with their own ideas and offer choices. These are building blocks for helping children develop self-agency, self-empowerment and self-esteem.

Children at this stage are also developing so many new neural pathways and physical abilities. Integrating crossing midline, bilateral movement, balance poses and lots of different types of movement (e.g. rolling, jumping, rocking, climbing, balancing) supports brain, sensory and motor development.

## Ages 7–8

At this stage, children are continuing to learn about the world around them and are building their sense of self as well as how they see themselves in relationship to others. They are able to be more accurate in following physical cues and instructions. They enjoy new challenges and have a strong sense of wanting to be seen and heard. They are more able to express what they are feeling *inside* their bodies. Opportunity to develop more interoceptive awareness and connection to emotion as well as healthy expression of emotion is important at this stage. Building self-regulation and communication skills is important. This is also an age when it is important to teach healthy boundaries, healthy expression of emotions and building more awareness of others and how their actions and behaviors impact not only themselves but those around them. Partner and group activities are a great way to teach these foundational skills.

## Ages 9–12

At this stage, children are beginning to navigate changes in their bodies, more awareness of their peers' opinions of them and more awareness and worry around how and where they "fit in." Many children may feel more shy about practicing yoga with their peers and may focus more on their performance and doing the poses "perfectly." It is so important at this stage to talk about how it's okay to make mistakes and how that helps build resiliency and new neural pathways in the brain. This is a great time to educate kids about their bodies and how their brains work. Giving them the *why* is so important for them to understand how yoga and mindfulness can support them in navigating stressful situations and help them to be mentally, emotionally and physically balanced. This is also a great time to explain how yoga can support learning, reducing anxiety and even helping them perform better in sports and other activities. Allowing them the opportunity to work together, problem solve and have autonomy is crucial.

Sun salutations, balancing poses, standing poses and core-building poses are great poses to work with for building self-confidence, self-empowerment and self-agency—standing in their truth! Partner poses are great poses for supporting connection, community and working together.

## Teens 13+

The teenage years are a time of great growth and great challenge. Physically, a significant amount of actual growth takes place as well as significant hormonal changes and changes in their bodies, moods and emotions. Because of hormonal changes and social and academic pressures, many teens will experience waves of confusing and distressing emotions. It's crucial during this stage to educate teens on what is happening in their brains and bodies and explain to them that being a teenager is like being a tidal wave—always moving and fluctuating. Teaching how yoga and mindfulness can be used as a tool to "ride the waves" of teenhood and help support their emotional, mental and physical wellbeing is critical.

Because of the awareness of and worry about their bodies, image of themselves and what others think of them, it is important to emphasize acceptance of different bodies, abilities and personalities and focus a lot of attention on activities to build self-esteem. Journaling, mantras, mudras and self-reflection activities will help teens build more self-awareness. Helping teens to connect more inwardly to their sensations and emotions will support them in building more awareness of their emotional wellbeing as well as letting their attention go more inward, rather than outward to a sometimes overwhelming outside world.

Having teens collaborate with you to develop their own sequences around a specific intention or focus can be helpful in building connection and asserting autonomy and self-agency. Teaching teens about yoga's physical benefits, which muscles are working, which muscles are stretching, along with its mental/emotional benefits gives them more of a sense of the *why*. Asking teens to identify which poses are their favorite and why will help them build more connection to their own personal experience and practice.

Teens can be very connected to music at this stage. Have them share some of their favorite songs and integrate their preferred music in your sessions.

Educating teens on simple and accessible self-regulation tools they can use throughout the day when feeling anxious, overwhelmed or stressed can be powerful in helping them develop coping strategies and build resilience.

Table 2.2 provides a guide to assist in understanding developmental considerations and challenges as well as specific practices and techniques to support children and teens at different ages and stages.

Table 2.2 Developing yoga sessions or classes for ages/stages

| Ages | Developmental considerations | Challenges | Types of poses/ practices | Techniques |
|---|---|---|---|---|
| 3–5 | • Short attention span<br>• Lack of self-control over emotions<br>• Difficulty with perspective taking (e.g. sharing, taking turns) | • Managing big emotions within a group or 1:1 setting<br>• Working with changing moods<br>• Transitions<br>• Personal space or boundaries within a group | • Animal poses along with animal sounds<br>• Use songs, games, stories and attention-grabbing activities<br>• Integrate art activities to correlate with poses | • Repetition<br>• Concrete language<br>• Give short and direct clues<br>• Focus on yoga "play" rather than "alignment" and getting the pose right |

| | | | |
|---|---|---|---|
| • Expectations and rules need to be frontloaded<br>• Use multi-modalities for teaching (e.g. visual, auditory, kinesthetic)<br>• Vivid imagination<br>• Rapidly developing brains<br>• Still developing language and communication skills | • Requiring a significant amount of attention<br>• Keeping them engaged<br>• Communication and processing<br>• Sharing<br>• Impulsivity<br>• Lack of attention skills | • Poses that support sensory processing and brain development<br>• Chants, singing, vowel chants<br>• Weave in the five senses | • Use a sing-songy voice and teach with energy and joy<br>• Attunement and co-regulation is very important at this stage<br>• Offer many opportunities for making choices<br>• Use stuffed animals and other visual props<br>• Teach through "cause" and "effect" |
| 6–8 | • Logic and reasoning increases<br>• Increased desire for independence<br>• Increased peer connection<br>• Building sense of self<br>• Increased focus and attention<br>• More able to follow instructions<br>• Brain is still building foundations for learning<br>• Need for structure and routine<br>• Development of empathy and perspective taking<br>• Imagination is expanding | • May be more aware of limitations or differences<br>• Want to be in charge<br>• Increase in testing boundaries<br>• More competitive<br>• Very focused on justice and fairness<br>• Sharing can still be challenging<br>• May show more "stubbornness" or defiance<br>• More sophisticated behaviors (desire to manipulate environment to get their needs met) | • Animal poses along with sounds<br>• Add facts about animals<br>• Yoga games with peers<br>• Partner and group poses<br>• Creating their own yoga stories<br>• Weave in the eight limbs and building empathy and connection<br>• Music, chanting, rhythm and songs<br>• Focus on self-regulation<br>• Begin exploring chakras in a simple way<br>• Build in simple explanations of the brain and anatomy<br>• Build in interoception<br>• Focus practices | • Begin with the simple variation and then offer more challenging options<br>• Emphasize effort rather than performance<br>• Provide opportunity to be a leader<br>• Offer choices<br>• Take turns letting them be a "yoga helper"<br>• Front-load rules and expectations<br>• Encourage them to share their ideas and be a part of the process in structuring classes |

*cont.*

| Ages | Developmental considerations | Challenges | Types of poses/ practices | Techniques |
|---|---|---|---|---|
| 9–12 | • Rapidly developing bodies<br>• Forging meaningful support relationships with peers and adults outside of family system<br>• May become more modest about body during this stage<br>• More interested in "skill mastery"<br>• More influenced by peer pressure and peer opinions<br>• May be more shy around peers<br>• Desire to be leaders and share their ideas and opinions | • May exhibit more self-consciousness around participating in classes with their peers<br>• May show increased anxiety around external pressures (e.g. peer, academic, sport, family)<br>• May "talk back" or lash out in emotional ways towards peers and adults<br>• Judgmental of peers<br>• Social isolation<br>• Challenges with self-esteem<br>• Difficulty taking responsibility for one's behavior | • Teach poses through categories/ resonating effects<br>• Share benefits and how poses impact the brain and body<br>• Self-inquiries (how does that feel in my body?)<br>• Chakras, chanting, mudras, mantras<br>• Incorporate music<br>• Weave in the Yamas and Niyamas (Eight Limbs)<br>• Challenge them to make up poses/ partner poses<br>• Add more challenging options for poses<br>• Teach the Sanskrit names of poses<br>• Focus on non-judgment and self-empowerment | • Emphasize the "experience" in the pose rather than how it looks<br>• Encourage exploring the poses in different ways<br>• Educate about anatomy, stress and the brain<br>• Teach simple self-regulation tools<br>• Discuss action, responsibility and consequences<br>• Provide opportunity to lead<br>• Allow them to choose poses and sequence poses<br>• Group/ teamwork<br>• Ask for input and ideas<br>• Create opportunities to share about emotions/ experiences |
| 13–18 | • Spike in growth<br>• Hormonal changes<br>• Mood swings<br>• Awkwardness with their bodies<br>• Increased physical skill and stamina<br>• Self-conscious | • Waves of mood and emotions<br>• More risk-taking behavior<br>• Problems can feel really big and overwhelming<br>• Physical pain in the body (growing pains) | • Partner poses that don't require looking right at each other (e.g. back-to-back breathing)<br>• Do poses and breathing with eyes closed or backs to one another<br>• Meditation practices | • Teach alignment-based practices<br>• Encourage exploration of the poses through using different variations and props<br>• Integrate confidence-building mantras and practices |

| | | | |
|---|---|---|---|
| • Greatly influenced by peers and peer opinions<br>• Desire to be their own person and make their own choices<br>• Pruning is happening in the brain, strengthening neural pathways | • Lack of sleep<br>• Anxiety/ depression<br>• Isolation<br>• Low self-esteem<br>• Can be impulsive<br>• Compare themselves to others<br>• Perfectionism<br>• Lack of reasoning and judgment when big emotions occur<br>• Feelings of being "out of control" | • Chakras, mudras, mantras<br>• Journaling<br>• Expressive arts<br>• Awareness of the senses (grounding and orienting practices)<br>• Breath control<br>• Sun salutations, strength- and stamina-building poses<br>• Somatic movement practices<br>• Build in yoga philosophy<br>• Teach about anatomy, brain development and fight/flight/freeze stress response<br>• Self-empowerment and self-agency<br>• Integrate favorite music/songs | • Emphasize the importance of repetition and practice<br>• Allow opportunities to make choices<br>• Avoid using mirrors for practice<br>• Encourage isolation of different muscles in the practice<br>• Interoception<br>• Self-inquiry (where do you feel the stretch or sensation?)<br>• Provide a "share box" where they can share their emotions, experiences in a safe way<br>• Educate about "growth mindset"<br>• Be an ally |

# Chapter 3

# The Autonomic Nervous System, Polyvagal Theory and Neuroception

The autonomic nervous system (ANS) is a division of the peripheral nervous system. It controls the conditions inside the body and has sometimes been referred to as the "visceral nervous system." The ANS automatically regulates the function of body systems without conscious effort. The ANS controls many different functions such as heart rate, digestion, respiratory rate and blood pressure. According to Stephen Porges' Polyvagal Theory, the ANS consists of three sequential systems or neural platforms that follow brain evolution (Porges, 2017).

Porges' theory developed out of his experiments with the vagus nerve. The vagus nerve serves as the parasympathetic branch of the nervous system, which is the down-regulating system. The parasympathetic branch of the nervous system balances the sympathetic nervous system (SNS), supporting rest, restoration and survival. Essentially, the parasympathetic nervous system (PNS) acts as the break for the sympathetic nervous system.

The SNS activates the fight/flight response during threat or when there is perceived danger. It essentially serves as an alarm system and elicits a rapid, involuntary mobilization response to stress or danger. When this alarm system goes off, the body actually prepares to fight or flee. The flow of blood moves towards the gross motor limbs, the adrenal glands release a surge of hormones, including adrenaline and cortisol, heart rate and blood pressure increase, and other "non-essential" functions for survival are suppressed in order to conserve energy, such as digestion and reproduction. The SNS has an important role in our overall functioning. It keeps us in balance by bringing *mobilization* to our system when needed. It's like pressing the gas pedal on a car to get it to move. If there was no gas, the car would not be able to function. The problem arises when the fight/flight response is always turned on or the gas pedal is constantly being pressed. The body's stress response system is meant to be limited, to fluctuate between sympathetic and parasympathetic in order to meet the particular need in the moment and then come back to a balanced state. When aroused, the system takes time to return to a resting state. Being in a perpetual state of fight/flight over an extended period of time can lead to physical, mental and emotional issues for children and teens. Children who are in fight/flight may present as:

- easily frustrated, angered or flustered
- impulsive
- having aggressive or acting-out behaviors
- very emotional
- oppositional or argumentative
- distracted, unfocused or having difficulty paying attention
- hyper
- fearful
- fidgety
- avoidant
- anxious, worried or overwhelmed.

The most primitive part of the ANS is the dorsal vagal complex (DVC), which dates back as far as 500 million years ago. Anatomically, the dorsal vagus is sub-diaphragmatic (below the diaphragm). The DVC is the unmyelinated branch of the vagus nerve and part of the parasympathetic nervous system. The dorsal vagal complex, when overloaded, is responsible for immobilization or *freeze*. This is what is considered the shut-down response often associated with trauma. Essentially, when there is a perceived life threat and the first survival response of fight/flight is not an option, the system goes into a freeze state in order to survive. The dorsal vagal state helps the body conserve oxygen and slows the use of energy. Think about a lizard when a dog is chasing it in the yard and it realizes it can't fight or flee; it will become very still and immobilized. When this freeze response occurs, the temperature in the body drops, respiration slows, heart rate decreases and the system goes into a state of energy conservation. This means there is not as much oxygen being produced to fuel the cells, not as much blood flowing to the internal organs and less energy moving towards thinking and memory.

Children who are in a dorsal vagal/freeze state may present as:

- withdrawn
- isolating from others
- zoned out
- having trouble with memory

- having difficulty focusing/learning
- apathetic
- having depressive energy
- lethargic
- numb
- immobilized/stuck
- disconnected
- shut down
- showing lack of emotion.

It's necessary to understand that the dorsal vagal system is not simply associated with the freeze response. The freeze/immobility response occurs when there are higher levels of dorsal activation. At low levels, the dorsal vagal system in combination with the ventral vagal system modulates ongoing activity of visceral function, experienced as pleasure, rest, restoration and wellbeing.

These functions include:

- supporting ambient digestion
- enhancing deep relaxation
- quiet connection with others (e.g. reading a book, nursing)
- shutting down systems to conserve energy when needed (time-limited) (Levin, n.d.a).

It's important to remember that both the fight/flight response and freeze response are survival responses, so when they are activated, it is not the optimal time for thinking, learning, communicating, reasoning and other higher-order processes. When children are in states of high sympathetic arousal or high dorsal activation, they are not able to access the higher brain. Daniel Siegel refers to this as the downstairs brain (brain stem, amygdala) and the upstairs brain (prefrontal cortex) (Siegel & Bryson, 2012). We first have to address children's downstairs brain (survival) before they can access their upstairs brain (growth, learning, communication and connection).

The ventral vagal complex (VVC) is also part of the parasympathetic nervous system. This branch is the most recent evolution and is only present in mammals. Porges refers to the VVC as the social engagement system. The VVC is the myelinated branch of the vagus nerve. "Myelination begins at birth and continues throughout childhood. Myelination facilitates growth, learning, social connection and the sense of touch" (Levine, n.d.a). Anatomically, the ventral vagus is supradiaphragmatic (above the diaphragm). The social engagement system is our face–heart connection. The vagus (heart) and nerves in the face and head connect to control:

- facial expression (emotional expression)
- eyelids (social gaze)
- middle ear (to hear human voice)
- mastication (ingestion, sucking)
- larynx, pharynx (vocalizing, swallowing, breathing)
- head turn and tilt (social gesture, orienting).

"Through these pathways you send and search for signs of welcome and signals of warning" (Dana, 2020).

Think about our social engagement systems and how we cue into facial expressions, gestures and people's voices in order to decipher between people who feel "safe" and people who we perceive may pose a threat. Now consider how we express ourselves through our facial expressions, voice and gestures when we are in a more regulated and connected state, and how that can directly impact whether a child experiences a felt sense of safety and connection with us.

As a society, we place such a strong emphasis on self-regulation, when, really, shifting to a relational culture of co-regulation—where we work towards mutual care, respect, attunement and understanding of one another and recognize our own impact our nervous system states have on those around us—follows the natural evolution of co-regulation before self-regulation.

## CO-REGULATION

"Babies are born with fully functioning dorsal vagal systems. The sympathetic system develops and begins to function only after birth. The caretaker acts as the ventral vagal (soothing) system until the baby's system is myelinated and can begin to regulate itself" (Levine, n.d.a). This is referred to as co-regulation. If a baby receives consistent care and attention from their caregivers and receives nourishing co-regulation, their nervous systems will develop in a healthy way. If babies' needs are not attended to and they do not have the support of co-regula-tion from their primary caregiver, their system may be stuck in more of the dorsal state or hypervigilance in the nervous system. This can affect the ways their brains develop and their ability to create secure attachment relationships throughout their lives. Essentially, a child's early attachment relationships greatly impact their nervous systems, the way they perceive the world and the way in which they move through the world. Secure and healthy attachment relationships provide a foundation of trust and safety, which in turn provides a sense of security for a child to move through the world with curiosity and connection. When a child has not experienced healthy and safe attachment relationships with a primary adult, they may tend to be more cautious, fearful or distrusting, and may perceive the world and the people in it as unsafe and even dangerous. Stephen Porges (2022) describes this as neuroception.

Children's neuroception is shaped by experience. For instance, if a child experienced ongoing neglect, abuse or other significant trauma, their brain becomes hardwired to look for danger and their perception can be that the people and environment around them are dangerous, even when they are not. Kathy Kain and Stephen Terrell describe this as "sticks and snakes" (Kain & Terrell, 2018). If we have experienced a lot of "snakes," which represent danger in early development, our brains will build up a memory catalog of snakes. Imagine taking a hike. As you are walking along the path, there is a stick, but your brain is hardwired that every snake is a snake and every stick is also a snake. So when you see this stick, your body's stress response becomes activated as if it were a snake, and this continues as you walk along the path. Essentially, our goal as the adult working with the child is to help them build up a memory catalog of more sticks than snakes, so their neuroception becomes more attuned to safety and connection than danger and threat. It's helpful to understand neuroception in relation to polyvagal theory. Here is a simple guide.

### Ventral Vagal: Neuroception of Safety

When a child is in a ventral vagal state, they are more attuned to safety and connection. There is more of a felt sense of safety, their nervous systems are more regulated, and they are more able to access the thinking and reasoning parts of the brain. When children experience a felt sense of safety, they are more willing to explore, engage, express and experience new things.

It's important to understand that the VVC does not work on its own. Its helpers are the SNS and the DVC. For instance, when a child is engaged in active play, is preparing for a race, to take a test or needs the energy and mobilization to engage in a task or social situation, the VVC and SNS work together in order to mobilize their systems so they can be both energized and connected at the same time. This is also true with the VVC and DVC relationship. For instance, when a baby is nursing or a child is snuggling up with their caregiver while reading a story, both the VVC and DVC are working together to offer this engaged, restful and connected experience.

### Fight/Flight: Neuroception of Danger

When a child is in fight/flight or sympathetic activation, they are more attuned to danger. Their alarm system is on and they will tend to be on high alert. They will be more apt to orient to danger and may feel more anxious, agitated or hypervigilant. This impacts their desire to explore the world and connect with others. Their dysregulation can often present as maladaptive behaviors that impact their attention, learning and social relationships with others.

## Freeze: Neuroception of Life Threat

When a child is in a high dorsal vagal state or freeze state, they are more attuned to life threat. This survival state can present as a child who is disconnected and disengaged. These are the children or teens who may not present as "acting out" but instead may appear as unemotional, apathetic and more passive.

It's important to understand that simply because a child is not acting out, it does not mean their nervous system is not in a high state of activation or overwhelm. Each nervous system state presents itself differently in terms of the impact it has on the system as a whole. This is referred to as allostatic load or what Stephen Porges calls "the cost of doing business" (Kain & Terrell, 2018).

Allostatic load refers to the cumulative burden of chronic stress on the physiological system or, simply put, "the wear and tear" on the body. When environmental challenges exceed a person's ability to cope and a person is in overwhelm for an extended period of time, allostatic overload ensues. Essentially, the neuroendocrine, cardiovascular, neuroenergetic and emotional responses become persistently activated, which in turn causes a breakdown in the body's systems and impacts physical, emotional and mental wellbeing (Wikipedia, 2022a). Think about having a bank account of energy reserves. Allostatic overload is essentially using up more in the bank account than is available. Specific nervous system states generate a higher allostatic load than others. For instance, when a child is in a state of high sympathetic activation or fight/flight for an extended period of time, there is a high allostatic load on the system. This makes sense because what we often associate with fight/flight is increased arousal and energy. It's also important to understand that high levels of dorsal activation or being in a freeze state more often than not also causes a high allostatic load. It requires a tremendous amount of energy to "suppress" the system. In fact, this increased energy conservation and immobilization response can require more energy than it does to just mobilize the system. Think of pressing the gas and the brake on a car at the same time. There is a tremendous amount of energy (gas) being used but the system is still immobilized or stuck. Imagine the "revving" of the engine while the brake is being pressed over an extended period of time. The engine would eventually give out. This high allostatic load over an extended period of time, due to increased dorsal vagal activity, can lead to more syndromal responses in the body. Some examples of syndromal response might include autoimmune conditions, unexplained chronic pain and other symptoms.

Effects of high allostatic load include:

- irritability
- inattention
- behavior issues
- weakened immune system
- chronic illness
- mental illness
- chronic pain
- digestive issues
- autoimmune conditions
- increased risk of heart conditions.

Examples of nervous systems states that have a lower allostatic load are the ventral vagal state and sympathetic states that are time-limited.

So let's talk about allostasis. Allostasis is the active process that leads to adaptation to a stressor (McEwan & Wingfield, 2007). Homeostasis is the regulation of physiological processes, whereby systems respond to the state of the body and the external environment (Billman, 2020). Our nervous system is constantly working to bring our bodies back to homeostasis. This role of the SNS is to turn on when mobilization or "action" is required, and the role of the PNS is to meet the SNS and bring it back to a balanced and restful state in order to allow for restoration and regeneration. Homeostasis is this beautiful dance between the SNS and PNS that responds according to the demands of the environment.

What causes the system to go awry is when there is an overload to the system and the body is not able to come back to homeostasis frequently enough to keep the system balanced and running efficiently. So how do we decrease allostatic load and support children's systems in coming back to balance or homeostasis? By helping them to increase their window of tolerance and build capacity in their nervous systems.

## Window of Tolerance

The window of tolerance is a concept created by Daniel Siegel to describe the "optimal arousal zone" of human beings (Siegel, 1999). When we are managing the stressors in life and are able to move back and forth between sympathetic and parasympathetic states in order to meet the demands of the experience, then we are in our "window of tolerance." For example, a child becomes upset that he didn't win a board game and yells, "It's not fair!" and pounds his fist on the table (sympathetic). The caregiver responds, "It can be hard not to win all the time, can't it?" and then offers a hug to the child. The child calms down and asks to play another game (parasympathetic). In this case, the child became upset and was able to express his emotion but was then able to calm down quickly and continue to engage in play. An example of the child being out of his window of tolerance would be if he were to have a complete meltdown and be inconsolable for hours about losing the game.

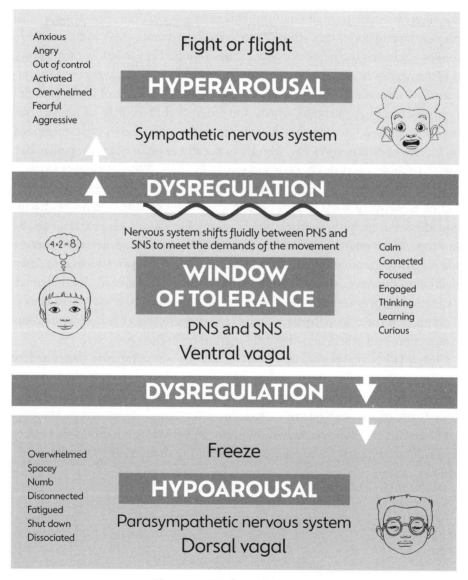

**Figure 3.1** Window of tolerance

Each of our windows of tolerance looks different. Some windows are wider with a lot of space and others are narrower. Much of this depends on a child's early experiences and whether or not they had a healthy and attuned connection with their primary caregiver. A child's ability to self-regulate is dependent on the co-regulation they received in their early formative years. If a child experiences trauma such as neglect or abuse, or their needs were not met by their primary caregiver, their nervous systems may become dysregulated or overwhelmed. This can also be the case for children who have sensory processing challenges or who are highly sensitive to their environment, as well as children who struggle with processing and communication. Their systems are more rigid and not as able to move between the nervous system states fluidly. Their window of tolerance is often narrower, and they may become "stuck" in a survival response or dys-regulated nervous system state. They may be stuck in more of a state of high sympathetic or hyperarousal, which is the fight/flight response, or high dorsal, hypoarousal, also known as the freeze response. Hyperarousal is characterized by excessive activation/energy, which can present as anxiety, anger, panic, fear, hypervigilance, overthinking and emotional flooding. When a child is stuck in this state of hypervigilance, it can be difficult for them to relax. It's as if the "on" button is always turned on. This impacts their sleep, attention, mood, behavior and physical functioning in their body systems. Hypoarousal is characterized by low tone, low arousal or shut-down energy. This response occurs when there is too much hyperarousal and the system goes into overwhelm and has to shut down in order to survive. In this state, a child may present as exhausted, disconnected, distracted, depressive, apathetic, mentally foggy, numb and even dissociated. This impacts their sleep (they may tend to oversleep), mood, behavior, learning, connection with others and physical functioning in their body systems.

Essentially, our aim is to support children and teens to increase their window of tolerance and build capacity for managing stressful and unexpected events—to be able to move with relative ease from sympathetic back to parasympathetic. This is the capacity to return to baseline after experiencing stress. We help children expand their window of tolerance by providing a container of safety and support, offering co-regulation and teaching them tools to regulate their nervous systems.

Chapter 4

# Sensory Processing and Neurodiversity: Autism, ADHD and Other Neuro Differences

## WHAT IS NEURODIVERSITY?

The term "neurodiversity" was first used in the late 1990s by Judy Singer, a sociologist who is also autistic (Neurodiversity Hub, n.d.). Neurodiversity emphasizes that the world is made up of individuals with different brain variations and there's no "normal" way of functioning, rather a spectrum of different ways of processing, learning, communicating, behaving, socializing and moving through the world. Neurodiversity focuses on celebrating neuro differences and recognizing the benefits and strengths of seeing and experiencing the world through a unique lens. Neurodiversity represents the full spectrum of both neurotypical and neurodivergent humans.

## NEURODIVERGENT VS NEUROTYPICAL

Several important terms are employed within the field of neurology, including the terms "neurodivergent" and "neurotypical."

Someone who is neurotypical has a brain that works according to the "normal" standards of our society. Anyone whose brain doesn't work according to those standards can be termed neurodivergent.

The neurodiversity movement sees the differences in brain function as normal variations in brain functionality (Tougaw, 2020). In this view, there is nothing "wrong" with children who have these differences and they don't need to be "fixed" or "cured," but instead accepted for who they are, supported by society and provided with the necessary supports in order for them to thrive.

Many brain variations fall under the category of neurodivergence to include:

- autism
- ADHD
- Down syndrome
- post-traumatic stress disorder (PTSD) and other mental health diagnosis (anxiety, depression, schizophrenia, bipolar)
- obsessive compulsive disorder (OCD)
- Tourette's syndrome
- sensory processing variations
- dyslexia
- dyscalculia
- dyspraxia
- epilepsy
- Parkinson's disease
- intellectual disability.

Over the years, I have had the honor of working with hundreds of children and teens who presented as neurodivergent, both in the school setting and one-on-one yoga therapy settings. What I often observed when working in the education system was that there was a tremendous amount of emphasis placed on the child's disability, inabilities and specific challenges. What I found to be most helpful and most impactful in the child's programming was really getting to know their unique preferences, learning styles, interests and strengths. This is particularly important in working therapeutically with a child or teen. Of course, it is necessary to know and understand a child's diagnosis and the challenges they face, but it is equally important to identify their strengths and build upon those strengths in their sessions. I think of their strengths and interests as foundational building blocks in addressing the challenges they face. It is our duty to gather all of the information so we are well informed and can support their specific needs, but we must always see and acknowledge each child or teen as a whole and perfect human being and honor their unique strengths and ways of moving through the world.

The deeper philosophy of yoga teaches that we are whole, perfect and beautiful just as we are, that we don't need "fixing" because we are not broken. To love and accept ourselves and recognize that we each have an important purpose in the world. Our responsibility as yoga therapists is to embody love and acceptance and support children in building self-confidence, self-esteem, self-acceptance and self-appreciation of their unique gifts, qualities and strengths. We can best do this by providing necessary supports for diverse brains and learning styles to thrive. Our differences are what make the world such an interesting, colorful, vibrant and compelling place.

Below is a reference to specific diagnoses and some of the challenges children or teens with these diagnoses may face, as well as the strengths they may present. Keep in mind that each individual child is different and unique and may or may not present with the outlined challenges or strengths. Information about each child's unique challenges and strengths should be gathered via an intake form as well as parent and child interview. Your first several sessions with the child will also provide a great deal of insightful information about both their challenges and strengths.

## AUTISM
### Common Challenges Autistic Children or Teens May Experience
### Challenges with Social Relationships and Communication

- Understanding social cues and social pragmatics (recognizing and making sense of facial expressions, gestures and social situations)
- Language processing
- Expressive and receptive language
- Processing verbal language and expressing their wants/needs
- Understanding their emotions and emotion of others
- Rigidity and strong need for predictability
- Hyperfocused interests
- Speech apraxia

### Emotional/Mental Health Challenges

- Anxiety
- Depression
- ADHD
- OCD

### Learning Challenges

- Focus/attention
- Memory
- Processing information
- Reading/writing
- Learning disabilities

### Sensory Processing Challenges

- Sensory overwhelm
- Sensory underwhelm
- Challenges with interoceptive awareness
- Challenges with eating
- Challenges with body awareness and connection to their body
- Alexithymia (difficulty identifying and expressing emotions)

### Motor Coordination Challenges

- Gross/fine motor skills
- Timing
- Coordination
- Balance
- Dyspraxia

### Physical Challenges

- Low muscle tone
- Hypermobility
- Epilepsy

### Health Challenges

- Digestive issues
- Sleep issues
- Chronic pain
- Autoimmune conditions

## Autistic Strengths and Important Qualities

- Visual skills
- Creative minds
- Attuned to deeper layers of consciousness
- Aware of environment
- Special interests
- Honest
- Resilient
- Intelligent
- Gifted

- Thinking outside of the box
- Unique
- Attention to detail
- Absorbing and retaining facts
- Observant
- Expertise in topics of interest
- Deep focus

## ADHD
## Common Challenges Children or Teens with ADHD May Experience
### Challenges with Social Relationships and Communication

- Difficulty with developing and maintaining social relationships
- Difficulty with social pragmatics

### Emotional/Mental Health Challenges

- Impulsivity
- Hyperarousal/hyperactivity
- Scattered thoughts
- Behavior challenges
- Low self-esteem
- Anxiety/depression

### Learning Challenges

- Difficulty with focus/attention
- Challenges with executive functioning
- Challenges with cognitive processing
- Difficulty with reading and/or writing

### Sensory Processing Challenges

- Lack of body awareness
- Lack of interoceptive awareness
- Difficulty identifying and communicating emotions
- Challenges with sensory integration
- Difficulty with self-regulation

### Motor Coordination Challenges

- Difficulty with coordinated movement
- Fine/gross motor challenges
- Hypermobility

### Health Challenges

- Autoimmune conditions
- Digestive issues
- Sleep issues
- Chronic pain

### ADHD Strengths and Important Qualities

- Hyperfocus
- Ingenuity
- Risk-raking
- Energetic
- Creative
- Persistent
- Passionate
- Out-of-the-box thinking
- Unique
- Resilient
- Motivated
- Full of personality
- Attention to detail
- Charismatic
- Social

## SPEECH AND MOTOR IMPAIRMENTS

Many of the children identified in this chapter as well as children with Down syndrome may struggle with speech and motor impairments. Yoga can be a great adjunct therapy in supporting children with speech and motor coordination challenges.

## What Is Praxis?

Praxis refers to when you want to do a movement and your brain tells your muscles what steps to take in order to accomplish the task.

## Motor Apraxia

Motor apraxia refers to difficulty with motor planning and coordination and is a neurological disorder characterized by loss of ability to execute or carry out skilled movements and gestures. Apraxia results from the dysfunction of the cerebral hemispheres of the brain, in particular the parietal lobe (National Institute of Neurological Disorders and Stroke, n.d.). Children's daily functioning, movement and speech can be greatly impacted by motor apraxia.

## Dyspraxia

Those with dyspraxia—also known as motor planning difficulties or perceptual-motor dysfunction—have difficulty with movement, coordination, judgment, processing, memory and sometimes other cognitive skills. Dyspraxia affects the body's immune and nervous systems. Gross and fine motor skills are impacted. Children with dyspraxia will often present with poor posture, balance and hand–eye coordination. They may also fatigue easily (Newman, 2017).

### Therapeutic Focus

If a child has motor apraxia or dyspraxia, work on step-by-step movement of poses, sequencing poses, balancing poses, crossing the midline, bilateral movements in poses, breathing exercises, chanting and mantras, yoga games, deep pressure and poses for proprioceptive and vestibular feedback, as well as poses that soothe the nervous system and strengthen the immune system. Incorporate patterning, repetition and rhythm. Provide accommodations and supports as well as variations of poses and practices to support their specific physical needs.

## Speech Apraxia

Childhood apraxia of speech (CAS) is a motor speech disorder that makes it difficult for children to speak. Children with the diagnosis of apraxia of speech generally have a good understanding of language and know what they want to say. However, they have difficulty learning or carrying out the complex sequenced movements that are necessary for intelligible speech (Cedars Sinai, n.d.). Children with CAS may also present with fine motor delays, sensory processing challenges, delayed language development and difficulty with reading and writing.

### Language Processing Disorder

Language processing disorder impacts a child's ability to process language and communicate verbally. Their expressive and receptive language processing can be impacted. Expressive language is the ability to effectively communicate wants, needs and thoughts. Receptive language is the ability to process and understand verbal communication.

Children with speech apraxia and language processing challenges may struggle with attention, learning, understanding and coping with the frustration of not being able to communicate effectively.

Yoga is a wonderful complementary therapy for children with speech difficulties. The practice of yoga can support speech and communication in these ways:

- opens the body and creates better posture for more diaphragmatic breathing
- extends the exhalation through breathing strategies, animal noises and chanting
- making different animal noises and sounds encourages different oral motor movements
- the practice of yoga can reduce stress and anxiety, which impacts our breathing, speech and communication
- the practice of yoga can support self-confidence and self-esteem
- gross motor development supports fine motor development. The phrase "hips before lips" refers to the importance of developing trunk stability and strengthening respiratory muscles, including the diaphragm and pelvic floor, in order to facilitate speech and communication.

#### Therapeutic Focus

If a child has speech apraxia or language processing challenges, use chanting, vocalizations, mantras, singing, breathing exercises, crossing the midline, bilateral movement, balancing poses, core-strengthening poses, practices that build self-esteem, proprioception and repetition in order to gain mastery. Incorporate patterning, repetition and rhythm.

### High Tone or Hypertonia

High tone or hypertonia is increased tension or muscle tone in the muscles which can cause stiffness and restricted mobility, and can lead to joint contractures (when a joint becomes frozen). Muscle tone is regulated by signals that travel from the brain to the nerves and tell them to contract. Hypertonia occurs when regions of the brain or spinal cord that control these signals are damaged (National Institute of Neurological Disorders and Stroke, n.d.). Hypertonia in children can be caused by cerebral palsy, traumatic birth injuries or injury to the spinal cord (Cerebral Palsy Guide, 2022).

### Therapeutic Focus

- Breathing practices, visualizations, chanting and singing that calm the nervous system
- Passive stretching using props and supports such as restorative poses
- Front body openers to support posture and breathing
- Focus on asanas that support functional movement
- Positive mantras and practices to build self-confidence and self-esteem
- Accessible mudras that support down-regulation of the nervous system

### Contraindications

- Avoid overstretching
- Be cautious with fatigue

## Hypermobility or Low Tone

Hypermobility and low tone can also be co-occurring with sensory processing challenges and neurodivergence.

See Chapter 5 for definition and therapeutic approaches.

## Positive Supports to Enhance Skills

One of the key elements in working with children who are neurodivergent is to get to know their unique strengths and challenges, and provide the necessary supports and accommodations that will set them up for success. Inclusion and accessibility are not only about modifying physical poses; they require identifying each individual child's learning, communication, physical, sensory and emotional needs. Only by gathering in-depth information about the child or teen can we best support them in their practice.

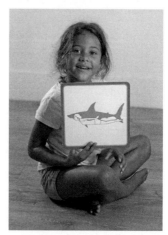

## Setting Them up for Success

- Use visual supports such as yoga pose cards, emotions cards, images of landscapes, etc. to support processing and understanding.
- Communicate in their "language" (e.g. sign language, gestures, visuals, written language, PECS, augmentative communication devices).

- Use direct and concrete language. Avoid too much verbal instruction.
- Model poses rather than only cueing verbally.
- Provide tactile supports to enhance body awareness and connection to body.
- Use visual schedules for predictability.
- Give auditory and visual cues for transitions.
- Provide props and variations to support different bodies.
- Create an environment of sensory safety.
- Teach to their strengths and skills.
- Integrate their preferred interests in your sessions.
- Provide choice whenever possible.

## SENSORY PROCESSING AND CHALLENGES

Sensory processing is how our brain takes in and digests internal and external information through our eight senses—the five senses we are familiar with (sight, sound, taste, touch, smell), our sixth and seventh senses (vestibular and proprioceptive systems) and our eighth sense (interoception). In fact, everything we know about the world around us begins with the information we take in through our sensory systems.

Sensory integration theory was developed by Jean Ayres, an occupational therapist with advanced training in neuroscience and educational psychology (Bundy & Murray, 2002). Ayres (1972, p.11) defines sensory integration as "the neurological process that organizes sensation from one's own body and from the environment and makes it possible to use the body effectively within the environment." Ayres' sensory integration theory emphasizes the relationship between our sensory processing systems and our behavior. The way in which children process sensory information greatly impacts the way in which they navigate the world. When a child's sensory system is out of balance, it can impact their movement, learning, emotional and physical regulation, behavior and relationships with the people and environment around them. Our sensory systems are complex and unique and shaped by our biology and experiences.

Let's begin with our five senses.

### Touch

Our sense of touch plays a significant role in our perceptual and emotional experience. The sense of touch is attributed to receptors in our skin, located throughout the body, that send signals to the brain in relation to pressure, temperature, light touch, vibration, pain, texture and other sensations. The sense of touch receives and processes information from both our internal and external environments. Children use their sense of touch to explore the world around them. They learn about their bodies, their environment and how to connect with others through touch. Recent studies suggest that nurturing touch during the early stages of development and throughout childhood from a primary caregiver is fundamental to a child's emotional and physical wellbeing (Field, 2010) and may aid in maturation of the somatosensory system (Carozza & Leong, 2021). In fact, welcomed and nourishing touch can not only calm us down and reduce our stress response, but it also increases the release of oxytocin, sometimes referred to as the "cuddle hormone." Oxytocin is a feel-good hormone that promotes feelings of trust, bonding and connection (Algoe, Kurtz & Grewen, 2017). Children with sensory processing challenges can present with high or low sensitivity to touch. Tactile defensiveness is a common symptom of sensory processing disorder (SPD). Children who experience tactile defensiveness have a hypersensitivity to touch. Heightened sensitivity can occur with certain clothing and fabrics, food textures, certain self-care tasks (e.g. brushing hair and teeth, showering, washing face/hands), receiving hugs or touch from others and experiencing certain textures in their environment.

## Sight

Our sense of sight also plays a key role in sensory perception. Having sight means the ability to see. Our visual system is responsible for tracking movement through the field of vision and regulates the interpretation of color, tint and sharpness of images, or what is referred to as visual perception. Problems with visual processing could include high sensitivity to light, color and movement in the visual environment, challenges with hand–eye coordination and difficulty with reading, writing, attention and learning. We also use our sense of sight to explore and learn about the world around us, to connect with others and to orient to safety and danger. The way we see the world and connect with others can be impacted by whether or not we experience a sense of safety.

## Hearing

Our sense of hearing or auditory perception is the ability to detect and process sound. The inner ear is a hollow cavity filled with a liquid and lined with tiny hair-like structures. When sound passes into the liquid of the inner ear, it applies pressure to the tiny hair-like structures and triggers a signal to the brain, which then interprets the sound (National Institute on Deafness and Other Communication Disorders, 2022). When a child experiences auditory processing disorder or challenges, they are not able to process auditory information correctly. This is due to the ears and brain not fully coordinating with one another. Difficulty with auditory processing affects a child's ability to process verbal language as well as interpret and discriminate different sounds.

Children who have auditory processing challenges can present as over-responsive or under-responsive to noise or sound. Children who are over-responsive or hypersensitive to sound may cover their ears in loud or unpredictable environments or refuse to go to certain places that feel noisy or overwhelming to them. Children who are under-responsive or hyposensitive to sound may present as not listening or being checked out. This can also be the case for children who are hypersensitive to sound because of overwhelm and inability to discriminate or focus on one sound in their environment. Imagine the overwhelm you would feel if you heard every sound in your environment, from people's voices to a person tapping on their desk to the sound of the fan in the room, and you were not able to tune sounds out in order to focus on the task at hand or one specific sound you needed to attend to in the moment. Or imagine if someone was talking to you and your brain wasn't able to isolate their voice from other sounds in the environment or process what they were saying. Then imagine a child being reprimanded because they are "not listening" or because they are presenting with behaviors in order to manage the frustration of not being able to process auditory information effectively. Our sense of hearing is directly connected to our vestibular sense. The hearing system and balance organs share a nerve pathway to the brain known as the vestibulocochlear nerve (Bordoni, Mankowski & Daly, 2022).

## Smell

Our sense of smell or olfaction is the sense through which smells or odors are perceived. Our sense of smell plays a vital role in detecting odors, identifying toxic substances and spoiled food, identifying dangerous scents such as fire or gasoline and discriminating between foods we like or dislike. When we sniff, the chemicals in the air are dissolved in mucus, odors are detected and signals are sent to the olfactory cortex where odor is perceived and processed (Bailey, 2021). The olfactory cortex is part of the limbic system, which is why our sense of smell plays such a vital role in memory and emotion. Our sense of smell is closely linked to our sense of taste. In fact, when we lose our ability to smell, how we taste food is greatly impacted. Children with sensory processing challenges can be over-responsive or under-responsive to smells. They may also present as picky eaters depending on their level of sensitivity to certain odors. Pleasant odors can induce feelings of calm, happiness and pleasure.

## Taste

Our sense of taste or gustatory system is responsible for the perception of taste and flavor. Taste buds in the back of our tongue help us perceive sweet, sour, salty, bitter and savory. Our gustatory sense helps to keep us safe from ingesting things that are toxic, spoiled or inedible. Along with our gustatory sense, we also rely on texture, temperature and our sense of smell in order to perceive flavor. Children with sensory processing challenges can be over-sensitive or under-sensitive to certain textures, temperatures, smells and flavors, which can affect their willingness to eat certain foods. Our gustatory sense is also directly connected to our proprioceptive sense. Often, children who are under-responsive to proprioceptive input may put things in their mouth, chew on items, bite objects, etc. in order to get oral motor input.

## Vestibular

Our vestibular system governs our sense of balance, gravitational security and movement. Tiny hair-like structures in our inner ear become stimulated with the movement of our head, which then signals our brain to work to maintain a sense of balance and gravitational security. Well-functioning vestibular systems provide a sense of stability and being "grounded" as well as a sense of spatial awareness. It's important to note that the visual system plays a significant role in a well-functioning vestibular system. The vestibular system and visual system work together by sending messages from the muscles in the eyes to the balance organs in the inner ear in order to facilitate balance.

An underdeveloped vestibular system in a child may present as:

- difficulty with balance, movement and coordination
- poor posture or low muscle tone
- constant movement or avoidance of movement
- fear or hypervigilance
- hyperactivity or fidgetiness
- inattentiveness
- difficulty with reading and writing.

### Therapeutic Focus

- Core strength and stability
- Balance
- Fluidity in movement
- Reduce anxiety or fear
- Increase focus and attention
- Encourage an increased sense of groundedness and feeling supported
- Increase confidence and a felt sense of "safety"

## Proprioception

Our proprioceptive system governs our connection to our body, what each body part is doing and where our bodies are in space. We have proprioceptors all over our bodies in the joints, muscles, tendons and skin that play a critical role in our movement and coordination. There are constant messages from our body to our brain and our brain back to our body that tell us how much force, pressure and strength to use when engaging in any type of movement. Our proprioceptive systems are always working to give us information about where our bodies are in relation to our environment (Lloyd, 2020). A well-functioning proprioceptive system allows for smooth, coordinated movement without having to use our eyes to track or plan how our body is going to move or work. A way to explore proprioception is to close our eyes and reach one arm with a pointer finger extended, then slowly bring the pointer finger to touch the nose, keeping the eyes closed. Our ability to touch our nose without actually using our vision as a guide is proprioception, an awareness of where our body is in space.

An underdeveloped proprioceptive system in a child may present as:

- lack of body awareness
- bumps into walls, objects or people
- difficulty with balance, movement and coordination
- poor posture or low muscle tone
- low energy
- frustration or seemingly unmotivated
- difficulty with writing
- difficulty with focus and attention
- seeks out deep pressure touch or avoids touch.

### Therapeutic Focus

- Improve body awareness and connection to body
- Develop core strength and stability
- Improve posture
- Increase smooth and coordinated movement of both sides of body
- Improve balance
- Increase stamina and energy
- Decrease frustration
- Increase focus and attention
- Encourage an increased sense of groundedness and feeling supported
- Increase confidence and a felt sense of "safety"

### Interoception

Our eighth sense, interoception, governs our ability to feel the sensations inside our bodies (e.g. hunger, fullness, need to use the bathroom, heartbeat, temperature, itchiness, sleepiness, irritability). Interoception is directly correlated to feelings and emotions. Essentially, interoception governs how we feel. Not only does interoception govern how we feel, but it also gives us a sense of self in relation to our BME or body–mind environment (Damasio, 2010; Craig, 2009). Antonio Damasio states: "Consciousness, much like our feelings, is based on a representation of the body and how it changes when reacting to certain stimuli. Self-image would be unthinkable without this representation" (Lenzen, 2015). Our experience in our bodies is constantly shifting in relation to the information we are taking in from our internal and external environments. This experience of self or how we feel in the world is also impacted by trauma and our neuroception of safety and danger. Essentially, our interoception (internal cues) is influenced by our exteroception (external cues) and vice versa. Now consider how both of these interrelate with proprioception (our perception of where our bodies are in space and what our bodies are doing in the world). Consider how these factors—exteroception, interoception and proprioception—influence our identity, sense of self, experience of "belonging" and how we behave and relate with others. Having a strong sense of self governs self-awareness, self-reflection and self-regulation.

Many children with sensory processing challenges may be hyposensitive (under-sensitive) or hypersensitive (over-sensitive) to sensory information. When a child has sensory processing difficulties, they may exhibit unexpected or maladaptive behaviors in an attempt to get a need met (e.g. avoid input, gain input, communicate their discomfort). What does this have to do with yoga? The wonderful thing about yoga postures is that each one can provide specific sensory input in order to help balance the sensory system. For instance, inversions (poses in which the head is below the heart) provide vestibular input while weight-bearing and tense/relax poses provide more proprioceptive input. Embodied practices such as movement, tapping, breathing and connecting to sensations in the body support increased interoception and connection to emotion.

## THE IMPACT OF TRAUMA AND NEGLECT ON A CHILD'S SENSORY PROCESSING SYSTEM

Just as it is important to understand sensory processing and how that impacts a child's learning, movement and behavior, it is also important to understand how trauma and neglect can impact a child's sensory processing system. According to Bessel van der Kolk (2015), sensory processing issues are considered to be clinically significant in children who have suffered abuse and trauma. Our sensory systems develop in relation to our experiences in early childhood. Early movement and exposure to sensory experiences (or lack of) affects brain development. Children's sensory systems develop through movement, play, positive interaction with others and being exposed to novel experiences. Early experiences that support a healthy sensory system include:

- nurturing, attunement and co-regulation from a caregiver (cuddles, eye contact, quiet connection)
- rhythmic movement
- play
- rich sensory experiences
- exposure to novel experiences
- tummy time
- opportunity for movement and to explore the environment
- time outside and in nature
- felt sense of safety with the caregiver and the environment.

These experiences are the foundation for children developing healthy sensory systems. When children lack these early experiences or have experienced developmental trauma, you may observe:

- hypervigilance—fight/flight
- shut down—freeze
- over-responsiveness or under-responsiveness to sensory experiences
- lack of body awareness
- delayed gross/fine motor skills
- difficulty with self-regulation, learning, behavior and social relationships
- lack of interoceptive awareness.

It's also important to note that children's sensory systems can be impacted not only by developmental trauma but an event such as a shock trauma. Some examples of shock traumas children may experience are a car accident, medical trauma, witnessing a traumatic event or a frightening fall. Shock traumas can also impact our sensory systems, particularly if the result of the trauma is a diagnosis of PTSD. Trauma changes the way our sensory systems work because our neuroception of danger increases and our nervous system states become more fixated in fight, flight or freeze. Being in these states of arousal or shut down can either increase or decrease our sensitivity to sensory stimuli.

I have a real-life experience related to a shock trauma and my sensory system. After I was in a near-death car accident and was diagnosed with PTSD, my visual processing became very hypersensitive to any unexpected movement in my field of vision, my hearing became extremely sensitive to noise, particularly unexpected noises, and, tactilely, I felt pain from any tags or seams in my clothing. It was a fascinating experience for me because I truly experienced what had been felt by many of the children I had worked with over the years who had sensory processing challenges or who experienced significant trauma. As I learned about trauma and how it impacts our sensory processing systems, I also gained a better understanding of my own unique sensory sensitivities I had experienced throughout my childhood and into adulthood. When we understand our sensory systems better, we can better understand the ways in which we can support balancing our sensory systems so we can be in our bodies and in the world with more comfort, confidence and connection.

## MULTI-SENSORY APPROACH

As I began integrating yoga practices in my classroom with my students and then in individual therapeutic yoga sessions, I found that taking a somatosensory approach was key, especially with children who presented with sensory processing challenges. It is my belief that understanding sensory processing and how it impacts a child's mood, behavior, learning, movement and interaction with others is essential in any work that emphasizes child development. We are complex sensory beings, and understanding our sensory systems can be both empowering and transformational. Tapping into the eight senses and encouraging children to explore their internal and external landscapes can support them in becoming familiar with their own sensory systems and sensory needs, and providing practices that support sensory integration can teach them how to balance their sensory systems. I often explain this to children and teens as learning to "pilot their own planes." Not only do they need to be aware of the external landscape (the weather conditions outside their plane), but they also have this big panel of buttons and knobs that they can learn to control and navigate in order to feel more balanced and integrated.

I'll share an anecdotal experience relating to movement and how it impacts children's learning and behavior. When I worked in the public school system, I was asked to create a behavior program for middle-school-aged kids who struggled to be in their mainstream classrooms due to high needs and challenging behaviors. The intention of the program was to provide the necessary supports to those kids in order to keep them in their community school and eventually transition them into mainstream classes, rather than sending them to a non-public school. The kids in my program were some of the most challenging kids in the district. All of them had some degree of sensory processing challenges and struggled in areas of communication, self-regulation, social skills and learning. I wove in a five-minute yoga break (yoga poses and breathing) followed by a ten-minute movement break of their choice between each period. You would have been amazed to see what a difference this made in their behaviors and ability to focus and learn! Some of the kids in my classroom were better regulated and better behaved than the kids in the mainstream classrooms. An added bonus was that my staff and I, their co-regulators, were getting in movement and breathing throughout the day so we could be the calm, grounded, energized and regulated adults they needed to help them succeed! This is my dream for all schools—that they include yoga, mindfulness and movement throughout the day in all classrooms. The schools would have nothing to lose and everything to gain.

**8 SENSES POEM**

*I have 8 senses, did you know?*
*And when they're balanced, I'm in the flow.*
*My 5 senses*
*Hearing, Taste, Touch, Smell and Sight*
*Help me learn about the world*
*What is wrong and what is right*
*I use my sight to see all around*
*My hearing, to listen to the sounds*
*My taste to choose what foods I like*
*My sense of smell, what's gross, what's nice?*
*My touch to feel from the outside in*
*My hidden senses*
*Vestibular and Proprioception*
*Vestibular helps me feel balanced and upright*
*Its helper is my sense of sight*
*Proprioception tells me where my body is in space*
*How my body is moving and where my hands and feet are placed*
*My eighth sense starts with the Letter "I"*
*Interoception—what I feel inside*
*What sensations do I feel?*
*When I laugh, stomp, cry or squeal*
*When I'm hungry or when I'm full*
*When I'm energetic or feeling dull*
*When my heart is beating fast*
*How my breath feels in my chest*

*My 8 Senses help me know myself*
*So I can balance my emotional health*
*Know what I'm feeling from the inside out*
*That's what my senses are all about*

Shawnee Thornton Hardy

## A SOMATOSENSORY APPROACH TO WELLBEING

I have found that the most effective way to enhance the child's experience of *embodiment* is by using a somatosensory approach, integrating *all* of the senses in their sessions and inviting them to explore their sense of self, through their visual, auditory, tactile, gustatory, olfactory, vestibular, proprioceptive and interoceptive senses.

### PAUSE AND REFLECT

Take a moment to reflect on your own unique sensory experience in the world. Are there certain senses that are more or less sensitive than others? How has that impacted the way in which you have experienced the world around you? Allow for compassion and kindness in your inquiry.

Invitation to journal your reflection.

As you move through the practices in the book, I encourage you to experience them in your own system.

## EXPERIENCING = EMBODYING

It is my experience as a yoga therapist and practitioner that in order to be authentic in our teaching and sharing of these practices, it's important for us to *feel* them in our own bodies. There is a bottom-up learning that happens and a deep embodied wisdom that comes from doing rather than thinking. Having experienced the practices in our own systems also gives us greater perspective and understanding of what children and teens may be experiencing. There is an embodied resonance that can only come from an internal felt sense of the practices.

## INTEGRATING THE EIGHT SENSES
### Visual: Sight
#### Eye Tracking

This eye-tracking exercise supports visual tracking. Visual tracking is important because it allows children to follow a moving object, scan their environment for information, accurately shift their eye gaze from one thing to another and direct hand movements. Eye tracking is a necessary developmental skill for reading, writing, fine motor skills and coordinated movement. Eye tracking can also support a child's nervous system regulation either by slowing down rapid eye movements that can occur in a fight/flight state and bringing more focus or by bringing more mobilization to a child's eyes that may be in a freeze state.

**Instructions:**

1. Use a finger puppet, pencil with a fun erasure or just your finger.
2. Tell the child you are going to move your finger and ask them to try to follow your finger with their eyes, without moving their head.
3. Begin in the center, at midline.
4. Movement of the finger should be slow throughout the tracking exercise.
5. Move your finger to the right, then back to the center.
6. Move your finger to the left, then back to the center.
7. Move your finger up, then back to the center.
8. Move your finger down, then back to the center.
9. Move your finger diagonally and up to the right, then back to the center.
10. Move your finger diagonally and down to the left, then back to the center.
11. Move your finger diagonally and up to the left, then back to the center.
12. Move your finger diagonally and down to the right, then back to the center.
13. Have the child check in and notice how their body feels.
14. It is important to track the child's nervous system as you do this exercise. If you see or they communicate any dysregulation from the activity, stop the activity.

#### Drishti

Drishti or focused gaze is a yogic practice that supports developing concentration, withdrawal from the senses and focusing inward. Many children with sensory processing challenges can be overwhelmed by sensory information and their experience with the outside world. Other children may struggle with attention, focus and connecting internally. Practicing drishti or one-point focus can support attention and down-regulation and is an accessible meditation practice for children. Drishti practice can be done simply sitting or standing and looking at something in front of them and is also encouraged during balancing poses to support balance and focus.

**Option:** Have the child choose an image or make their own drishti to put on the wall in front of them, or have them focus on something that is already right in front of them.

**Instructions:**

1. Invite the child to look at their drishti image or something in front of them, right in line with their eyes.
2. Encourage them to focus on that image or object.
3. It can be helpful to have a period of time that you encourage them to focus.
4. Have the child check in and notice how their body feels.
5. The time focusing on the object or image can increase as the child develops their ability to focus.
6. Integrate focusing on the drishti image or object while practicing balancing poses.

## Orienting

Orienting is a natural survival behavior that we see in the animal world and that we also do as humans in order to orient to safety or danger. Visual orienting, particularly to safety, can support regulation, attention and awareness of the present moment.

1. Invite the child to look around their space and see if they notice something that is pleasant or brings a feeling of calm, goodness or connection.
2. Invite the child to describe the color, shape, texture and anything else they notice about that object.
3. Invite the child to notice how they feel in their body when they look at that object.

## Color Discrimination and Orienting

1. Place different-colored objects around the room.

2.  Ask the child to find a "blue" object.
3.  Once they locate the object, ask them to describe the object to you (e.g. shape, texture).
4.  Ask the child how their body feels when they look at the colored object.
5.  Repeat for other colors.

### Palming

Children who are hypersensitive to visual input or who are more hypervigilant in their nervous systems tend to have overactive visual processing. Palming allows the eyes to rest and provides an experience of warmth and comfort to the eyes.

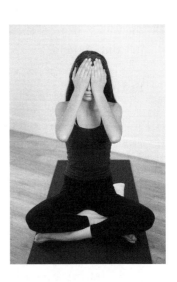

**Instructions:**

1.  Have the child rub their hands together until they feel warmth in their palms.
2.  Invite them to bring their palms to their eyes and rest their eyes gently in their palms.
3.  Let them know they can remove their palms when they are ready.
4.  Invite them to notice how their eyes and body feels.

### Using visual aids (e.g. yoga cards, images)

Children who struggle with visual processing, attention, focus, language processing and communication benefit most from visual aids. Using yoga pose cards, breathing cards, visuals of colors, images, etc. will support them with understanding, focus, communication, memory and imagination.

## Auditory: Hearing

### Sound bowls

Sound bowls are a method for working with our more subtle body energy (pranamaya kosha) and can be differentiated according to each child's individual vibratory rate, preferences and needs. In his book *Healing Sounds: The Power of Harmonics* (2022), Goldman states, "In alignment with this concept of sound, every organ, bone and tissue in your body has its own separate resonant frequency. Together they make up a composite frequency, a harmonic that is your own personal vibratory rate" (p.14).

According to Goldman, the rhythms of the body can be altered through sound, which is referred to as entrainment. This describes "the ability of the more powerful rhythmic vibrations of another object to cause them to synchronize their rhythms with the first object. Through sound it is possible to change the rhythms of our brainwaves, as well as our heartbeat and respiration" (2022, p.14).

Using a sound bowl can also be a wonderful way to integrate auditory input. Each sound bowl will have a different tone or emphasize a different chakra. I have found the best decibel of sound to begin with when introducing to children who have auditory sensitivities are the base sound or deeper tones such as the root or heart chakra. Of course, each child will respond differently to each chakra sound as each sound carries a unique vibration and each child's system has their own unique vibratory makeup. One way to introduce singing bowls and the different sounds to children who have auditory sensitivity is to allow them to play the singing bowl first. This promotes self-agency and a sense of predictability.

### Heart/Belly Listening
**Instructions:**

1. Introduce the sound of the singing bowl.
2. Ask the child how that sound feels to their ears.
3. Once you have a sound that they are comfortable with, invite the child to take one hand on their heart and one hand on their belly.
4. Invite the child to close their eyes or keep them softly open with their gaze down.
5. Explain to the child that you are going to play the singing bowl and they are going to listen for the sound until they can't hear the sound anymore.
6. Tell them once they don't hear the sound anymore, to open their eyes and raise their hand.
7. Have the child check in and notice how their body feels.
8. Option: Play sound bowls while the child is in savasana or a resting pose.

### Sound Discrimination
**Instructions:**

1. Make a playlist of different nature sounds.
2. Tell the child, "I am going to play some nature sounds and you can guess what the sound is."
3. Invite the child to close their eyes or keep them softly open.
4. Play a nature sound.
5. Ask the child, "What do you think that sound was?"

6. Repeat for several nature sounds.
7. Option: Play a nature song that has many different nature sounds in it.
8. As the child listens to the song, have them say each nature sound they hear as they listen.
9. Have the child check in and notice how their body feels.

## Head Wrap

**Note**: It's best to use an Iyengar head wrap for this activity. This activity can support allowing the child's auditory system to rest and restore, particularly children who have heightened sensitivity to sound.

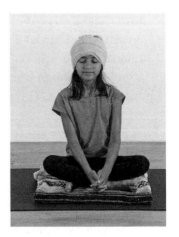

**Instructions:**

1. Option: Have a bolster and blanket set up for relaxation after the head wrap is applied.
2. Tell the child you are going to wrap their ears in a head wrap.
3. Begin wrapping by placing the edge of the head wrap over one ear.
4. Wrap around the back of the head near the occiput, then across the forehead.
5. Wrap around the opposite ear.
6. Be sure the wrap is snug but not too tight.
7. As you begin wrapping, ask the child how the pressure feels and adjust accordingly.
8. Continue to wrap until you are close to the end of the wrap.
9. Tuck the edge of the wrap inside.
10. Have the child lie done on a bolster or a mat and let their ears have a rest.
11. Have the child sit up when they are ready.
12. Unwrap the head wrap.
13. Have the child check in and notice how their body feels.

## Chanting

Chanting is a wonderful way to get auditory input. Not only does chanting provide auditory input but it also down-regulates the nervous system by offering a vibrational experience to the vagus nerve. Chanting also extends the exhalation, which elicits more of a parasympathetic response. Each sound has a unique vibration and can be felt in different areas of the body. Chanting is also a great practice to enhance speech and communication. Chanting is a meditation practice that builds focus and concentration. Exploring chanting with children and the vibration they feel in their body also supports building interoceptive awareness. A wonderful way to introduce chanting is through letter chanting. As the child explores the sounds, invite them to notice where they feel vibration or sensation in their body.

*Letter Sounds (Short and Long Vowels): A, E, I, O, U*

- Short A—Ahhh
- Long A—Ayyyy
- Short E—Ehhh
- Long E—Eeee
- Short I—Ihhh
- Long I—Iiii
- Short O—Awww
- Long O—Ohhh
- Short U—Uhhh
- Long U—Ewww

*Sound of Om (Aum)*
Om is the sacred sound of the universe. Breaking the Om chant into its three sound components can be a helpful way to teach children. Practice each sound separately, then have the child put the sounds together in a complete Om.

- A—Ahhhh
- Oh—Ohhhh
- M—Mmmm

## Sound Tuning
Another way to incorporate sound and chanting with children is through sound tuning with musical notes. Each note and sound connects to a specific chakra (see Table 4.1). As you explore the sounds, invite them to notice where they feel vibration or sensation in their body. You can also explore chanting the seed sound for each chakra listed in Chapter 1.

Table 4.1. Note and Sound for Each Chakra

| Note | Sound | Chakra |
|---|---|---|
| C | Uh | Root |
| D | Ooh | Sacral |

*cont.*

| Note | Sound | Chakra |
|------|-------|--------|
| E | Ho | Solar Plexus |
| F | Ahh | Heart |
| G | Eh | Throat |
| A | Ee | Third Eye |
| B | Silence | Crown |

### Lokah Samastah Sukhino Bhavantu

"May all beings everywhere be happy and free."

This is a beautiful chant that is accessible to children and encourages compassion for themselves and others in the world. It can be helpful to have the child think of someone they want to send love and compassion to as they sing the chant.

I often teach Sanskrit chants through call and response. Breaking the chant up into single words, then doing the whole chant together helps with learning and memory.

### Call and Response
**Instructions:**

1. *Lokah*—have child repeat.
2. *Samastah*—have child repeat.
3. *Sukhino*—have child repeat.
4. *Bhavantu*—have child repeat.
5. Do this 2–3 more times.
6. To enhance the auditory experience, attention and mind–body connection, you can incorporate tapping the thighs and clapping hands as you chant together.

    | Tap thighs | Clap hands |
    |------------|------------|
    | *Lo* | *Kah* |
    | *Sama* | *Stah* |
    | *Sukhi* | *No* |
    | *Bhavan* | *Tu* |

7. Sing the full chant together, repeating the entire phrase several times: *Lokah samastah sukhino bhavantu, lokah samastah sukhino bhavantu, lokah samastah sukhino bhavantu.*
8. Check in and have the child notice how their body feels after doing the chant.

### Bee Breath or Hum Breath (Bhramari Pranayama)

Bhramari is a humming practice named after the black bumble bee in India. The Sanskrit translation of Bhramari is "big black bee." I refer to this breath as Bee Breath or Humming Breath with children. Benefits of this humming practice include reduced anxiety and improved focus. It can also provide relief from tension, anger and agitation. Along with other chanting and sound practices, humming can also facilitate improved speech and communication. I have found that Bee Breath both eases anxiety and provides a sense of calm alertness with children. Bee Breath also provides soothing auditory input, stimulates the vagus nerve and can support interoceptive awareness when attention is brought to where the child feels the vibration of the breath in their body.

**Instructions:**

1. Ask the child what sound a bee makes. Demonstrate the hum sound to the child.
2. Encourage the child to breathe a natural breath in.
3. Invite the child to make the hum sound with lips closed.
4. Invite them to notice where they feel the vibration or sensation in their body when they do the breath.
5. Encourage them to hum until they are at the end of their exhalation without straining.
6. Repeat 3–5 times.
7. Check in and have the child notice how their body feels after doing Bee Breath.

### Call and Response Singing

Singing is a wonderful way to integrate auditory input. Singing also supports nervous system regulation, ventral vagal connection, communication and activation of the throat chakra. Call and response is a wonderful way to introduce new songs to help with focus and memory.

### Fanga Alafia

Fanga (pronounced *Funga*) Alafia (pronounced *Ah-la-fee-ah*) is a greeting song sung throughout parts of West Africa. *Fanga* means "talking drum," *Alafia* means "good health" or "peace," and *Ase* (pronounced *Ashay*) translates to "thank you" in Yoruba, a West African language (Powell, 2019). Not only is it a fun song to sing, but it also has a message of welcoming and good health.

**Instructions:**

1. Have the child repeat each phrase.
2. *Fanga* (pronounced *Funga*) *Alafia*—child repeats.
3. *Ase Ase* (pronounced *Ashay Ashay*)—child repeats.
4. *Fanga Alafia*—child repeats.
5. *Ase Ase*—child repeats.
6. *Ase Ase*—child repeats.
7. *Ase Ase*—child repeats.
8. *Fanga Alafia*—child repeats.
9. *Ase Ase*—child repeats.
10. Invite the child to sing the whole song together with you.
11. Option: Have the child clap hands and tap the floor along with the lyrics in order to enhance rhythm and body connection.

### Listening to Music

Listening to relaxing music during the yoga session can help facilitate down-regulation and give the child's mind something to focus on during savasana. Music can be used not only to facilitate down=regulation but to bring more energy and alertness to a child's system. Music is also a powerful resource for both children and teenagers. Having them share some of their favorite songs when doing their intake and integrating them into your sessions can help build connection. Not only does music provide auditory input that can be both soothing and resourcing, but research shows that music accesses all areas of the brain, facilitating whole-brain integration. In one particular study, using functional magnetic resonance imaging (fMRI), Finnish researchers found that listening to music recruits not only the auditory areas of the brain, but also employs large-scale neural networks such as the emotional, motor and creative areas of the brain (Alluri *et al.*, 2012). It is important to note that children who have heightened auditory sensitivity may be distracted by music and could even become dysregulated with certain songs or types of music. Each child will present differently as to whether they can tolerate music in their sessions or not.

## Tactile: Touch

### Tactile Box

**Instructions:**

1. Gather items with different textures to explore. Examples: shell, smooth stone, rough rock, cotton ball, feather.
2. Place them in a box or basket.

3.  Invite the child to choose an item.
4.  Ask the child to describe what the item feels like.
5.  Option: Integrate the other senses into this activity (notice the texture, color, shape and smell—there may even be a sound they can explore with the item).
6.  To enhance interoceptive awareness, you may inquire how the child's body feels as they explore the texture and other senses connected to the item.
7.  You can promote agency by asking the child whether they like or don't like the texture of the item.
8.  Continue to explore the other items in the box.

### Firestarter
**Instructions:**

1.  Begin by sharing that long ago when humans needed to start a fire, they would rub two sticks together.
2.  Invite them to do Firestarter with their hands, imaging that their hands are sticks.
3.  Have them rub their hands together quickly until they begin to feel warmth and heat in their hands.
4.  Have them pause and notice what sensations they feel in their hands.

### Self-Hug
Self-Hug encourages self-love, provides deep pressure input and also crosses the midline.

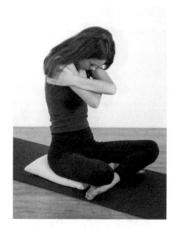

**Instructions:**

1.  Talk about the importance of self-love and that when we feel like we need a hug, we can give ourselves a hug.
2.  Have the child open their arms wide, filling their arms with love.
3.  Tell them to wiggle the fingers of their right hand and cross their right arm over their left.
4.  Then wrap their arms around themselves and give themselves some love.
5.  Encourage the child to use whatever pressure feels best to them.
6.  Have them open their arms wide again, filling their arms with love.

7. Tell them to wiggle the fingers of their left had and cross their left arm over their right.

8. Then wrap their arms around themselves and give themselves more love.

9. Have the child check in and notice how their body feels.

## Arms Squeezes

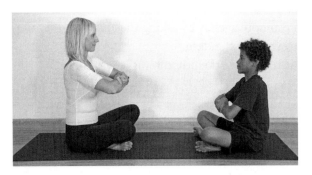

Arms squeezes provide proprioceptive input, midline crossing and deep pressure touch. This can be an easily accessible practice for the child to do throughout the day for sensory input and self-regulation. Self-contact can be tremendously resourcing and can also bring more experience of embodiment and connection to the body.

**Instructions:**

1. Have the child cross their arms and bring their hands to their opposite shoulders.

2. Invite them to begin massaging their arms from the shoulders, moving down their arms to their elbows, then to the wrists and ending with massaging their hands.

3. Encourage them to explore the amount of pressure that feels best to them.

4. Have them massage from the hands back up to the shoulders.

5. Have the child check in and notice how their body feels.

## Olfactory: Smell
### Essential Oils (on Cotton Ball)
Essential oils can be a nice way to explore the sense of smell. Essential oils will have varying effects on a child's nervous system. Children with heightened sensitivity to smell will respond differently to essential oils, so it is important to

introduce them with intention and in a safe way. A safe way to introduce essential oil smells is using a cotton ball. Place the cotton balls in ziplock baggies, then add a tiny bit of essential oil, shaking the cotton balls around in the bag so the oil reaches the cotton balls evenly. Allow the cotton balls to dry. Each bag will hold a different scent. Here are a few scents I use regularly and their common effects. It is recommended any time that you use essential oils in a therapeutic manner that you use therapeutic-grade oils.

- Lavender—calming
- Peppermint—invigorating
- Orange—mood lifting
- Lemon—energizing

**Instructions:**

1. Choose a cotton ball with a scent and invite the child to hold the cotton ball and smell it.
2. Have the child try to guess the scent.
3. Have the child share if they like the scent or not.
4. Check in and have the child notice how that scent makes them feel in their body.
5. After exploring all the scents, ask the child which one was their favorite.
6. Incorporate their favorite scents in your sessions.

### Scented Playdough
A fun way to connect with the sense of smell as well as tactile sense is through scented playdough. Make the playdough—recipe at www.youngliving.com/blog/essential-oil-playdough-recipe—adding different scents to each playdough ball.

**Instructions:**

1. Have the child choose one of the playdough balls.
2. Invite them to smell the playdough ball and guess the scent.
3. Have the child share if they like the scent or not.
4. If it is a scent they like, invite them to explore the texture of the playdough with their hands, making whatever shapes they want.
5. Option: Make animal shapes from the playdough and then do the animal pose!
6. Check in and have the child notice how that scent and texture makes them feel in their body.

7.  After exploring all the scents, ask the child which one was their favorite.
8.  Incorporate their favorite scents with playdough in your sessions.

### Scented Markers

I like using this activity as an exploration of the sensory and emotional experience of pleasure and disgust or like and dislike. Our sense of smell is directly connected to the limbic system, the emotional centers of our brain, including the amygdala and hippocampus. The hippocampus is also the filing system of our brain, which is why we can so often tie a certain scent to a memory of an experience we've had in the past. When we experience pleasant smells, we may feel pleasure or goodness, and when we experience an unpleasant smell, we may feel disgust or dislike. These are important emotions to explore, particularly when it comes to self-agency and boundary work. A child's ability to express like and dislike is foundational in setting healthy boundaries and having agency.

**Materials:** Silly Scents Washable Markers. I like using these markers because they have both icky smells and pleasant smells. You can purchase Silly Scents Sweet and Silly Scents Stinky Washable Markers.

**Instructions:**

1.  Have two cards, one that says "sweet" or "pleasant" and another that says "stinky" or "icky."
2.  Mix the markers together and have the child choose one.
3.  Invite the child to smell the marker and let you know whether it smells pleasant or icky (you can interchange the language with "sweet" or "stinky"), then have them place the marker on the correct category.
4.  After the child smells the scent and shares how it smells, invite them to notice how they feel in their body after smelling the scent.
5.  Repeat until the child smells each marker.
6.  End the activity with the child choosing their favorite scent, smelling it and noticing how they feel in their body as they smell the scent.

### Gustatory: Taste

One way to connect with our gustatory sense is through oral motor activities, including breathing activities.

### Straw Breathing

**Materials:** A straw, a colored scarf.

**Instructions:**

1. Have the child hold the straw in one hand and put the palm of their other hand in front of the straw.
2. Invite them to see if they can breathe air with their straw onto their palm.
3. Option: Hold a colored scarf in your hand and have them blow on the scarf through their straw. I call this "Scarves Blowing in the Wind Breath".
4. Repeat 2–3 times.
5. Check in and have the child notice how their body feels after doing Straw Breathing.

### Feather Breathing
**Materials:** Colored soft feathers.

**Instructions:**

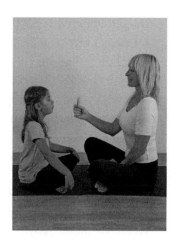

1. Have the child choose a feather they like.
2. Invite them to look at the feather, to feel the feather and to describe to you what it looks like and feels like.
3. Have them hold the feather up in front of their mouth and blow softly on the feather.
4. Repeat 2–3 times.
5. Check in and have the child notice how their body feels after doing Feather Breathing.

### Letter Chants
Letter chants are a wonderful way to explore oral motor movements. As you do the letter chants with the child, encourage them to overexaggerate the movements of the mouth as they practice the different sounds. (See 'Chanting' in the 'Auditory: Hearing' section.)

Check in after doing the vowel chants and have the child notice how their body feels.

### Taste the Fruit
Getting children to explore different textures and tastes of food offers gustatory input. Remember that our gustatory sense, taste, and our olfactory sense, smell, are interconnected. Each child will respond differently to the smell, texture and taste of the food item they are exploring.

**Materials:** Assortment of sliced fruits.

**Instructions:**

1.  Have the child choose a fruit they want to taste.
2.  Invite them to smell the fruit and notice if the fruit smells good or icky.
3.  If the fruit smells good to them, invite them to take a taste.
4.  Ask them to share how the fruit tasted and felt. Sweet or sour? Crunchy or mushy?
5.  Ask if they liked or disliked the taste of the fruit.
6.  Check in and have the child notice how their body feels.
7.  Repeat for the other fruit items.

### Mindful Hydration

Drinking water can be a great way to bring some regulation to the nervous system. I often find that a mindful sip or drink of water throughout the day really supports my ability to focus, not to mention the importance of good hydration for our physical wellbeing! According to Harvard School of Public Health (2018), maintaining optimal hydration is crucial for regulating body temperature, lubricating joints, preventing infections, delivering nutrients to cells and keeping organs functioning properly. They also report that being well hydrated improves sleep quality, cognition and mood. Mindful hydration can be a great way to get gustatory input while also hydrating and nourishing our bodies and minds. Drinking water from a straw can also facilitate enhanced input. I like to begin yoga sessions by having children and teens take mindful sips of water at the start of our sessions and throughout.

**Instructions:**

1.  Give the child a glass of cool water.
2.  Talk about the importance of hydration and how drinking water throughout the day helps us hydrate our muscles, tissues and bones, helps us with eliminating toxins from our bodies and keeps our minds and bodies alert and well balanced.
3.  Invite them to take a sip of the water or drink the water through a straw and swish it around in their mouth, noticing how that feels for them.
4.  Invite them to notice the sensation of swallowing their water and feeling it move down their throats and into their tummies.
5.  Check in and have the child notice how their body feels after drinking the water.

6. Repeat a few times, sipping the water mindfully and noticing how it feels in their body.

### Crunchy vs Chewy Snacks

The texture of our food can bring more calm or energy to our systems and provide oral motor input. The following suggestions can be offered to parents to help regulate their child's energy states and provide gustatory input in a healthy way:

- **Calming:** Chewy foods such as dried fruit, dates, bagels, cheese, granola bars and raisins.
- **Energizing:** Crunchy foods such as carrot sticks, sliced apples, pretzels, banana chips and nuts.

## The Two Hidden Senses: Vestibular and Proprioception

### Vestibular Input

Vestibular input is often used to stimulate a child's system, leaving them energized and alert. Each child will present differently in their response to vestibular input. Some children will have a high threshold for vestibular input—these are the children who will typically seek out vestibular input. Other children will have a low threshold for vestibular input and will tend to avoid it altogether. The children who are constantly seeking out this type of input through spinning, rocking, fidgeting in their chairs, etc. are communicating to us that they need frequent movement throughout the day in order to have the capacity to focus and learn. It's no wonder children are struggling with learning and behavior in schools! The education system has managed to remove the very thing that is essential to regulation and learning: frequent opportunity for movement! It is also important for those children who are avoidant of vestibular input to provide movement that offers vestibular input in order to bring energy and alertness to their systems. The thing to keep in mind is that we must provide this input differently based on their threshold and tolerance for vestibular input. It's important to note that it is long-lasting and more stimulating than proprioceptive input. Here are a few things to consider when integrating movement that provides vestibular input:

- Introduce vestibular input slowly and with intention. Notice how their systems respond to the input and adjust accordingly.
- Provide props to bring the ground closer to enhance a felt sense of safety and support for those children who have a lower threshold or are more fearful.
- Ground before and ground after. In order to avoid leaving a child in

a disorganized state, always do a grounding practice before and after integrating vestibular input. Giving deep pressure and proprioceptive input are the most effective ways to help ground after vestibular input.

• Provide vestibular input throughout the day in order to support regulation and bring energy and alertness to the child's systems.

### Practices for Vestibular Input

• Inversions
• Standing and balancing poses
• Movement with rocking, swaying, bouncing, etc.
• Visual processing activities (see Visual: Sight Activities)

See Table 4.2 below for specific pose suggestions.

Table 4.2 Vestibular poses

| Inversions | Standing | Balancing | Movement (e.g. rocking, swaying, bouncing) |
|---|---|---|---|
| Giraffe | Mountain | Tree | River |
| Rabbit | Warrior I | Half Moon | Cookie Dough Mixer |
| Down Dog | Warrior II | Teetering Star | Rock-a-Bye Baby |
| Rag Doll | Triangle | Eagle | Jumping Frog |
| Gorilla | Chair | Flamingo | Rowing Boat |
| Spider Legs up the Wall | Star | | Washing Machine |
| | | | Rock and Roll |
| | | | Happy Baby |
| | | | Sunrise to Sunset |

### Proprioceptive Input

There is growing evidence that balance, movement and proprioceptive input can play an important role in managing anxiety. Maintaining balance requires input from both the proprioceptive and vestibular systems, which have a direct pathway to the parts of the brain that modulate the autonomic nervous system, the system that controls the stress response. Research suggests that increased balance, movement and proprioceptive input can reduce sympathetic activation in the nervous system, down-regulate the stress response and reduce anxiety. Researchers at Tel Aviv University have correlated lack of balance with increased levels of anxiety (Bart *et al.*, 2009). The study, conducted by Dr. Orit Bart in collaboration with TAU researchers, investigated the anxiety–balance connection in young children for the first time. Dr. Bart tracked children between the ages of 5 and 7 who had been diagnosed with both problems to see how treatment would affect each disorder.

After a 12-week intervention of sensory-motor integration, the children in Dr. Bart's study improved their balance skills. She reported that anxiety reduced to normal levels in the children who were part of the study. She also reported that as their balance and anxiety improved, the children's self-esteem also increased. This confirms the importance of building in balancing practices in children's daily routines. If their bodies are out of balance, so too their minds.

### Practices for Proprioceptive Input

- Weight bearing
- Balancing poses
- Poses on belly
- Container poses (forward bends)
- Tense/relax
- Deep pressure
- Tapping

See Table 4.3 for specific pose suggestions.

Table 4.3 Proprioception poses

| Weight-bearing | Standing | Balancing | Prone | Forward bends | Tense/relax |
| --- | --- | --- | --- | --- | --- |
| Table | Mountain | Tree | Cobra | Child's | Orange Juice Squeeze |
| Cat | Warrior I | Half Moon | Shark | Rock | Self-Hug |
| Cow | Warrior II | Teetering Star | Superhero | Rabbit | Arm Squeezes |
| Plank | Triangle | Eagle | Crocodile | Puppy | Show Me Ten |
| Down Dog | Chair | Flamingo | | Turtle | Sponge |
| Standing | Star | | | Sponge | Progressive Relaxation |
| Balancing | | | | Monkey Toes | |

### A Behavioral Perspective

I come from a behavioral perspective. Having worked as an educational and behavioral specialist for years, my job was to observe a child's behavior in the context of their environment while also taking into consideration their individual needs and challenges. Unless it is our scope of practice, it is not our job to "diagnose" a child with sensory processing disorder (SPD). However, we can view the child through a behavioral lens and observe their behaviors that may give us insight into their sensory imbalances and needs. This will give us meaningful information on how to develop a therapeutic protocol that is appropriate for their specific sensory needs. Bear in mind that SPD is not a current diagnosis in the *Diagnostic and Statistical Manual of Mental Disorders* (DSM-5); however, it was once a diagnosis and is often used for children who have sensory processing challenges that significantly impact their daily life. If the child sees an occupational therapist, it can be wonderful to connect with them and work collaboratively together to support the child. However, many children don't have access to resources such as occupational therapy. By strengthening our own observational skills, gathering information from caregivers and from other support professionals and understanding the behaviors of children who have sensory processing challenges, we can develop protocols that integrate tools and practices to support them in balancing their sensory systems.

I'll give an example of the correlation between observation and identifying a child's sensory needs. There was a young boy in my program, age 11, who was struggling in his classroom environment. I was told he was always "acting out" and "disrupting" his other classmates, and the teacher wanted him removed from the class. Prior to him entering my program, I went for a classroom observation. I noticed right away that he was very unaware of his own body. He would stomp loudly when he walked through the classroom and slam his book on his desk. He would also bump into his classmates and get into their personal space, which did not help his social relationships with his peers. The teacher said he was always stomping and slamming things, always purposely "trying to get attention," and it was driving her crazy. We ultimately decided that the best thing for the student would be to come to my program, as he was not showing a lot of success in his current placement. You will hear me make this statement throughout the book: *Behind every behavior is a need*. It was clear that one of his needs was proprioceptive input. One of the factors of having a well-developed proprioceptive system is knowing what amount of force to use in your body for specific tasks such as walking, placing a book on a desk, holding a pencil, etc. Another factor is having a sense of where your body is in terms of its proximity to others. He was showing observable behaviors that suggested his proprioceptive system was unbalanced. He is an example of a child who would be referred to as a sensory seeker. In order for his brain to register his body and its movements, he would do things with more force. He bumped into his peers because his brain was not registering exactly where his body was in space. He was not "acting out" on purpose with these behaviors; he was just trying to get a need met. So my question was: "How can I help him get his needs met and also support him in being part of a classroom environment where he could thrive academically and socially?"

1.  Offering proprioceptive input throughout the day to support increased body awareness. This was provided through yoga practices and other activities.
2.  Supporting him in building more awareness around his body in relation to his environment. This involved integrating mindfulness practices and activities that included both vestibular and proprioceptive input.
3.  Facilitating understanding and compassion among his peers.
4.  Offering a container of support, safety and understanding so he felt that he was wanted, understood and cared for.

One year later and I can tell you that he was a different kid, more regulated, more confident, more connected to his body and more connected to his peers. As I think of him, it makes me smile in my heart because *he* did the work in learning to pilot his own plane; he just needed the right support and guidance to do so. Pilots who fly planes don't do it alone; they have the support of air traffic control to help them navigate their journey safely. Perhaps we can consider ourselves air traffic controllers, helping children and teens navigate their bodies, hearts and brains so they move through the world with less turbulence and more ease.

## SUPPORTING PHYSICAL, SOCIAL-EMOTIONAL AND COGNITIVE DEVELOPMENT OF THE INDIVIDUAL CHILD

The instructions provided in the following poses include language for younger children or children and teens who respond to more playful language. The language should be adapted to meet the social-emotional, cognitive and developmental needs of the child. The amount of language you use will vary, depending on the child's ability to process language, level of attention and communication style. The amount of time the child stays in the pose will depend on their age, level of attention, stamina and physical capacity. Each asana has a child-friendly name along with the traditional Sanskrit name.

### Supporting All Bodies and Abilities

You will find that children and teens who come to you for therapy will present with a wide range of bodies and abilities. The first yama, ahimsa, emphasizes non-harm. As adults, it is our responsibility to accommodate the needs of the child or teen and provide the necessary supports to keep them safe. We also want to emphasize self-love and self-acceptance. Helping the child to love themselves and their body just as they are while exploring practices that bring more confidence, balance and ease to their systems. When we are teaching asanas to children, the emphasis should not be on them doing the pose right or getting their bodies to look a certain way in the pose. We want them to explore the shapes and movements in their bodies and begin to discern:

- How does this pose feel in my body?
- What poses help me feel calm, relaxed, energized, focused, strong, confident, connected?
- What do I notice is happening in my body when I do this pose?
- What poses do I like or dislike?
- What do I notice before and after doing the pose?

In providing the appropriate props, variations of poses, individualized cues and the accommodations and supports that set them up for success, we make the practices accessible and inclusive to children and teens of all brains, bodies and abilities. T.K.V. Desikachar (1999, p.31) said, "Anybody can breathe, therefore anybody can practice yoga," reminding us that yoga is for every*body*, regardless of physical challenges or limitations. Every asana can be adapted to meet individual physical needs.

## Making Asana Inclusive and Accessible

- Focus on the essence of the pose. What is its resonating effect, and how can that be offered through variations that are supportive to the individual body? For instance, Cat and Cow can be practiced seated in a chair rather than in a weight-bearing position on the floor. The essence of the poses is mobility of the spine, moving from extension to flexion of the spine. The resonating effect of mobilization and energy to the spine and nervous system can still be experienced as a seated variation.
- Positions of poses can include being seated in a chair, standing or lying down.
- Supports might include using a block, chair, wall or floor for safety, stability and grounding, and exploring the poses in different ways to meet the physical needs of the individual.
- Variations of poses might include:
  - having the feet wider apart to provide a wider base of support for those with gravitational insecurity, instability or larger bodies

- allowing the arms to be wider apart to accommodate for shoulder issues, mobility or larger bodies
- bending the knees in forward bends to accommodate tight hamstrings, high tone or hypermobility.
- Props might include wooden dowels, blocks, bolsters, bean bags and blankets to accommodate various physical needs and provide tactile cues.
- Connection to the body and exploring shape and movement can be facilitated through visualization, breath and sound if there are limitations with movement and physical poses are not as accessible.
- Teach the most accessible variation of the pose first, then give options for the child to explore other variations that may be more challenging for them. Set them up for success!

## POSES FOR VESTIBULAR AND PROPRIOCEPTIVE INPUT
### Inversions

**Contraindications for inversions:** heart conditions, high blood pressure, glaucoma, detached retina, hiatal hernia, seizure disorder, TBI (traumatic brain injury). Caution with vestibular imbalance. Caution with spinal issues or injuries (including osteoporosis) with forward bends.

**Supports:** Use blocks, a chair or wall to provide more subtle vestibular input to support balance and grounding.

### Giraffe (Prasarita Padottanasana)
**Additional contraindications:** Hamstring injury; be aware of hypermobility.

**Benefits:** Stretches hamstrings, calves, ankles and spine, releases tension in shoulders and upper back, supports healthy digestion, calms the mind, provides vestibular and proprioceptive input.

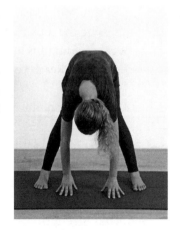

**Instructions:**

1. Begin standing with toes pointing forward.
2. Step your feet out wide.
3. Reach your hands up and get tall, as if you're growing your long giraffe neck.

4. Breathe in.
5. Breathe out and bring your hands towards the floor.
6. Bend knees if needed.
7. If you're a thirsty giraffe, you can slurp up some water.
8. Breathe in with your tongue on the roof of your mouth.
9. Breathe out through your mouth.

### Rabbit Pose (Sasangasana)

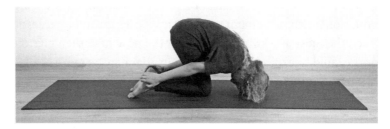

**Additional contraindications:** Spinal issues or injuries, atlanto-axial instability.

**Benefits:** Stretches the spine, upper back and shoulders, supports healthy digestion, calms the mind, provides vestibular and proprioceptive input.

**Instructions:**

1. Stand on your knees.
2. Breathe in and reach your hands up.
3. Breathe out and bend forward.
4. Bring your forearms and elbows to the mat.
5. Bring the top of your head to the mat.
6. Keep your hips lifted.
7. Option: Reach your hands back towards your heels if your neck feels okay.
8. Wag your bunny tail back and forth.

### Down Dog (Adho Mukha Svanasana)
**Additional contraindications:** Shoulder, arm, wrist, knee or ankle injuries; be aware of hypermobility.

**Benefits:** Strengthens arms, shoulders and legs, stretches the hamstrings, calves, ankles and spine, calms the mind, provides vestibular and proprioceptive input.

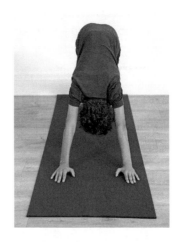

**Instructions:**

1. Come onto your hands and knees.
2. Tuck your toes.
3. Press into your hands.
4. Lift your hips up and back.
5. Stretch your spine like a dog.
6. Bend knees if needed.
7. Breathe in, breathe out.
8. Wag your doggy tail back and forth.
9. What sound does a doggy make?

### Rag Doll or Woody/Jessie from *Toy Story* (Uttanasana)

**Additional contraindications:** Hamstring injury; be aware of hypermobility.

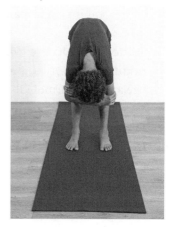

**Benefits:** Stretches the hips, hamstrings and calves, relieves tension in the spine, neck and upper back, strengthens the thighs and knees, supports healthy digestion, calms the mind, provides vestibular and proprioceptive input.

**Instructions:**

1. Stand with feet hip-width apart.
2. Bend forward from the hips.
3. Bend knees if needed.
4. Keep your legs active.
5. Let arms and head hang like a floppy doll.
6. Option to hold opposite elbows and sway back and forth.
7. Breathe in, breathe out.
8. Come up very slowly.
9. Option: Press hands on thighs to support coming up to standing.

### Gorilla (Uttanasana)

**Additional contraindications:** Hamstring injury; be aware of hypermobility.

**Benefits:** Stretches the hips, hamstrings and calves, relieves tension in the spine, neck and upper back, strengthens the thighs and knees, supports healthy diges-tion, calms the mind, provides vestibular and proprioceptive input.

**Instructions:**

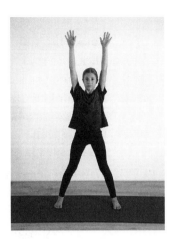

1. Stand with feet hip-width apart.
2. Reach your hands up as if you're reaching for a banana.
3. Bend forward from the hips.
4. Bend knees if needed.
5. Keep your legs active.
6. Pound your fists on the ground like a gorilla.
7. What sound does a gorilla make?
8. Breathe in, breathe out.
9. Come up very slowly.
10. Option: Press hands on thighs to support coming up to standing.

### Spider Legs up the Wall (Vipartita Karani)

**Additional contraindications:** Hamstring injury; beware of hypermobility.

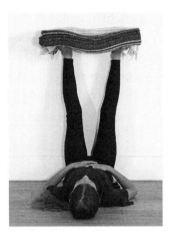

**Benefits:** Stretches the hamstrings, improves circulation, supports healthy digestion, relieves insomnia, provides vestibular and proprioceptive input.

**Instructions:**

1. Sit with one hip against the wall.
2. Lean back on your hands.
3. Walk your feet up the wall like a spider until your back is flat on the floor.
4. Palms face up.
5. Bend knees if needed.
6. Let yourself rest just like a busy spider rests in its web at the end of the day.
7. Option: Do Daddy Long Legs Breath. Place the hands on the belly and breathe in, filling up the belly like a daddy long legs belly, breathe out, letting the air out of your spider belly. Repeat 2–3 times.
8. Option: Add some grounding to the pose by placing a folded blanket on the feet or belly.

## Standing and Balancing Poses

**Contraindications for standing and balancing poses:** Injury to the pelvis, leg, knee, ankle or foot; be aware of hypermobility and neurological conditions that impact balance.

**Supports:** Use blocks, a chair, a wall or practice poses lying on the floor to support balance, stability and grounding.

### Mountain (Tadasana)

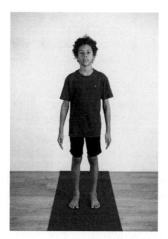 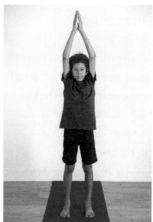

**Benefits:** Improves posture, strengthens legs, strengthens core, supports attention and focus, grounds the nervous system, provides vestibular and proprioceptive input.

**Instructions:**

1. Stand with your feet hip-width apart.
2. Point your toes forward.
3. Press your feet into the floor.
4. Reach your hands up towards the ceiling.
5. Option: Bring palms together above the head to make a mountain peak.
6. Gaze forward.
7. Breathe in, breathe out.
8. Stand strong and stable like a mountain.

### Tree (Vrksasana)

**Benefits:** Strengthens the legs and upper body, strengthens core, stretches the hips, improves posture, supports balance, supports attention and focus, provides vestibular and proprioceptive input.

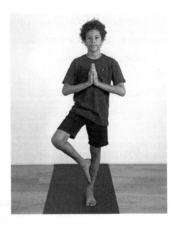

**Instructions:**

1. Stand with your feet together or a bit apart.
2. Point your toes forward.
3. Tap your right leg.
4. Bring your right heel to the inside of your ankle with your toes on the floor.
5. Press your standing leg into the ground.
6. Bring your palms together at your heart center.
7. Stand tall like a tree.
8. Gaze in front of you.
9. Breathe in, breathe out.
10. Stay here or reach your arms up as if you're growing the branches of your tree. Stand strong and grounded like a tree.
11. Repeat on the other side.
12. Option: Explore variations such as placing the foot on the inside of the shin or upper thigh.

### Warrior I (Virabhadrasana I)

**Benefits:** Strengthens the legs and upper body, strengthens core, stretches the hamstrings, calves, ankles and hips, improves posture, supports attention and focus, provides vestibular and proprioceptive input.

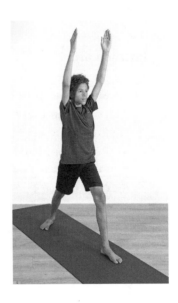

**Instructions:**

1. Stand at the front of your mat.
2. Bring feet hip-width apart.
3. Step your right foot back.
4. Point your back toes out slightly.
5. Bend your front knee just above or behind the ankle.
6. Press your feet into the floor.

7. Reach your hands up towards the ceiling.
8. Breathe in, breathe out.
9. Stand strong and brave like a warrior.
10. Come back to the front of the mat.
11. Repeat on the opposite side.

### Warrior II (Virabhadrasana II)

**Benefits:** Strengthens the legs and upper body, stretches the hamstrings, calves, ankles and hips, improves posture, supports attention and focus, provides vestibular and proprioceptive input.

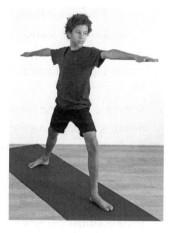

**Instructions:**

1. Stand in the center of your mat, facing the long edge.
2. Step your feet out wide.
3. Point your toes forward.
4. Tap your right leg.
5. Turn your right foot out to the side.
6. Bend your right knee.
7. Keep your knee above the ankle or just behind.
8. Press your feet into the ground.
9. Make your upper body tall.
10. Reach your arms out to the side at shoulder height, palms facing down.
11. Look towards your right hand and gaze at the tips of the fingers.
12. Breathe in, breathe out.
13. Stand with courage and strength, like a warrior.
14. Point both toes forward again.
15. Repeat on the opposite side.

### Airplane (Virabhadrasana III)

**Benefits:** Strengthens the legs and upper body, strengthens the core, stretches the hips, supports balance, supports attention and focus, provides vestibular and proprioceptive input.

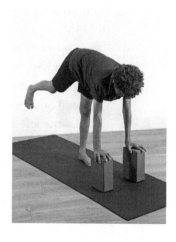

**Instructions:**

1. Stand with your feet slightly apart.

2. Tap your right leg.
3. Step your right foot back.
4. Reach your arms out wide like airplane wings.
5. Lean forward.
6. Lift your right leg up.
7. Gaze forward and down towards the floor.
8. Breathe in, breathe out.
9. Bring your right foot down.
10. Come to standing.
11. Repeat on the opposite side.
12. Option: Explore this pose using blocks for support.

### Triangle (Trikonasana)

**Benefits:** Strengthens the legs and upper body, stretches the hamstrings, calves, ankles and hips, stretches the spine, strengthens core, supports attention and focus, provides vestibular and proprioceptive input.

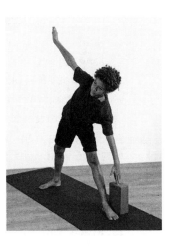

**Instructions:**

1. Stand in the center of your mat (sideways on the mat, facing the long edge).
2. Step your feet out wide.
3. Point your toes forward.
4. Tap your right leg.
5. Turn your right foot out to the side.
6. Make your upper body tall.
7. Reach your arms out to the side at shoulder height, palms facing forward.
8. Bring your right hand down towards the ground, resting it on your right shin or a block.
9. Reach your left arm up towards the ceiling.
10. Keep your back leg straight.
11. Option: Bend your front knee slightly if needed.
12. Option: Look forward, look down at the ground or block or look up towards the left hand.
13. Breathe in, breathe out.
14. Stand strong and sturdy like a pyramid.
15. Point both toes forward again.
16. Repeat on the opposite side.

### Half Moon (Ardha Chandrasana)

**Benefits:** Strengthens the legs, glutes and spine, stretches the upper body, stretches the hamstrings, calves and ankles, strengthens core, supports attention and focus, provides vestibular and proprioceptive input.

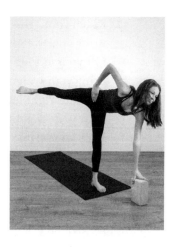

**Instructions:**

1. Stand in the center of your mat (sideways on mat, facing the long edge).
2. Hold a block.
3. Step your feet out wide.
4. Point your toes forward.
5. Tap your right leg.
6. Turn your right foot out to the side.
7. Bend your right knee softly.
8. Bring the block forward with your right hand and place in line with your shoulder.
9. Begin to straighten your right leg.
10. Lift your left leg.
11. Keep the inside of your left foot parallel to the ground.
12. Take your left hand to your left hip.
13. Option: Keep your hand on your hip or reach it towards the ceiling.
14. Your gaze can be neutral, down towards block or up towards left hand.
15. Breathe in, breathe out.
16. Stand cool and solid like the moon.
17. Come down slowly.
18. Repeat on the opposite side.

### Teetering Star (Utthita Tadasana)

**Benefits:** Strengthens the legs, ankles, shoulders and arms, strengthens core, improves posture, supports balance, provides vestibular and proprioceptive input.

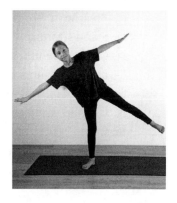

**Instructions:**

1. Stand in the center of your mat, facing the long edge.
2. Step your feet out wide.

3. Point your toes forward.
4. Reach your arms out to the side at shoulder height, palms facing down.
5. Bring your weight into your right leg.
6. Lift your left leg, keeping it out wide.
7. Bring your weight into your left leg.
8. Lift your right leg, keeping it out wide.
9. Shift your weight back and forth between your right and left legs.
10. Keep your arms out wide.
11. Breathe in, breathe out.
12. Rock back and forth like a teetering star!

### Eagle (Garudasana)

**Benefits:** Stretches the hips, thighs, shoulders and upper back, strengthens the legs, ankles and core, supports balance, supports attention, focus and whole-brain integration, provides vestibular and proprioceptive input.

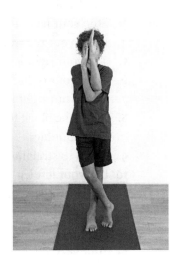

**Instructions:**

1. Stand with feet slightly apart.
2. Point your toes forward.
3. Tap your right leg.
4. Cross your right leg over your left.
5. Bring your right toes to the ground.
6. Reach your arms out wide, as if you're spreading your eagle wings.
7. Wiggle your left fingers.
8. Cross your left arm over your right.
9. Give yourself an eagle hug!
10. Gaze forward.
11. Breathe in, breathe out.
12. Stand strong and focused like an eagle.
13. Option: Bend the elbows and bring the backs of the hands together or bring the palms together.
14. Option: Lift the right foot and wrap around the ankle.
15. Unwind your arms and legs.
16. Come back to standing with your toes pointing forward.
17. Repeat on the opposite side.

### Flamingo

**Benefits:** Strengthens the legs, knees, ankles and core, stretches the quadriceps, improves posture, supports balance, attention and focus, provides vestibular and proprioceptive input.

**Instructions:**

1. Stand with your feet slightly apart.
2. Point your toes forward.
3. Tap your right leg.
4. Lift your right foot and bend your knee.
5. Stand strong on your left leg.
6. Reach your arms out wide at shoulder height, palms facing down, as if you're spreading your pink flamingo wings.
7. Gaze forward.
8. Breathe in, breathe out.
9. Be like a flamingo standing on one leg!
10. Option: Bring your right heel towards the buttocks and hold the ankle.
11. Repeat on the other side.

### Chair or Lightning Bolt (Utkatasana)

**Benefits:** Strengthens hips, legs, knees, ankles, core, shoulders and arms, stretches upper back and chest, provides vestibular and proprioceptive input.

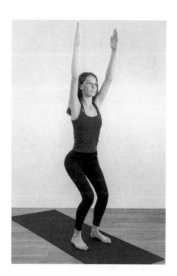

**Instructions:**

1. Stand with feet hip-width apart.
2. Bend your knees and sit back as if you're going to sit in a chair.
3. Keep your knees behind your toes, weight towards your heels.
4. Keep your chest lifted.
5. Breathe in.
6. Reach your arms forward, then up like a lightning bolt.
7. Breathe out.
8. Option: Make the "chhh" sound on the exhalation.

### Movement with Rocking, Swaying, Bouncing, etc.

Movements such as rocking, swaying and bouncing provide a great deal of vestibular input. As mentioned earlier, vestibular movement can be more energizing and alerting. It is also long-lasting and sometimes the effects of the input might not be observed until several hours later. It is important to track the child's nervous system response to the movements and integrate slowly with children who may become overwhelmed by vestibular input. Avoid more rapid vestibular input if the child presents as dizzy, disoriented, nauseous, dysregulated, overwhelmed or aversive to the movements, or shows psychological signs of distress such as dilated pupils, sweating or agitation. Always integrate proprioceptive input and grounding before and after doing these movements. If a child presents as over-responsive to vestibular input or shows signs of gravitational in security, begin with the more static asanas such as inversions with supports that give the nervous system a feeling of stability and security.

**Precautions:** Exercise caution in doing these practices with injuries to the hips, knees, legs, ankles and shoulders as well as any spinal issues or injuries. Do not do rapid movements if the child has seizures, a headache, TBI, spasticity or hypertonia.

### River

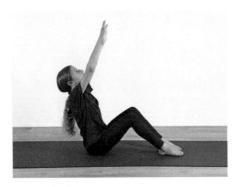 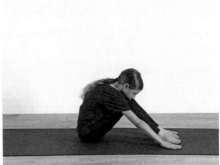

**Benefits:** Strengthens core, upper back and shoulders, stretches the front body, stimulates digestion, provides rhythmic movement for down-regulation, supports bilateral integration, provides vestibular input.

**Instructions:**

1. Begin seated with your knees bent and feet on the floor.
2. Imagine a boat on the river moving up and down on the water.

3. Breathe in.
4. Reach your hands up to the ceiling.
5. Breathe out.
6. Bring your hands down towards the ground.
7. Repeat 4–5 times.

### Cookie Dough Mixer

**Benefits:** Increases spinal mobility, stretches the hips, strengthens core, stimulates digestion, provides rhythmic movement for down-regulation, provides vestibular input.

**Instructions:**

1. Begin seated with your legs crossed.
2. Imagine a cookie dough mixer moving in a circle to mix the dough.
3. Bring your hands on your knees.
4. Breathe in.
5. Bring your belly forward and lean to the right.
6. Breathe out.
7. Round your back and lean to the left.
8. Repeat four more times.
9. Move your body in a circular motion.
10. Uncross your legs and cross the opposite leg on top.
11. Switch to the opposite direction.
12. Do five times.

### Rock-a-Bye Baby

**Benefits:** Stretches the spine and hips, strengthens the shoulders, upper back and core, provides rhythmic movement for down-regulation, supports bilateral integration, provides vestibular input.

**Instructions:**

1. Begin seated with your legs crossed.
2. Breathe in.
3. Reach your left hand up and over to the right.
4. Breathe out and bring your left hand down.
5. Breathe in.
6. Reach your right hand up and over to the left.
7. Breathe out and bring your right hand down.

8. Continue reaching opposite hands up and over, rocking back and forth with the movement and breath.
9. Option: Sing "Rock-a-Bye Baby" song, substituting the child's name.

### Leaping Frog

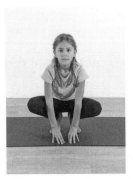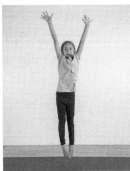

**Benefits:** Strengthens the hips, knees, legs, core and ankles, stretches the hips, provides proprioceptive and vestibular input.

**Instructions:**

1. Begin standing.
2. Crouch down into a squat with your knees out wide.
3. Lift your heels.
4. Place your hands on the ground between your legs.
5. Squat like a frog getting ready to leap from lily pad to lily pad.
6. Breathe in.
7. Leap like a frog.
8. Breathe out saying, "ha!" and stick out your tongue like a frog catching a fly to eat.
9. Repeat 4–5 times.

### Rowing Boat
**Benefits:** Stretches and strengthens the upper back, shoulders and arms, strengthens core, energizes, stimulates digestion, supports bilateral integration, provides vestibular input.

**Instructions:**

1. Begin seated with your knees bent, feet on the floor.

2.  Imagine you are on a rowing team, rowing a boat.
3.  Breathe in.
4.  Bring your hands back towards your body, elbows to your side.
5.  Lean back.
6.  Breathe out.
7.  Reach your hands forward and lean forward.
8.  Option: Make the sound "ha!" on the exhalation.
9.  Repeat 4–5 times.

### Washing Machine

**Benefits:** Increases spinal rotation, strengthens core, energizes, stimulates digestion, provides vestibular input.

**Instructions:**

1.  Stand with your feet wider than hip-width apart.
2.  Point your toes forward.
3.  Keep your knees bent slightly.
4.  Take your hands to your hips.
5.  Think about the movement and sound a washing machine makes.
6.  Breathe in.
7.  Breathe out and make the "ch" sound.
8.  Turn your upper body towards the right.
9.  Breathe in.
10. Come back to the center.
11. Breathe out and make the "ch" sound.
12. Turn your upper body towards the left.
13. Repeat several times rotating back and forth.

### Rock and Roll

**Benefits:** Strengthens core, energizes, stimulates digestion, provides vestibular input.

**Instructions:**

1.  Begin seated with your knees bent, feet on floor.
2.  Breathe in.
3.  Come onto your back, drawing your knees towards your body and your feet back towards your head.
4.  Rock forward onto your bottom with your knees bent, feet on the floor.
5.  Reach your hands forward.

6. Breathe out making the "ha" sound.
7. Repeat several times.

### Happy Baby (Ananda Balasana)

**Benefits:** Strengthens core, stretches the hips, stimulates digestion, provides rhythmic movement for down-regulation, provides vestibular input.

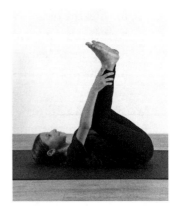

**Instructions:**

1. Lie on your back.
2. Bend your knees.
3. Bring them out wide.
4. Bring your hands to the backs of your thighs, back of knees, shins, ankles or feet.
5. Breathe in.
6. Breathe out and rock towards the right.
7. Come back to the center.
8. Breathe in.
9. Breathe out and rock towards the left.
10. Come back to the center.
11. Continue to rock side to side, like a happy baby!

### Sunrise to Sunset

**Benefits:** Improves posture, strengthens shoulders, arms and core, stretches the spine, stimulates digestion, provides vestibular input.

**Instructions:**

1. Stand with your feet hip-width apart or wider.
2. Point your toes forward.
3. Breathe in.
4. Reach your hands up to the ceiling.
5. Face your palms forward.
6. Imagine the sun rising.
7. Breathe out.
8. Bring your hands down towards the ground.
9. Bend forward.
10. Imagine the sun setting.
11. Repeat reaching the hands up and bringing them down, mimicking the sun rising and setting.

## Weight Bearing

Weight-bearing poses provide a significant amount of proprioceptive input. Weight bearing simply means supporting the body's weight through the extremities. Standing and balancing poses are examples of weight bearing through the legs. It is also important to do practices where there is weight bearing through the arms. Anytime the body is in a weight-bearing position, there is extra input to the joints and muscles that give us more of a felt sense of connection to our body. These weight-bearing poses strengthen the hands, wrists, elbows, shoulders, neck and core muscles—all muscles that are important for both gross and fine motor activities. Weight-bearing poses also support maintaining good bone density. Weight-bearing poses can be both energizing and grounding.

Table

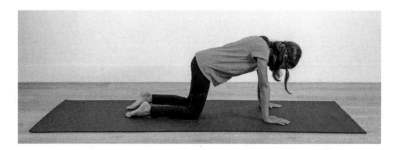

**Benefits:** Strengthens the upper body and core, provides proprioceptive input.

**Contraindications:** Injury to the shoulders, arms, wrists or knees, caution with hypermobility in the elbows and wrists.

**Supports:** Place a folded blanket under the knees. See variations in Chapter 5.

**Instructions:**

1. Come onto your hands and knees.
2. Place your shoulders over your wrists.
3. Place your hips over your knees.
4. Keep your neck long.
5. Look down at the mat.
6. Press your hands into the mat.
7. Breathe in.
8. Breathe out and hug your belly button in towards your spine.
9. Hold the pose sturdy and strong like a table.

### Cat (Bitilasana)

**Benefits:** Strengthens the upper body and core, stretches the spine, provides proprioceptive input.

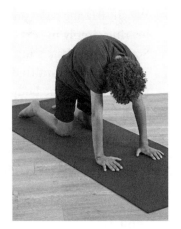

**Contraindications:** Injury to the shoulders, arms, wrists or knees, caution with spinal injuries or issues, avoid extreme cervical flexion if there is atlantoaxial instability, caution with hypermobility in the elbows and wrists.

**Supports:** Place a folded blanket under the knees. See variations in Chapter 5.

**Instructions:**

1. Come onto your hands and knees.
2. Place your shoulders over your wrists.
3. Place your hips over your knees.
4. Breathe in.
5. Press your hands into the mat.
6. Round your spine.
7. Breathe out.
8. Look towards your belly button.
9. Arch your back like a cat.
10. Option: Hiss like a cat on the exhalation.

### Cow (Marjaryasana)

**Benefits:** Strengthens the upper body, back and core, stretches the front body and the spine, provides proprioceptive input.

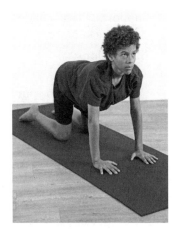

**Contraindications:** Injury to the shoulders, arms, wrists or knees, caution with spinal injuries or issues, avoid extreme cervical extension if there is atlantoaxial instability, caution with hypermobility in the elbows and wrists.

**Supports:** Place a folded blanket under the knees. See variations in Chapter 5.

**Instructions:**

1. Come onto your hands and knees.
2. Place your shoulders over your wrists.
3. Place your hips over your knees.
4. Drop your belly.
5. Press your hands into the mat.
6. Draw your chest forward.
7. Breathe in.
8. Breathe out.
9. Look up with your eyes, like a cow looking up at the sky.
10. Option: Make the "moo" sound on the exhalation.

### Plank (Kumbhakasana)

**Benefits:** Strengthens the upper body and core, energizes, provides proprioceptive input.

**Contraindications:** Injury to the shoulders, arms, wrists or knees, caution with hypermobility in the elbows and wrists.

**Supports:** Place a folded blanket under the knees. See variations in Chapter 5.

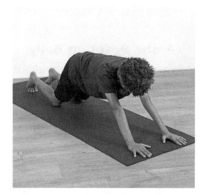

**Instructions:**

1. Come onto your hands and knees.
2. Place your shoulders over your wrists.
3. Place your hips over your knees.
4. Walk your right hand forward.
5. Walk your left hand forward.
6. Keep walking your hands forward until your hips are in front of your knees.
7. Press your hands into the mat.
8. Keep your neck long.
9. Gaze down at the mat.
10. Breathe in.
11. Breathe out.
12. Hug your belly button in towards your spine.
13. Hold the pose strong and sturdy like a pirate's plank.

14. Option: On exhalation, make the "arghhhh" sound like the sound a
    pirate makes.

### Down Dog (see "Inversions" section in "Poses for Vestibular and Proprioceptive Input")

**Benefits:** Strengthens the upper body and core, stretches the hamstrings, calves, ankles and spine, calms the mind, provides proprioceptive input.

**Contraindications:** Injury to the shoulders, arms, wrists or hamstrings, caution with spinal injuries or issues, caution with hypermobility in the elbows, wrists and knees.

## Standing Balancing Poses

**Supports:** Place a block under the forehead to add a more calming effect. See variations in Chapter 5.

## Prone Poses on Belly

Poses on the belly provide proprioceptive input and can feel grounding for the nervous system.

### Cobra (Bhujangasana)

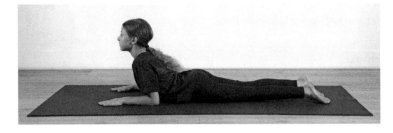

**Contraindications:** Caution with spinal issues or injuries, avoid extreme extension of the cervical spine with atlantoaxial instability.

**Benefits:** Strengthens the spinal extensors and core, opens the front body, stimulates digestion, provides proprioceptive input.

**Instructions:**

1. Lie on your belly.
2. Bring your hands under your shoulders, palms on the mat.

3. Place the tops of your feet on mat, toes pointing back.
4. Hug your elbows in towards your side body.
5. Breathe out.
6. Breathe in.
7. Press your palms down.
8. Lift your shoulders and chest.
9. Gaze forward.
10. Breathe out.
11. Imagine you are a snake lifting its head and hissing.
12. Option: On exhalation, make the "tsss" sound, like a snake hissing.

### Shark (Salabhasana)

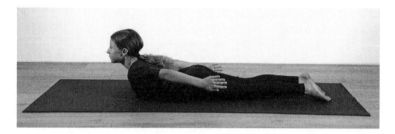

**Contraindications:** Caution with spinal issues or injuries, avoid extreme extension of the cervical spine with atlantoaxial instability.

**Benefits:** Strengthens the spinal extensors and core, opens the front body, stimulates digestion, provides proprioceptive input.

**Instructions:**

1. Lie on your belly.
2. Place the tops of your feet on mat, toes pointing back.
3. Press the tops of your feet into the mat.
4. Breathe out.
5. Breathe in.
6. Lift your chest and shoulders.
7. Reach your arms back towards your feet.
8. Breathe out.
9. Imagine you are a shark swimming in the ocean.

### Superhero

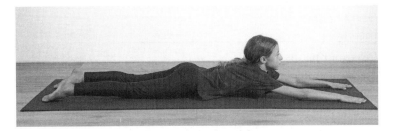

**Contraindications:** Caution with spinal issues or injuries, avoid extreme extension of the cervical spine with atlantoaxial instability.

**Benefits:** Strengthens the spinal extensors and core, opens the front body, stimulates digestion, provides proprioceptive input.

**Instructions:**

1. Lie on your belly.
2. Place the tops of your feet on mat, toes pointing back.
3. Reach your arms forward.
4. Place your palms on the mat.
5. Lift your chest and shoulders.
6. Breathe in.
7. Breathe out.
8. Option: Lift arms and legs.
9. Breathe in.
10. Breathe out.
11. Imagine you are a superhero flying in the sky.

### Sleepy Crocodile (Makarasana)

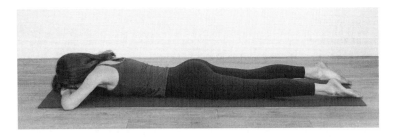

**Contraindications:** Shoulder injury, caution with spinal issues or injuries.

**Benefits:** Strengthens the spinal extensors and core, stimulates digestion, calms the mind, provides proprioceptive input.

**Instructions:**

1. Lie on your belly.
2. Place the tops of your feet on mat, toes pointing back.
3. Bring your forearms to the mat.
4. Bend your elbows.
5. Rest your forehead on your arms.
6. Breathe into your crocodile belly.
7. Feel your belly filling with air.
8. Breathe out slowly.
9. Rest like a sleepy crocodile.

## Forward Bends (Container Poses)

I refer to forward bends as container poses because there is a closing in, a moving inward physically, energetically and emotionally. Because the body is literally contracting, there is a significant amount of proprioceptive input. Forward bends can be soothing to the nervous system and calming to the mind and body.

### Child's Pose (Balasana)

**Contraindications:** Injury to the hips, knees, ankles or shoulders, caution with spinal injuries or issues, including osteoporosis.

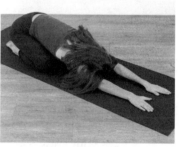

**Benefits:** Stretches the hips, quads, shoulders, arms and spine, stimulates digestion, calms the mind, provides proprioceptive input.

**Supports:** Place a block under your forehead if it doesn't reach the mat, bring your knees in closer, place a folded blanket under your knees, place a folded blanket on top of your calves if your bottom is lifted.

**Instructions:**

1. Come onto your hands and knees.
2. Sit your bottom back towards your heels.
3. Spread your knees wide.

4. Bring your forehead to the mat.
5. Reach your arms forward, palms facing down on the mat.
6. Breathe in.
7. Breathe out.

### Rock

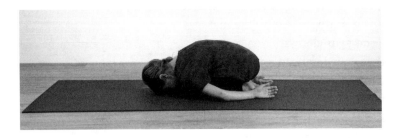

**Contraindications:** Injury to the hips, knees, ankles, or shoulders, caution with spinal injuries or issues, including osteoporosis.

**Benefits:** Stretches the hips, upper back and spine, stimulates digestion, calms the mind, provides proprioceptive input.

**Supports:** Place a block under the forehead if it doesn't reach the mat, place a folded blanket under the knees, place a folded blanket on top of the calves if the bottom is lifted, keep the arms reaching forward rather than back.

**Instructions:**

1. Come onto your hands and knees.
2. Sit your bottom back towards your heels.
3. Bring your forehead to the mat.
4. Reach your hands back towards your heels.
5. Let your arms rest.
6. Breathe in.
7. Breathe out.
8. Be still and grounded like a rock.

### Rabbit
See earlier in the chapter.

### Puppy (Uttana Shishosana)

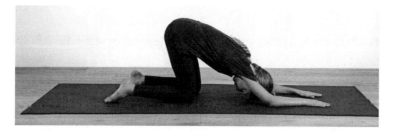

**Contraindications:** Injury to the knees or shoulders, caution with spinal injuries or issues, including osteoporosis.

**Benefits:** Stretches the shoulders, upper back, arms and spine, opens the front body, stimulates digestion, calms the mind, provides proprioceptive input.

**Supports:** Place a folded blanket under the knees, place a block under the forehead if the forehead doesn't reach the mat.

**Instructions:**

1. Come onto your hands and knees.
2. Bend your elbows and come onto your forearms.
3. Bring your forehead to the mat.
4. Keep your hips high.
5. Reach your hands forward towards the front of the mat.
6. Breathe in.
7. Breathe out.
8. Option: Wag your puppy tail and make a puppy sound.

### Turtle (Kurmasana)

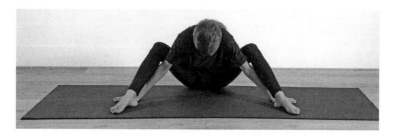

**Contraindications:** Caution with spinal injuries or issues, including osteoporosis, avoid extreme cervical flexion with atlantoaxial instability.

**Benefits:** Stretches the hips and upper back, calms the mind, provides proprioceptive input.

**Supports:** Place stacked blocks under the forehead to increase the calming effect.

**Instructions:**

1. Begin seated with your knees bent, feet on the floor.
2. Bring your feet and knees out wide.
3. Reach your arms up.
4. Bring your hands down to the mat between your legs.
5. Look back towards your belly button like a turtle bringing its head inside its shell.
6. Breathe in.
7. Breathe out.
8. Option: Bring your arms under your knees.
9. Option: Lift your head up on the exhalation and say "hellooo."

### Sponge

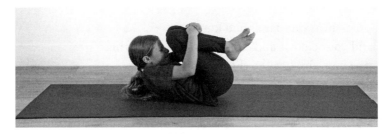

**Contraindications:** Caution with spinal injuries or issues, including osteoporosis, avoid extreme cervical flexion with atlantoaxial instability.

**Benefits:** Stretches the spine, strengthens core, releases tension, provides proprioceptive input.

**Supports:** Keep your head on the ground to avoid cervical flexion.

**Instructions:**

1. Lie on your back.
2. Hug your knees in towards your chest.
3. Wrap your arms around your knees.

4.  Bring your forehead towards your knees.
5.  Squeeze all the muscles in your body.
6.  Scrunch the muscles in your face.
7.  Imagine squeezing any icky, mucky stuff from the day out of your sponge.
8.  Breathe in.
9.  Breathe out.
10. Release and let your arms, legs and head relax on the mat.

### Tense/Relax

Tense-and-relax practices fit into the category of progressive muscle relaxation, a deep relaxation technique that has been effectively used to control stress and anxiety and relieve insomnia (Toussaint *et al.*, 2021; Simon *et al.*, 2021). The technique of progressive muscle relaxation was first described by Edmund Jacobson in the 1930s and is based on his premise that mental calmness is a natural result of physical relaxation (Stoppler, 2005). Progressive muscle relaxation supports down-regulation of the nervous system by first tensing the muscles, which gives a signal to the brain that stress is present, then by relaxing the muscles, which lets the brain know that everything is okay. Tensing then relaxing the muscles also supports increased interoceptive awareness by really feeling what it's like to be tense, then what it feels like for the muscles to be relaxed. I find that these practices support children and teens in recognizing what tension and relaxation feel like in their bodies. I also like to use tense-and-relax practices with children and teens as a way to help them imagine squeezing uncomfortable energy or emotions from their bodies and for proprioceptive input to support body awareness.

### Orange Juice Squeeze

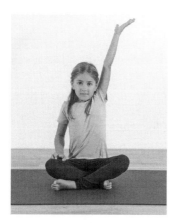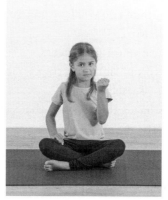

**Benefits:** Relieves tension and stress, supports healthy expression of emotion, supports bilateral integration, provides proprioceptive input.

**Instructions:**

1. Can be done seated on the floor, in a chair or standing.
2. Wiggle your right fingers.
3. Reach your right hand up.
4. Breathe in.
5. Imagine picking an orange.
6. Breathe out.
7. Bring your hand down.
8. Squeeze your hand into a fist.
9. Imagine you're squeezing orange juice from an orange.
10. Repeat two more times on the right side.
11. Option: Have the child or teen imagine squeezing tension or an emotion from their body.
12. Repeat on the opposite side.
13. Option: Alternate back and forth between the left and right.

### Self-Hug

**Benefits:** Relieves tension and stress, encourages self-love, offers self-contact, supports whole-brain integration, provides proprioceptive input.

**Instructions:**

1. Can be done seated on the floor, in a chair or standing.
2. Reach your arms out wide.
3. How much do you love yourself?
4. THIS MUCH!
5. Wiggle your right fingers.
6. Cross your right arm over your left.
7. Give yourself a hug.
8. You decide the pressure that's best for you.
9. Breathe in.
10. Breathe out.
11. Say the mantra: I am so loveable.
12. Repeat on the opposite side, left arm on top of the right.
13. Say the mantra: I am love.
14. Option: Have the child or teen imagine they are hugging a person or pet whom they love or is a resource to them.

### Arm Squeezes

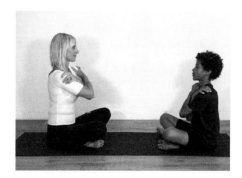 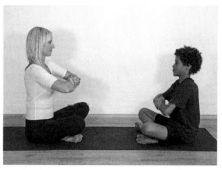

**Benefits:** Provides deep pressure touch, offers self-contact, supports whole-brain integration, provides proprioceptive input.

**Instructions:**

1. Can be done seated on the floor, in a chair or standing.
2. Bring your arms out wide.
3. Wiggle your right-hand fingers.
4. Cross your right arm on top of your left.
5. Bring your hands to your shoulders.
6. Begin squeezing your shoulders.
7. You decide the pressure that's best for you.
8. Move from the shoulders all the way to your wrists, then your hands.
9. Breathe in.
10. Breathe out.
11. Squeeze your hands, wrists and all the way back to your shoulders.
12. Repeat on the opposite side, left arm on top of the right.

### Show Me Ten

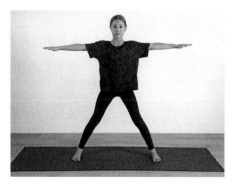 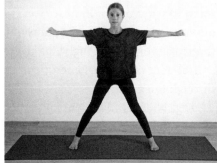

**Benefits:** Stretches and strengthens the hands, relieves tension and stress, provides proprioceptive input.

**Instructions:**

1. Can be done seated on the floor, in a chair or standing.
2. Breathe in.
3. Spread your fingers wide.
4. Show me ten!
5. Breathe out.
6. Squeeze your fists together.
7. Repeat 3–4 times.

### Sponge
See earlier in the chapter.

## Progressive Relaxation or Yoga Nidra Practice for Children

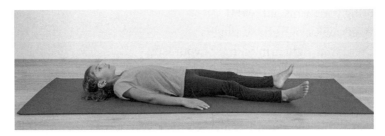

A parent shares with you during the intake process that when it comes to their bedtime routine, their child is fidgety, anxious, worried and can't seem to wind down. When children struggle with bedtime and sleep, there's often a lot more going on beneath the surface.

They may have built-up energy in the body that needs releasing, and their nervous systems may be stuck in a hypervigilant state that makes it difficult for them to wind down. In order to actually get "rest" during sleep, we want our nervous systems to be in a parasympathetic state or "rest and digest," rather than in a sympathetic (fight/flight) state. Many children who have active minds and/or a lot of internal energy can struggle with getting to sleep and sleeping through the night.

Yoga Nidra is an ancient mind–body practice. One study on the effectiveness of Yoga Nidra on stress, sleep and wellbeing showed lower stress, higher wellbeing and improved sleep quality (Moszeik *et al.*, 2020). The best way to describe it to children and teens is that it is a deep rest practice that will help quiet the mind and calm the body.

Some of the benefits of this modified Yoga Nidra practice or *progressive relaxation* for kids is that it supports more body awareness and interoceptive awareness (awareness of the internal senses), helps release built-up tension or energy in the body, offers proprioceptive input for grounding and soothing the nervous system and can bring about a sense of calm and relaxation to support with reduced stress and better sleep.

### Yoga Nidra (Progressive Relaxation) Practice Designed for Children Prior to Bedtime with Guided Imagery and Moon Meditation

**Instructions:** Pre-pose preparation: Have the child watch the adult while seated. Describe what the words "clench," "tense," "squeeze" or "tighten" mean. Show the child how to clench, tense, squeeze or tighten the muscles in their body (e.g. adult squeezes fingers into a fist and says, "I squeeze my fingers"). Count to 5 as you squeeze your fists and then release your fingers and say, "I relax my fingers." Repeat one or two more examples with different body parts for the child. Soothing music turned down low may be helpful in creating a calm and relaxing environment.

**Note:** The suggestion is to do this in bed prior to turning out the light for sleep, but this practice can be done on a mat, blanket on floor, couch or bed or seated in a chair.

1. Lie on your back in bed.
2. Place your feet wide apart.
3. Place your arms wide apart.
4. Feel the contact of your body with your bed.
5. Feel how the bed supports you.
6. Clench your toes and hold "1, 2, 3, 4, 5."
7. Exhale.
8. Relax your toes.
9. Squeeze your legs together for "1, 2, 3, 4, 5."
10. Exhale.
11. Relax your legs.
12. Squeeze your butt muscles for "1, 2, 3, 4, 5."
13. Exhale.
14. Relax your butt muscles.
15. Tighten your belly muscles for "1, 2, 3, 4, 5."
16. Exhale.

17. Relax your belly muscles.
18. Squeeze your elbows tight to your side body for "1, 2, 3, 4, 5."
19. Exhale.
20. Relax your arms.
21. Squeeze your fingers tight into fist for "1, 2, 3, 4, 5."
22. Exhale.
23. Relax your fingers.
24. Shrug your shoulders up to your ears and hold for "1, 2, 3, 4, 5."
25. Exhale.
26. Relax your shoulders.
27. Smile big with your lips closed for "1, 2, 3, 4, 5."
28. Exhale.
29. Relax your lips.
30. Close your eyes and squeeze them tight for "1, 2, 3, 4, 5."
31. Squeeze out any worried thoughts.
32. Exhale.
33. Relax your eyes.
34. Feel the heaviness of your body relaxing into your bed.

### Guided Imagery Following Progressive Relaxation Practice

"Imagine lying on the beach beneath the moon. The warm glow of the moon shining down on you. Your body is relaxed. Your towel is soft and cozy. Your body is relaxed. You see the color of the blue ocean. Your body is relaxed. You hear the quiet sounds of the waves…shhhhh, shhhh, shhhh…your body is relaxed. The waves carry away any worries. Your body is relaxed. Your body begins to feel heavy. Your body is relaxed. You feel the weight of your body sink into your bed. Your body is relaxed. The glow of the moon surrounding you. Your body is relaxed. Your mind and body are still and quiet, like the moon. Your body and mind are relaxed. Allowing the glow of the moon to hold and comfort you.. Your body is relaxed."

### What Is Stimming?

Stimming—or self-stimulatory behaviors—is repetitive body movements or noises that serve to help individuals regulate their sensory and nervous systems. Some of the more observable stims are hand flapping, finger flicking, rocking, jumping, spinning and twirling. There can also be more subtle stims such as wiggling toes, rubbing fingers together or tapping fingers. For a long time, stimming has received a bad rap. Stims have been thought of as maladaptive behaviors that need to be suppressed in order for the individual who is stimming to fit into "normal" societal expectations of behavior. Rather than thinking of stims as maladaptive behaviors, I consider stimming to be both intuitive and supportive to the individual, barring self-injurious behaviors that cause self-inflicted harm. When we look at stimming as a means for self-soothing and self-regulation, we see it with an entirely different lens. In fact, we all have ways that we move our bodies in order to self-soothe or self-regulate. Some of us tap our pens on our lap or the table when we're feeling antsy or nervous. Others might pick at their nails when they're feeling anxious. You may observe someone pacing back and forth when they're about to give a speech or jumping up and down when feeling excited. You might find yourself rocking back and forth in order to relax. These movements or "behaviors" are natural impulses that arise in response to certain stimuli, sensations or emotions. In an online educational blog about autism, an autisitic person describes how taking away his ability to stim takes away his coping mechanisms that allow him to function throughout the day (Ambitious About Autism, n.d.). It's important to come back to the reminder that *behind every behavior is a need*. Stimming is a means for individuals to balance their sensory systems, cope with stress and self-regulate.

## Savasana and Stim Toys

Stimming can provide movement and sensory input that is calming and regulating to the child. Providing stim toys during savasana can be a wonderful way not only to support the child with meeting their sensory and nervous system needs, but also to give them something on which to place their attention, helping them stay in savasana for longer. For many children who have sensory challenges and struggle with an ability to "be still" for long periods of time, providing stim toys during their relaxation pose can support their ability to "settle" in their savasana. Being calm does not have to mean that we must be still. If a child's body needs movement and stimming in order to feel calm and grounded, then we want to attempt to meet that need. Many stim toys or stim items can provide sensory input that is soothing to the nervous system.

### Suggested Stim Toys for Savasana

Give the child the option to lie on their belly or their back during savasana and choose a stim toy or item they prefer to explore. Invite the child to bring their own stim toy or item to incorporate in their resting pose.

- **Glitter jars:** Have the child lie on their belly or back, shake the glitter jar, then watch the glitter settle. This provides visual input.
- **Tactile objects:** Have a selection of tactile objects for the child to choose from to hold and explore during savasana.

- **Fidget balls:** Offering a variety of fidget balls to squeeze and touch provides tactile and proprioceptive input.
- **Pipe cleaners:** Giving the child pipe cleaners to twist and make into shapes provides visual and tactile input. You can invite the child to make shapes of the animals they embodied in their poses if that is developmentally appropriate and accessible for them.
- **Push pop bubble fidgets:** The child can push the bubbles during savasana, which provides tactile, visual and auditory input.
- **Sensory chew necklaces:** If the child tends to chew on items, a sensory chew necklace can be a great item to provide proprioceptive and oral-motor input.
- **Weighted plush animals:** A weighted plush animal can provide tactile, visual and proprioceptive input.
- **Scented playdough:** As the child is lying on their belly in savasana, they can create shapes with scented playdough. Scented playdough provides tactile, visual and olfactory input.

### Deep Pressure

Deep pressure is based on sensory integration theory and was initially developed by Jean Ayres (1972). Deep pressure is widely used in occupational therapy, particularly with autistic individuals and those who have sensory processing challenges (Lang *et al.*, 2012). Deep pressure has been found to reduce symptoms of stress and anxiety, improve performance in school and offer a calming and rewarding experience (Losiniski, Sanders & Wiseman, 2016). Temple Grandin, a well-known autistic adult, researcher, advocate and author of many books on her experience as an autistic person, recognized her need for deep pressure touch and designed a hugging machine that could provide the input she craved to regulate her nervous system. She reported that the effects of the hugging machine were reduced anxiety, increased calm and a greater capacity for touch from others. In fact, the children's book, *How to Build a Hug: Temple Grandin and Her Amazing Squeeze Machine*, tells the story of how Temple came to build her hug machine. (Guglielmo, Tourville & Potter, 2018).

Adding weight to the body or deep pressure touch can support down-regulating the nervous system and enhance a felt sense of groundedness. There are many ways to integrate deep pressure in a yoga therapy session. Keep in mind when integrating any type of sensory input to start with less input for shorter periods and slowly increase, depending on the response from the child.

## Burrito Wrap

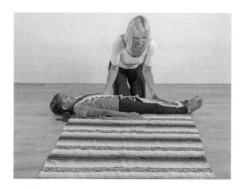
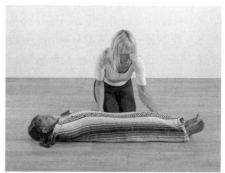
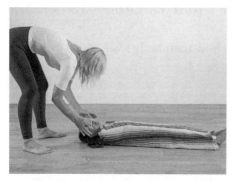
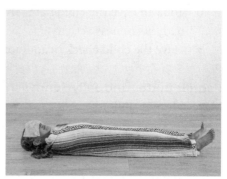

**Materials:** Blanket or yoga mat.

**Instructions:**

1. Have the child lie on the edge of the blanket or yoga mat with their arms by their sides.
2. Tell them you are going to roll them up like a burrito.
3. Roll them in the yoga mat or blanket until they are rolled up and facing upward.
4. Option: Place a folded blanket on the belly and a lightly weighted eye pillow on the eyes for increased proprioceptive input.
5. Let the child decide when they want to come out of the burrito.
6. Slowly unroll them from the yoga mat or blanket.
7. Have the child check in and notice how their body feels.

## Steamroller
**Materials:** Medium-size exercise or therapy ball.

**Instructions:**

1. Have the child lie on their back.
2. Tell them the ball is going to be like a steamroller on their body.
3. Begin at the feet and move upward (avoid the head and neck and private area, and be cautious on the stomach), rolling the ball on their body with gentle pressure, increasing the pressure to the child's desire. Some will want lighter pressure; some will want more pressure.
4. With younger children, making the sound of a steamroller can increase engagement and enjoyment of the activity.
5. Have the child lie on their belly and do the same on their back.
6. You can have the child name the body parts you roll the ball on for a body awareness activity.
7. Have the child check in and notice how their body feels.

### Peanut Butter and Jelly Sandwich
**Materials:** Two pillows.

**Instructions:**

1. Tell the child you're going to make them into a peanut butter and jelly sandwich.
2. Have them lie with their trunk and belly on a pillow (bottom slice of bread).
3. Place the other pillow (top slice of bread) on their back side and apply pressure, beginning with light pressure, then gradually increasing pressure to the child's desire.
4. Have the child check in and notice how their body feels.

## Weight-Bearing Poses

- Table Pose
- Cat/Cow
- Plank
- Balancing poses

## Pushing, Pulling, Lifting Heavier Objects
### Wall Pushes
**Instructions:**

1. Have the child come to a wall and push on the wall with the pressure that feels best to them. Tell them to imagine they are trying to push the wall down.
2. You can also explore Wall Dog, a variation of Down Dog at the wall.

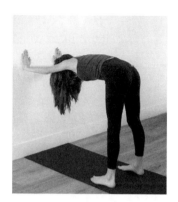

### Tug-o-War
**Instructions:**

1. Have the child bend both elbows with palms facing in towards their body.
2. Reverse the right hand so palm is facing out, with thumb down.
3. Clasp the fingers together.
4. Breathe in.
5. Breathe out and tug, pulling on the fingers.
6. Switch sides and do the same on the other side.
7. Repeat 2–3 times.

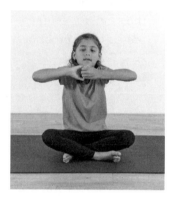

### Bear Walks
**Instructions:**

1. Tell the child they're going to pretend to walk like a bear.
2. Have them come onto their hands and feet and walk around like a bear.
3. You can invite the child to growl like a bear if they would like.

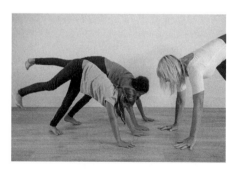

### Carrying or Lifting Yoga Mats and Bolsters

- Have the child help with carrying heavier objects during set-up or clean-up in sessions.
- Have the child imagine they are a weightlifter; they can explore lifting items like a weightlifter, for example, lifting a bolster above the head like weights.
- Use weighted items on the body such as blankets, pillows and light sand bags in restorative poses.

### Anchor Pose

I call this Anchor Pose because the weight of the sandbags on the different parts of the body supports anchoring and grounding the nervous system. The placement of the sandbags on the body provides deep pressure and proprioceptive input.

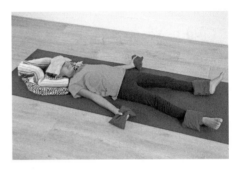

**Instructions:**

1. Have the child lie on their back in savasana with their palms face up.
2. Place the small sand bags or eye pillows on their body, making sure to communicate where you are placing them so they know what to expect.
3. Place a sand bag on one ankle, then the other.
4. Place a sandbag on the palm of one hand.
5. Be sure the fingers are not flat; they should almost be gently holding the beanbag without effort.
6. Place the sandbag on the opposite palm.
7. Option: Place a folded blanket on the child's belly if that is comfortable for them.
8. Place a light eye pillow on their eyes.
9. Notice how their nervous system responds.
10. The desired outcome is that they are able to settle in the pose and have an experience of feeling grounded.

### Tapping/Tactile Supports

Tapping the body provides proprioceptive input which can support brain–body connection. When we encourage children to tap a body part that they will be moving or use tactile supports to provide proprioceptive feedback, it facilitates increased body awareness, connection to their body parts and improved interoceptive awareness.

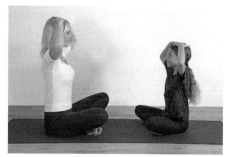

Tactile supports that offer proprioceptive input and bring awareness to certain areas of the body can facilitate greater body awareness and connection. These include:

- blocks
- blankets
- bean bags
- sand bags
- eye pillows
- straps
- wooden dowels.

## THE EIGTH SENSE: INTEROCEPTION

### What is Interoceptive Awareness?

Interoception is the sense of the body's internal state. This can be both conscious and nonconscious. Signals are relayed from the body to specific subregions of the brain including the brain stem, thalamus, insula, somatosensory and anterior cingulate cortex, allowing for a nuanced representation of the physiological state of the body. This is important for maintaining homeostatic conditions in the body and facilitating self-awareness (Wikipedia, 2022b). Interoception helps us understand how we "feel" on the inside and is directly correlated to understanding and regulating our sensory experiences, arousal states and emotions.

Since interoception can be both conscious and nonconscious, interoceptive awareness refers to the consciousness and awareness of body-based sensations and emotions such as hunger, fullness, rapid heartbeat, irritability, anger, etc. Interoceptive awareness is key to developing self-awareness, self-regulation and a felt sense of embodiment.

## Building Interoception

Our level of interoceptive awareness depends on many factors, including how our sensory systems are organized, our nervous system state and what experiences we have had that may have impacted our connection to our bodies. Research suggests that disturbances of interoception occur frequently in psychiatric conditions such as PTSD, anxiety disorders, major depressive disorders, anorexia, bulimia, OCD and autism (Brewer, Murphy & Bird, 2021). This includes over-responsiveness to physiological sensations in the body as well as under-responsiveness.

### Sensation Vocabulary

Part of building interoceptive awareness is teaching children sensation vocabulary that can help them to describe what they are feeling. I often refer to the term "front loading" when teaching children new skills, especially children who may struggle with language and communication. We have to front-load or teach the words first before a child can actually use the words to communicate. I also encourage adults to teach children and teens body parts vocabulary and where the parts are prior to teaching them poses. Building vocabulary is a prerequisite to developing skills such as learning yoga poses and expressing what they feel and where they feel the sensation in their body. Figure 4.1 shows a few sensation vocabulary words along with images that can be taught in order to help children describe their "inner experience." I developed visual sensation cards and a somatic movement curriculum to support children and teens with communicating the "felt sense" in their bodies. There were three main reasons for creating these visuals.

1.  Children who are in a high stress or activated state have less access to the parts of the brain that are responsible for language and communication.
2.  Some children communicate and process information more effectively when given visual images.
3.  Visual images support memory retention.

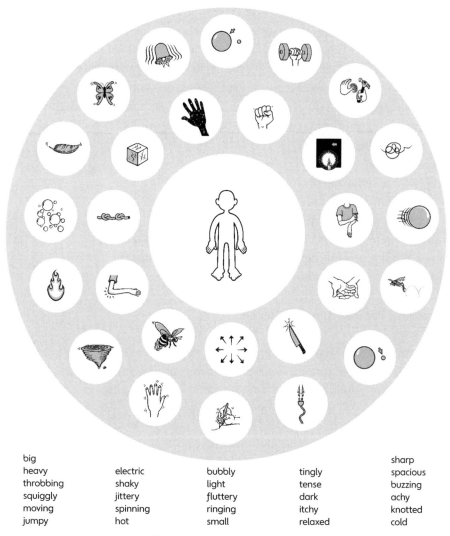

| big | | | | sharp |
| heavy | electric | bubbly | tingly | spacious |
| throbbing | shaky | light | tense | buzzing |
| squiggly | jittery | fluttery | dark | achy |
| moving | spinning | ringing | itchy | knotted |
| jumpy | hot | small | relaxed | cold |

**Figure 4.1** My body sensations

### Body Check

Once a child has been taught sensation vocabulary and is able to use descriptive words to communicate what they are feeling in their body, beginning and ending a session with a body check is a great way to get them to tune in to their sensations as well as check in before and after their session to see if they notice any shifts or changes. Figure 4.1 shows an image of the body check that is part of the My Body Sensations curriculum, a program designed to help children learn how to identify what they feel in their bodies. I often begin the session by asking the child what they notice in their body in the moment or to discuss what they feel in their body when experiencing a specific emotion such as anxiety or anger.

Offering different-colored markers or crayons for the child to use as they do their body check gives them choice and can also serve as a means to describe their sensations. For instance, I give children red for hot, blue for cold. As the child describes the sensation, they may draw their own image that represents that sensation or they may use the images on the sensation cards to draw on the body. You can inquire where they feel that sensation in their body and have them draw the sensation image in that area of the body. Below are some specific inquiries I use for the sensation "tense."

- What sensation do you notice in your body?
- Where do you notice feeling tense?
- How would you describe what tense feels like?
- Is there a color, shape or image that comes to mind?
- What is something that might make you feel tense?
- Is there an emotion you connect to feeling tense?

### Exploring the Felt Sense of Tense

1. Squeeze your hands into tight fists.
2. What do you notice in your body as you squeeze your hands?
3. Now relax your hands.
4. What do you notice in your body now?

What I found to be so fascinating as I learned more about the vagus nerve and the physiological responses that are happening all of the time in our bodies is that the sensation or physiological response precedes the emotion. In fact, 80 percent of the information connecting our brain and body via the vagus nerve is *afferent*, meaning we experience a physiological change in the body, sensory fibers carry that information to the brain, then we have a cognitive or emotional response to that sensation (Foley & DuBois, 1937; Asala & Bower, 1986). Teaching children to notice what is happening inside their bodies can provide a foundation for emotional awareness and regulation.

### Emotions

I have often found that when adults ask children how they feel, the child's answer may be "sad," "mad," "frustrated," etc., but the conversation stops there instead of inquiring further about what they are experiencing in their bodies in connection to that emotion. Or the adults themselves don't feel comfortable with the child expressing emotion, so they either tell the child to suppress the emotion or attempt to appease the child in order to get the child to stop behaving in whatever way they are behaving (remember, behind every behavior is a need). As a child, I was not allowed to express my emotions. If I complained, I was ungrateful. If I showed sadness, I was whiny. And there was absolutely no option to express anger. I moved through life feeling that anger was a bad emotion and I shouldn't and couldn't be angry with people. Because I was around a lot of angry energy, I struggled with being around others who were expressing anger. Expressing how I felt was not safe, so I learned that my feelings were a burden, that they were not okay and that I could be harmed or love could be withheld from me unless I held my emotions in. As an adult, I know now that I was greatly impacted by suppressing my emotions in this way. I was diagnosed with Hashimoto's thyroiditis or hypothyroidism when I was 26 years old. It's not a surprise that my throat chakra was out of balance from suppressing so many things I wanted or needed to communicate to others but didn't feel safe enough or empowered enough to do so. Anger is a healthy emotion for us to feel. If we are attuned to feelings of anger, we can recognize when our boundaries have been ruptured or when someone has done something to us that is not okay. As an adult in my 40s, I am just now learning how to acknowledge and express my anger and show healthy aggression. It has been liberating, and so much of that suppressed energy in my body has begun to be freed up. What a beautiful thing to be feeling more spaciousness and also a felt sense of agency and power to be able to express my wants, needs and feelings without fear. This is the beauty and honor of teaching these practices to children and teens. We can teach them that it is important and necessary to connect with and express their emotions in healthy ways so they can have balanced throat chakras and move through the world in a more honest and empowered way.

## Emotions Breaths

A wonderful way to explore emotions with children is through emotions breaths. As we practice the emotions breaths, we support children in identifying the emotion, identifying the sensations connected to the emotion and exploring healthy ways to express or release difficult emotions.

## Adam — Dragon Breath

When I was working as an educational/behavioral specialist in a behavior program composed of middle and high school teens with autism, learning and communication differences and sensory processing challenges, I integrated yoga and mindfulness practices throughout the day to support my students with developing more self-awareness and self-regulation skills. Many of the teens in my program had experienced significant developmental trauma, and one of the main challenges for a majority of them was identifying and expressing their emotions in a healthy way. An autistic boy—we'll call him Adam—who had experienced severe abuse and neglect would often display angry and aggressive outbursts. He struggled to cope with feelings of frustration that would arise throughout the day. He developed a pattern of running out of the classroom or absconding from the school when he became angry or frustrated, which posed a safety threat for him, his peers and the adults in the program.

Through observation, I could see that he could easily be triggered into a fight/flight response and that his reactions and actions were survival responses to perceived threat and danger. His neuroception of the world around him was that people were out to get him and that he couldn't trust the adults in his life to keep him safe. He and I developed a connected relationship; my primary focus was to be a consistent and predictable base of support for him. I could see when he was in his fight/flight response, there was no verbal reasoning or cognitive processing that could happen in that moment of dysregulation.

As I mentioned earlier, I integrated yoga throughout the day in the program, teaching emotions breaths, taking yoga movement breaks and encouraging my students to use those practices as tools to support their self-regulation. Adam loved Dragon Breath. We would breathe in our anger or frustration and breathe out our dragon's breath to let go of the anger, to breathe out the fire. We also talked about what it felt like in our bodies when we felt angry or frustrated, and his response would be "I feel hot, like I'm on fire." One day, Adam and I came up with a plan for when he began to feel angry or frustrated. I made a Dragon Breath card for him. It was a picture of a dragon breathing fire glued to a popsicle stick. When he started to feel that heat begin in his body, he could just hold up his Dragon Breath card without speaking, go outside in a designated spot and do his dragon breaths until he felt calm and ready to return. After deciding on this strategy together, he began using his Dragon Breath card when he started to feel frustrated or angry. The result was a significant reduction in aggressive and absconding behaviors. There are several reasons why I think this strategy was a success:

- He didn't have to use verbal language to request a break, which can be difficult and even impossible when a child is acting from their survival brain.
- Our solution was a collaborative effort and he felt he had choice and self-agency in deciding on a strategy that worked for him.
- He felt a sense of control and self-empowerment, which is what is taken away when a child experiences abuse or trauma.
- He was given a healthy way to express his anger rather than being told not to feel angry. Doing Dragon Breath allowed him to actually release the activation and energy in his body rather than suppress it.
- He and I had a connection in which he developed a felt sense of trust and predictability.

### All Emotions Are Okay

What I have found in exploring emotions with children through breath and movement is that in bringing curiosity and inquiry to their experience of emotions, we help validate to children that all emotions are okay. We all feel anger, sadness, frustration, love, joy, etc. These are human emotions that we all share, and no emotion is a bad emotion. Our emotions are there to communicate to us what we are feeling, and our emotions are what make us such dynamic, complex and intuitive beings.

### Exploring and Expressing Emotions Through Movement and Breath

#### Color Breathing

Integrating breath and visualization can support bringing calming energy into our nervous system and releasing tension or stuck energy from our nervous system. Color breathing is a fun practice to work with breath and visualization.

**Materials:** Colored scarves or colored cards.

#### Calming the Nervous System
**Instructions:**

1. Have the child choose a colored scarf or colored card that brings them a feeling of calm.
2. Have them imagine breathing that color into their nostrils and filling their body with that calming color as they breathe in.
3. Have them imagine breathing that calming color out to others as they breathe out.
4. Repeat three times.

#### Welcoming Joy
**Instructions:**

1. Have the child choose a colored scarf or colored card that brings them a feeling of joy.
2. Have them imagine breathing that color into their nostrils and filling their body with that joyful color as they breathe in.
3. Then have them imagine breathing that joyful color out to others as they breathe out.
4. Repeat three times.
5. You can change the emotion they would like to welcome (e.g. love, courage).

### Releasing Difficult Emotions
**Instructions:**

1. Have the child identify a difficult emotion they may be feeling or feel sometimes.
2. Have them choose a color that represents that emotion.
3. Have them breathe in and grab that color with their hands.
4. Have them breathe out with an open mouth breath and release that color and emotion with their hands.

## Anger

Anger is a complex emotion. When we experience anger, other feelings may underlie it such as hurt, feelings of injustice, a felt sense that our boundaries have been ruptured, a protective response or fight energy that has been suppressed.

### Healthy Aggression

Often, what happens with children when they feel angry and are unable to manage this big emotion is they may "act out." This could show up as aggression towards themselves or others, tantrums, yelling, impatience and impulsivity. They'll often experience what I refer to as the "shame loop" (see Figure 4.2). They feel angry, they lash out, the adult responds by shaming them for acting out and then they shut down and suppress their emotional energy. This suppression of their fight energy can lead to explosive episodes, rage, emotional dysregulation, sleep issues, social issues and physical ailments.

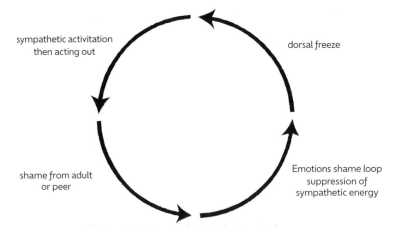

sympathetic activitation
then acting out

dorsal freeze

shame from adult
or peer

Emotions shame loop
suppression of
sympathetic energy

**Allowing for discharge of sympathetic arousal energy**
When we are not able to have completion of defensive responses or discharge of
fight/flight energy, our system goes into immobilization or freeze

Figure 4.2 The shame loop

We want children to learn to express anger in healthy ways, or what is referred to as "healthy aggression." Healthy aggression supports children with setting healthy boundaries, self-control, self-empowerment and releasing the stuck survival energy from their bodies. We want them to learn healthy ways to express their anger so they don't lash out inward toward themselves or outward toward others.

### Emotions Breaths to Release Anger and Support Healthy Aggression

As you encourage children to explore the emotions breaths, it's important to also encourage them to identify where they may feel that emotion and how that emotion feels in their body. Below is a script you can use to explore body sensations and emotions with children. You can also explore this using the body check along with emotions breaths.

"Do you ever feel angry? What do you notice in your body when you feel angry? Where do you feel anger in your body? What is something that makes you feel angry? We're going to do some breaths to help release some of that anger."

### Lion's Breath
**Instructions:**

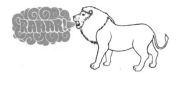

1. Think about an angry lion roaring.
2. Bring your hands up towards your face like you're raising your lion paws.
3. Breathe in through your nose.
4. Breathe out, stick out your tongue and go haaaaaaa!
5. Let out all that anger.
6. Feel your feet on the earth.
7. Notice how your body feels after letting out your anger.

### Choo-Choo Breath
This is also a great breath practice to work with flight energy.

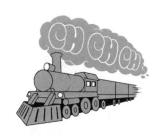

**Instructions:**

1. Think about the steam coming out of a choo-choo train.
2. Take your hands by your side and start moving one then the other in a circle like choo-choo train wheels.

3. Start making the sound "ch, ch, ch, ch," like a choo-choo train makes.

4. Keep moving your hands like a choo-choo train wheels and making the "ch" sound.

5. You can make the train go as fast as you want by speeding up your hands and "ch" sound.

6. Slow it down.

7. Feel your feet on the earth.

8. Notice how your body feels after letting all of that steam and anger out of your body.

## Volcano Breath
**Instructions:**

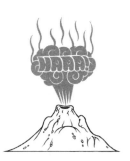

1. Think about a volcano.

2. What does a volcano do? Yes, it erupts and lets all of the heat and hot lava out.

3. Stand strong like a volcano and notice your feet on the earth.

4. Think about something that makes you feel angry.

5. Reach your hands forward, breathe in and grab your anger as you bring your fists towards your body.

6. Breathe out as you reach your arms up and out and go "chhhhhhhhhh," letting all of the heat and anger out of your body.

7. Feel your feet on the earth.

8. Notice how your body feels after letting all of that heat and anger out of your body.

## Dragon Breath
**Instructions:**

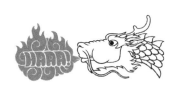

1. What do dragons do when they feel angry? Yes! They breathe fire.

2. We're going to let our anger out of our bodies by breathing fire, just like a dragon.

3. Stand with your feet planted on the floor.

4. Breathe in and reach your arms up like dragon wings.

5. Breathe out and reach your arms (dragon wings) down and say "haaaaaa!"

6. Feel your feet on the earth.

7. Notice how you feel after letting all of that fire and heat out of your body.

**Boxer Breath**
**Instructions:**

1. Think about a boxer punching a boxing bag and letting their anger out.
2. Put your boxing gloves on.
3. Stand with your legs wide apart and bend your knees.
4. Imagine punching the boxing bag as you punch with your right and left hands.
5. As you punch, go "huh!" with each punch.
6. You can speed up your punching and your breath.
7. Then slow it down.
8. Feel your feet on the earth.
9. Notice how your body feels after letting all of that anger out of your body.

**TODAY I FEEL MAD**

*Today I'm feeling very mad*
*But feeling mad is not all bad*
*When I feel mad, my cheeks get flushed*
*My heart races and my mind feels rushed*
*My muscles tense and I feel hot*
*My belly feels like it's in a knot*
*Behind the mad is often hurt*
*I want to kick and stomp the dirt*
*I want to yell and scream and hit*
*But doing that won't help one bit*
*At times I feel like I might explode*
*But there are ways to shift my mode*
*To get that tension and anger out*
*I can find ways to move about*
*Run and jump and squirm around*
*Make the Lion, Choo-Coo or Volcano Breath sound*
*Be like a boxer with Boxer Breath*
*Get it all out then take a rest*
*Check in with my body and feel the release*
*Notice my feet on the floor beneath*
*Soon my muscles will begin to relax*

*All that anger will surely pass*
*Suddenly, I won't feel mad*
*Instead, I'll feel oh so glad*
*Glad for all the feelings I feel*
*Because ALL feelings are important and real*

Shawnee Thornton Hardy

## Frustration

### I Don't Know, Let It Go Breath

I'll share a little story about one of my students and "I Don't Know, Let It Go Breath." He was a perfectionist and always wanted to get everything right. He would become frustrated if he didn't know the answer to a math problem or couldn't get his drawing just perfect. He would act this emotion out by banging his fists on the desk or banging his fists on his thighs. We talked about how not doing things just right made him feel frustrated and that he could do "I Don't Know, Let It Go Breath" to let some of that frustration out. We talked about how it was okay to not know the answer or get everything just right, and that when we make mistakes, we build new pathways in our brains. Over the course of the month, when he began to get frustrated, I would show him an image of "I Don't Know, Let It Go Breath" and we would do it together. After a couple of months, he began doing it on his own! Eventually, the banging on the table and his thighs diminished and he had this wonderful self-regulation tool to help him cope with his frustration. There is magic in these practices—I have seen it with my own eyes!

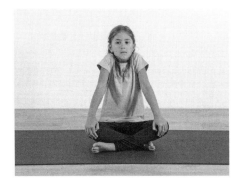 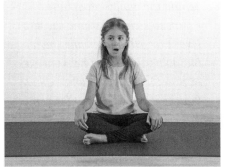

**Instructions:**

1. Sometimes we might get frustrated because we don't know how to do something or want to do something just right. When we get frustrated, we can do "I Don't Know, Let It Go Breath."

2. Breathe in and shrug shoulders up to ears, then say, "I don't know."
3. Breathe out, relax shoulders, then say, "Let it go."
4. Repeat three times.
5. Notice how your body feels after letting your frustration out.

## Fear/Worry
### Let It Go Breath

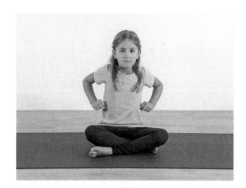 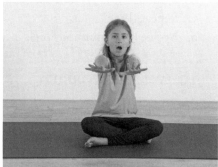

**Instructions:**

1. Think of something that makes you feel worried.
2. Reach your hands forward.
3. Breathe in and grab your worries, then bring your hands back towards your body.
4. Breathe out. Reach your hands out like you're tossing a worry ball and say "haaaaaa!"
5. Repeat three times.
6. Say, "bye worry!"
7. Notice how your body feels after letting your fear or worry out.

### Snake Breath
**Instructions:**

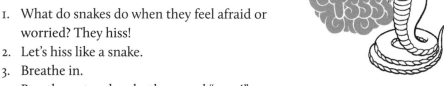

1. What do snakes do when they feel afraid or worried? They hiss!
2. Let's hiss like a snake.
3. Breathe in.
4. Breathe out and make the sound "tssss!"
5. Repeat three times.

Notice how your body feels after letting your fear or worry out.

## Cat Breath
**Instructions:**

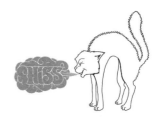

1. What do cats do when they feel afraid or worried? They hiss!
2. Let's hiss like a cat.
3. Breathe in.
4. Breathe out and make the "hisss" sound.
5. Repeat three times.
6. Notice how your body feels after letting your fear or worry out.

### TODAY I FEEL WORRIED

*Today I'm feeling very worried*
*My tummy aches*
*And my mind feels hurried*
*I feel tightness in my chest*
*And find it hard to take a breath*
*Everything feels so large*
*My amygdala is definitely in charge*
*I worry about lots of things*
*So many sensations my worries bring*
*A knot in my belly*
*Aches in my bones*
*Shaky hands and scrunched-up toes*
*My worries create a worry ball*
*Growing big in no time at all*
*I can let my worries go*
*And feel better from head to toe*
*I can do "let it go breath"*
*Put my tools to the test*
*Breathe them in, then blow them out*
*Move my body and run about*
*Hiss like a cat or even a snake*
*Give my body a little shake*
*Notice the present, the here and now*
*Place my hand on my heart and take a bow*
*Now my frontal lobe is online*
*The worries begin to fade with time*
*They may come but they'll also go*

*And I'll be glad for this, you know*
*Glad for all the feelings I feel*
*Because ALL feelings are important and real*

Shawnee Thornton Hardy

## Sadness

One important factor in feeling sadness is allowing ourselves to cry and release that energy from our bodies. Clinical psychologist Stephen Sideroff, PhD, states that "crying activates the body in a healthy way" (Govender, 2015). Research backs this theory. Studies have found higher levels of stress hormones in emotional tears as well as mood-regulating manganese (Messmer, 2009). When we cry, we release these stress hormones from our bodies. Crying can also alleviate tension and tightness around the muscles of the eyes and in the face. Sideroff also notes that "crying activates the parasympathetic nervous system and restores the body to a state of balance." Our society has a complicated relationship with crying. There is a general sense that crying is a sign of weakness and there is often shame attached to crying. I think of nature and how it releases its tears through rain. I use this analogy with children, telling them that even Mother Nature cries, that it's healthy to let that energy move through and out. It is not healthy to suppress any emotion, including sadness. Sometimes we may feel sadness and not have tears, but it is still important to acknowledge our sadness and move some of that stuck energy from our bodies in healthy ways. We explore this by practicing Rainforest Breath. As children do the "shhh" sound, it extends their exhalation and elicits the parasympathetic response, bringing a calming effect.

### Rainforest Breath

**Materials:** Rainforest stick (you can also do the practice without a rainforest stick if necessary).

**Instructions:**

1.  Play the rainforest stick and tell the child to listen to the sound of the rain.
2.  Tell them that when it rains, it is Mother Nature's way of letting out her sadness.
3.  Invite them to think of something that makes them feel sad.
4.  Invite them to make the sound of rain with their breath.
5.  Breathing in.
6.  Breathing out and making the sound "shhh."

7.  Letting all of their sadness out.
8.  Check in and have them notice how their body feels after doing Rainforest Breath.

### Bunny Breath

Somatic Experiencing is a body-oriented therapy for healing trauma and other stress disorders. One of its primary concepts is pendulation. Noticing difficult sensations and emotions *and* also being able to connect with feelings of okayness, goodness and even joy. The opposite of sadness is joy. Bunny Breath is a playful breath that often elicits laughter and silliness. Simply doing something that makes us smile or laugh can shift our energy from sadness to joy. There are also short and rapid inhalations with Bunny Breath that can elicit more of a sympathetic response that can bring energy and mobilization to a more stagnant or shut-down nervous system. Joy and laughter also have the same effect!

**Instructions:**

1.  Tell the child they are going to breathe like bunnies and do Bunny Breath.
2.  Invite them to think of a fruit or vegetable they want to sniff in the garden.
3.  Have them bring their hands up towards their ears and make bunny paws.
4.  Demonstrate the breath to them first.
5.  Breathe in through the nose several times, sniffing rapidly.
6.  Breathe out with an open mouth and go "awww"—like that fruit or vegetable smelled so good.
7.  Have the child do Bunny Breath three times.
8.  Check in and have them notice how their body feels after doing Bunny Breath.

### Bee Breath

Bee Breath can also be an energizing and invigorating breath practice that brings a feeling of joy and vitality. See earlier in the chapter for instructions.

### Self-Hug

Sometimes when we feel down, just offering ourselves a hug can boost our spirits. Self-Hug offers an experience of self-contact which can feel nurturing and resourcing. See earlier in the chapter for instructions.

## Breath of Joy

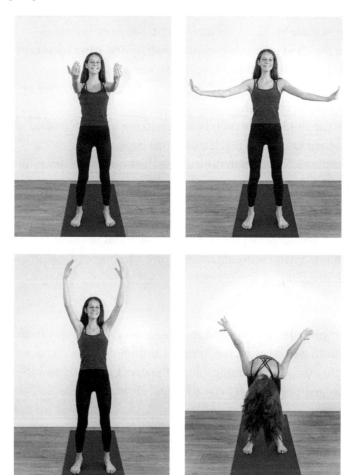

Breath of Joy is a three-part breathing technique that was introduced in the early 1970s by yoga teacher Lila Osterman from the Kripalu tradition (Weintraub, 2010). This breath awakes the whole body and can bring vitality, mobilization, energy and joy to one's system. The three-part inhalation elicits a sympathetic response, and the forceful exhalation releases built-up tension. Not to mention that it is called the Breath of Joy, so the nature of the breath is meant to connect with our inner joyful energy.

**Instructions:**

1.  Begin by having the child stand with feet apart, noticing their feet on the earth.

2. Invite them to think about something that brings them joy.
3. Have the child inhale one-third of lung capacity and swing arms up in front of their body at shoulder height, palms facing up.
4. Have the child inhale two-thirds capacity and wing their arms out to the side at shoulder height, palms facing up.
5. Have the child inhale to full capacity, swinging their arms up overhead, palms facing each other.
6. Have the child exhale their breath, making a "haaaa" sound as they bend their knees and reach their arms back.
7. Check in and have them notice how their body feels after doing Breath of Joy.

### Arm Squeezes

Arm squeezes provide deep pressure input which can be calming to the nervous system as well as giving self-contact, eliciting a feeling of comfort and support. See earlier in the chapter for instructions.

### Palming

Palming can provide comfort and rest to an overwhelmed system. When we experience sadness, we often feel tension around our eyes. By gently covering and supporting the eyes, palming allows the eyes to be held and the sadness to be acknowledged. See section "Visual: Sight" for instructions.

### Head/Jaw Massage

Often sadness brings tension in the head and jaw. A self-administered head and jaw massage can release built-up tension, soothe the nervous system and support more ventral vagal connection.

**Instructions:**

1. Invite the child to take their hands to the top of their heads and massage it with their fingers, using their thumbs to rub the back of their heads near their occiput.
2. Have them move their fingers to their forehead and along the tops of their eyebrows and temples.
3. Then just below their eyes on the bony part, moving towards their cheek bones.
4. Then encourage them to take their hands to the mandible, where the jawbone connects to the skull, and massage with their fingers.

5. Encourage them to move their hands down the jawline to the chin, massaging with whatever pressure feels best to them.
6. Check in and have them notice how their body feels.

### Lavender Oil Facial Savasana

When we feel sadness and suppress our sadness, we may continue to hold tension in our eyes, face, jaw and back of skull. Lavender Oil Facial Savasana can help release tension, and the nurturing care and touch can give the child a felt sense of connection, support and attunement. When we feel sadness, it can feel nurturing and nourishing to be cared for. As always with touch, it is important to have informed consent and to already have a foundation of trust and connection with the child. Not all children will respond positively to the smell of lavender oil. The best way to know if the scent is okay for them is to put a drop of the oil on a cotton ball and have them smell and see how they respond. Only use therapeutic-grade oils diluted with a carrier oil when integrating essential oils in your session. As you are doing the Facial Savasana, track the child's nervous system as well as your own.

**Instructions:**

1. Begin with setting the child up in a restorative savasana with a blanket under their head and a rolled blanket under their knees.
2. Place a small drop of essential oil on your palm.
3. Rub your palms together, creating warmth in your hands.
4. Gently bring your hands to the back of the child's head near the occipital ridge and use your fingers to massage gently.
5. Bring your hands to the child's forehead and rest them there gently for a moment. Breathe slowly. Share your calm, co-regulated energy with them.
6. Use your thumbs to trace the tops of the eyebrows down to the temples with gentle pressure.
7. Take your pointer fingers to the center just below the nose where the sinus passages are and trace along the passages up to the temples with gentle pressure.
8. Bring your thumbs and pointer fingers to the bottom of the jaw, pointer fingers on the front of the jaw and thumbs on the back. Trace the fingers up towards the mandible with gentle pressure.
9. Place a light eye pillow on the child's eyes.

### Koala Cuddle

Koala Cuddle is an example of a restorative pose that can provide a feeling of comfort and ease to a child's nervous system. Sometimes when we're sad, a little self-care and self-soothing might be just what we need.

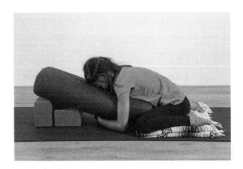

**Instructions:**

1. Place one end of a rectangular bolster on a block so the end is lifted.
2. Place a folded blanket in front of the opposite side that is down on the floor.
3. Have the child sit on the blanket with their knees out wide.
4. You may need to adjust the bolster so it comes right between their legs and is under their belly.
5. Have the child rest their forehead on the bolster and wrap their arms around the bolster as if they are giving their bolster a Koala Cuddle.
6. Allow them to rest in Koala Cuddle for as long as they desire.
7. Check in and have them notice how they feel after doing Koala Cuddle.

**TODAY I FEEL SAD**

*Today I'm feeling a bit sad*
*But feeling sad is not all bad*
*Sometimes I may want to cry*
*Just like the rain falls from the sky*
*If I allow my tears to fall*
*I'll feel better in no time at all*
*Tears are good for my heart and soul*
*I won't hold them in*
*I'll just let them roll*
*Every tear that I shed*
*Soothes my heart and clears my head*
*Some of the sensations I might feel*
*A lump in my throat, a heavy chest*
*Watery eyes, like my head is being pressed*
*So when I get that feeling of gloom*
*Here are things I can do in my room*

*Cozy up in something warm*
*And shelter down for the storm*
*Read a book that sparks some joy*
*Or play with my favorite toy*
*Dance or sing or just lie down*
*Let myself feel my frown*
*Move my body, do Bunny Breath*
*Give my body a little rest*
*Wrap my arms around myself*
*And remember that FEELING is good for my health*
*Being sad is not so bad*
*The sad will pass and soon I'll be glad*
*Glad for all the feelings I feel*
*Because ALL feelings are important and real*

Shawnee Thornton Hardy

## Anxiety

- Grounding
- Orienting
- Extended Exhalation
- Wave Breath
- Balloon Belly Breath
- Anchor Breath
- Self-Hug

 **TODAY I FEEL ANXIOUS**

*Today I'm feeling anxious*
*A revving inside me like a bus*
*So many thoughts swirling around*
*Feeling like I can't slow down*
*My heart is racing really fast*
*I wonder if this feeling will pass*
*My throat feels like it's closing up*
*And all I want is for it to stop*
*But I know that we all feel this way*
*At different times on different days*

*And there are things that I can do*
*To feel better and move this through*
*First I can simply feel the ground*
*Use my eyes to look around*
*Find something that looks nice to me*
*And focus on it for the count of three*
*Then I can take a mindful breath*
*Into my belly and then my chest*
*Breathe it out with pursed lips*
*Take my time, not rush a bit*
*Let my breath come and go*
*Breathing out oh so slow*
*Like a wave moving in and out*
*This feeling will pass I have no doubt*
*I can use my tools to feel less anxious*
*To ground my body and feel less stressed*
*What a gift it is to feel*
*Because ALL feelings are important and real*

Shawnee Thornton Hardy

## Joy/Happiness

- Breath of Joy
- Bee Breath
- Sunrise/Sunset
- Solar Plexus Chakra
- Happy Chant—Weee! (raise arms and make the sound "weee!")
- Sun Salutation
- Singing/Dancing
- Rainbow Breath

### Rainbow Breath

Using visualization and imagery can be a wonderful way to shift one's mood and nervous system state. Think of a time you were outside and saw a rainbow in the sky. It almost surely elicits a feeling of joy and happiness. Rainbow Breath involves not only visualization but also expansive movement in the upper body, which can bring more energy and vitality to the mind and body.

**Instructions:**

1. Spread your fingers wide with palms facing forward in front of your heart center.
2. Imagine your fingers are painted with the colors of the rainbow (red, orange, yellow, green, blue, indigo and violet).
3. Breathe in through your nose.
4. Breathe out and bring your hands up and out, making the arch of a rainbow.
5. Repeat 3–4 times.
6. Check in and notice how your body feels after doing Rainbow Breath.

**TODAY I FEEL HAPPY**

*Today I'm feeling happiness*
*A warm sensation in my chest*
*My body's filled with fuzziness*
*Like chirping birdies in their nest*
*I want to dance and skip about*
*Sing and twirl and laugh it out*
*My belly feels so bubbly*
*I'm buzzing round like a bee*
*Smiling, hopping, joyfully*
*This feeling feels good to me*
*Like sunshine on a summer day*
*When I can just play and play*
*So many things that bring me joy*
*My special place*
*My favorite toy*
*A cuddle, hug or cool high five*
*The things that make me feel alive*
*My friends, my pets, my family*
*Always bring me back to me*
*Remind me of the times in life*
*That feel carefree and free of strife*
*Some ways to describe happiness*
*The color yellow*
*A treasure chest*
*A rainbow that comes after rain*
*The honking of a choo-choo train*

*A big star shining bright*
*Standing in the sunlight*
*Watching a candle glow*
*Just being in the flow*
*I know this feeling may pass*
*Because life sometimes moves so fast*
*But that's OK*
*It will come again*
*It's just a matter of "when"*
*I'm so grateful for the feelings I feel*
*Because ALL feelings are important and real*

Shawnee Thornton Hardy

## Pride

- Star
- Mountain
- Airplane
- Solar Plexus Chakra
- Warrior poses
- Floating on a Cloud
- Bear Walk (walk on all fours)/Roar (like a bear)
- Open Mouth Breath
- Front Body Openers

### TODAY I FEEL PROUD

*Today I'm feeling oh so proud*
*Like I'm floating on a cloud*
*I stand up tall with arms out wide*
*It feels so good to feel my pride*
*An open feeling in my chest*
*A deep sigh in my breath*
*Strength and power in my bones*
*Feeling grounded in my toes*
*I reach my crown up to the sky*
*Like I could fly so very high*
*My body feels so energized*
*My muscles strong in my thighs*

*I hold my belly in my hands*
*And say the words, I can I can*
*I can do anything!*
*I want to shout and dance and sing*
*I feel like a star shining bright*
*Standing strong with all my might*
*Like a warrior, bold and brave*
*Or a courageous bear in its cave*
*Nothing can bring me down*
*I just want to jump around*
*Skip and hop and move about*
*Shout all of my pride out*
*When I feel this thing called pride*
*I feel sensations inside*
*Warmth in my heart*
*And buzzing in my head*
*No frown on my face*
*Only smiles instead*
*Rosy cheeks and bubbles all around*
*My head up high*
*And my feet on the ground*
*It feels so good to be proud of me*
*All the things I can do and be*
*This feeling of pride may come and go*
*But I'M ENOUGH, this I know*
*I'm grateful for the feelings I feel*
*Because ALL feelings are important and real*

Shawnee Thornton Hardy

# Chapter 5

# Down Syndrome and Hypermobility

## DOWN SYNDROME

Down syndrome is a genetic condition in which a baby is born with a full or partial extra copy of chromosome 21. This extra chromosome alters a child's course of development and causes the characteristics associated with Down syndrome. Some common characteristics of Down syndrome include the following.

### Physical

- Decreased or low muscle tone (hypotonia)
- Ligament laxity
- Hypermobility
- Decreased proprioception
- Difficulty with postural stability
- Risk of atlantoaxial instability
- Flat feet
- Vision problems (strabismus)
- Hearing problems
- Heart abnormalities
- Thyroid issues
- Digestive issues
- Respiratory problems
- Delayed fine/gross motor development
- Limited body awareness
- Sensory processing challenges
- Issues with motor planning and motor coordination
- Compromised immune system
- Scoliosis

## Cognitive

- Intellectual or cognitive disability (varying degrees)
- Delayed speech and language development
- Slower processing time
- Learning difficulties
- Challenges with working memory
- Shortened attention span
- Increased risk of epilepsy

## Social/Emotional

- Impulsivity
- Challenges with self-regulation
- Challenges with social communication
- Difficulty with perspective taking
- Increased risk of anxiety/depression and OCD
- Co-occurring conditions such as autism and ADHD
- Low self-esteem

Understanding the common challenges of Down syndrome is important in knowing how to develop a therapeutic approach that is both safe and supportive to the child; however, it is equally important to consider the strengths and unique qualities of a child with Down syndrome in order to best support them in shining their beautiful lights for the world to see. Each child with Down syndrome will have their own individual strengths, qualities and interests. Some of these may include:

- sociable
- cheerful
- affectionate
- friendly
- expressive
- willful
- playful
- imaginative
- dynamic
- creative
- loving
- determined
- helpful.

## WHAT IS HYPERMOBILITY?

Hypermobility is both a genetic and acquired condition that affects the body's connective tissue. Hypermobility of the joints occurs when the connective tissue holding a joint together, mainly ligaments and the joint capsule, are too loose. Often, weak muscles around the joint also contribute to hypermobility.

When someone has hypermobile joints, their joints can move beyond the normal range of motion. This puts a tremendous amount of strain on the tendons, which attach muscle to bone, and the ligaments, which connect bones to each other at the joint. This constant and repeated movement beyond the normal range of motion can lead to injury such as joint dislocation and ligament strains and tears. It can also result in arthritis of the joint and chronic joint pain. Research has also shown a link between anxiety, increased interoceptive sensitivity to changes in internal bodily arousal and hypermobility (Mallorquí-Bagué *et al.*, 2014).

One of the characteristics of Down syndrome is hypermobility. Hypermobility is not limited to children with Down syndrome and can be a common characteristic associated with other movement disorders and neurological differences such as autism, ADHD and sensory processing challenges. Any child or teen can be born with or develop hypermobility.

All too often, flexibility is emphasized in the practice of yoga, but when it comes to hypermobility, the emphasis is just the opposite.

### Therapeutic Focus

- Use more strengthening and stabilizing poses to develop strength in the surrounding muscles that support the joints.
- Incorporate poses that provide deep pressure and proprioceptive feedback.
- Integrate poses that soothe the nervous system.
- Integrate weight-bearing poses and poses for core strength.
- Integrate pranayama/breathing practices to support respiration and emotional/physical regulation.
- Provide opportunities for rest throughout the session.
- Provide variations and supports to avoid hyperextension/locking of joints. Encourage sustaining a soft bend in knees and elbows in the weight-bearing positions.

### Precautions

- Avoid overstretching
- Modify weight-bearing poses

## Atlantoaxial Instability

Atlantoaxial instability (AAI) is a condition that affects the bones in the upper spine or neck under the base of the skull. The joint between the first cervical vertebra, Atlas and the second cervical vertebra, Axis, is called the atlantoaxial joint. In people with Down syndrome, the ligaments (connective tissue between the bones) are "lax" or floppy. This can result in AAI where the bones are less stable and can damage the spinal cord (Massachusetts General Hospital, 2019). AAI affects 10–20 percent of individuals with Down syndrome and is mostly asymptomatic (Ali *et al.*, 2006). Most children with Down syndrome are screened by the age of 3 for AAI, so you would be able to gather this information in their intake form under medical conditions. However, due to laxity in their ligaments, it is best to follow the precautions listed below as if they have AAI, regardless of whether it's included in the intake as a medical diagnosis.

### Precautions

- Avoid extreme flexion or extension of the cervical spine
- Avoid extreme rotation of the cervical spine
- Avoid compression of the cervical spine

## Hypotonia/Low Tone

Muscle tone is defined by the amount of tension in our muscles when they're at rest. Those with normal muscle tone will have a slight bit of engagement in the muscles even at rest. Low muscle tone is used to describe muscles that are floppy or weak. It is also referred to as hypotonia. Children with low muscle tone may have increased flexibility, poor posture and get tired easily. The low muscle tone also affects how they interpret sensory input coming in through their muscles and joints (Bruni, 2016). It's important to note that you can't actually change "tone"; however, you can work with children therapeutically to improve strength, stability, coordination and muscular endurance in order to reduce the impact of hypotonia.

### Therapeutic Focus

- Use more muscle-strengthening and stabilizing poses, focusing on areas of the body that are the weakest
- Do active movements to activate the muscles
- Include core strengtheners
- Incorporate poses that provide deep pressure and proprioceptive feedback
- Integrate poses that soothe the nervous system

## Precautions

- Be cautious of fatigue
- Provide supports for stability
- Watch for locking of joints

# THERAPEUTIC CONSIDERATIONS AND SUGGESTIONS FOR CHILDREN AND TEENS WITH DOWN SYNDROME

## Proximal to Distal

Proximal to distal means "from near to far." Physical development starts at the center (proximal) with the head and trunk and moves outward (distal) to the arms and legs, then fingers and toes. Gross motor strength and development is necessary for well-developed fine motor skills. Proximal gross motor strength, control and stability is a prerequisite and lays the foundation for distal motor control, coordination and fine motor skills. Children with Down syndrome can often lack strength in their postural muscles and because of low tone and hypermobility, they tend to lack strength and stability in general. When working therapeutically with children or teens with Down syndrome, it's important to assess and develop their therapeutic protocol proximally to distally. For instance, if a child with Down syndrome struggles with fine motor skills, you would address the gross motor strength and development first.

## Body Awareness, Proprioception and Interoception

Children with Down syndrome tend to struggle with body awareness. There are several reasons for this. One is difficulty with sensory integration and the signals between the brain and body as to where they are in space. Remember that I shared earlier about our proprioceptive systems and what can occur when our proprioceptive systems are out of balance. There is a general sense of not knowing where your body is in space or what your body is doing. This can greatly impact movement, coordination and the experience of embodiment. Children and teens with Down syndrome often have co-occurring sensory processing challenges. Remember, interoceptive awareness is the ability to feel the sensations happening inside our bodies. This can also be due to sensory integration challenges. Children and teens with Down syndrome experience both of these challenges.

## Activities to Support Body Awareness, Proprioception and Interoception

### Tapping Body Parts

Some children with Down syndrome may struggle with identifying body parts. Tapping their body parts provides proprioceptive input and connection to them.

This is a foundational skill in teaching yoga postures to children. We want to help them build the vocabulary and connection to their body and body parts prior to expecting them to be able to follow verbal cues for asana and movement.

### Tactile Cues
Using tactile cues that provide proprioceptive input to the body can support that brain–body connection. As we explore the asanas in this chapter, you will see the tactile cues used to enhance body awareness.

### Weighted Pressure
Weighted or deep pressure provides a great deal of proprioceptive input to the sensory system. It supports grounding the nervous system and experiencing a greater sense of embodiment. Weighted pressure can also help decrease anxiety and enhance sleep (Ekholm, Spulber & Adler, 2020).

## Strength, Stability, Balance, Focus and Self-Esteem (Posture)
Children and teens with Down syndrome are naturally flexible due to the laxity in their ligaments. The focus in therapeutic yoga is cultivating the opposite. Because of their extreme flexibility, we want to focus on strength and stability rather than flexibility. We also want to emphasize balance, focus, attention and building their self-confidence and self-esteem.

Children and teens with Down syndrome often stand with their toes pointing out rather than forward. This can be due to weakness in their adductors as well as hypotonia, which causes laxity and weakness in their legs. They often present with poor posture including a posterior pelvic tilt, rounded trunk and head resting back on the shoulders. It is common for individuals with Down syndrome to struggle with balance and to present with floppiness, clumsiness and awkward or uncoordinated movement patterns. Core weakness is also present and is a contributing factor to their problems with posture, movement, coordination, attention and self-esteem.

As we explore asanas with children and teens with Down syndrome, it's helpful to use visual and tactile cues to support body awareness, focus, improved posture and engagement of specific muscles.

## Standing and Balancing Poses
These asanas promote balance, focus, strength, stability and self-confidence.

**Precautions:** Be cautious with hypermobility, balance issues, fatigue and seizure disorders.

## Mountain (block feet and between thighs)

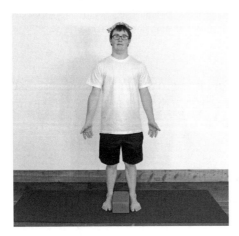 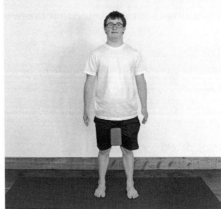

**Instructions:**

1. Tell the child they are going to be a mountain. Mountains are strong and stable.
2. Have the child stand with feet hip-width apart or wider depending on their need for a wider base of support.
3. Option: Place a block between their feet in order to teach standing with the toes pointed forward as well as bringing mind–body connection to their feet.
4. Option: Once they have their feet pointing forward, have them bring the block between their thighs.
5. Have them stand with palms facing forward.
6. Encourage them to squeeze the block between their thighs, engaging their leg muscles and standing strong and tall like a mountain.
7. Option: Place a bean bag on their head and tell them to press their head into the bean bag to encourage upright posture.
8. Encourage breathing in through the nose and out through the nose or mouth.
9. Mantra: "I am strong and stable like a mountain."
10. Check in and have them notice how their body feels after doing Mountain Pose.
11. Option: Do a chair variation if the child struggles with standing.

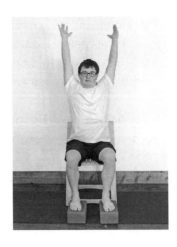

## Tree (toe on floor, block under foot, wooden dowel hands, chair/wall/floor)

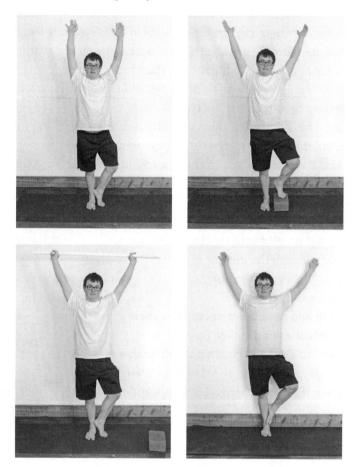

**Instructions:**

1. Tell the child they are going to be a tree. Trees stay rooted in the ground even when the wind blows. They are strong and resilient.
2. Have them stand with feet hip-width apart, toes pointing forward.
3. Have them look down at their feet and check that their toes are pointing forward.
4. Encourage them to bring awareness to their feet. Tell them their feet are like tree roots.
5. Tell them to tap their right leg, then bring their right heel to the inside of their left ankle. Toes on the floor like a kickstand.
6. Option: Place a block between their feet (wider) to facilitate toes

pointing forward and to help with balance. Instead of the ankle coming to the heel, they would bring their toes to the block with the knee pointed outward, pressing their toes to the block.

7. Encourage them to engage the muscles in their standing leg, thinking of their standing leg like the trunk of a tree, strong and sturdy.

8. Invite them to bring their palms to their heart center.

9. Option: They can grow their branches and reach their arms up, expressing their own unique tree.

10. Option: Use a dowel for them to hold on to when reaching their arms up in order to facilitate muscle engagement.

11. Option: Place a bean bag on their head and tell them press their head into the bean bag to encourage upright posture and lengthening the spine.

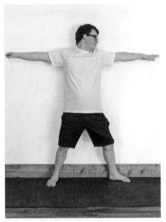

12. Have them gaze forward.

13. Encourage breathing in through the nose and out through the nose or mouth.

14. Mantra: "I am grounded like a tree."

15. Repeat on the other side.

16. Check in and have them notice how their body feels after doing Tree Pose.

17. Option: Do Tree Pose against a wall, with a chair in front to facilitate balance, or seated in a chair if the child struggles with standing or balancing.

### Warrior I (back heel lifted on wall)
**Instructions:**

1. Tell the child they are going to do Warrior I Pose. Warriors are strong and brave, and they help other people.

2. It can be helpful to practice this pose using the wall for stability.

3. Have the child step their right leg back and place the heel on the wall.

4. Tell them to bend their front knee, making sure their knee is above or just behind their ankle.

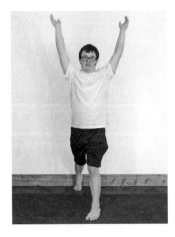

5. Encourage them to press their heel against the wall as they push their front foot firmly to the floor.
6. Option: Have a chair in front of them to hold on to to support balance or they can reach their arms up, coming into their strong Warrior I Pose.
7. They gaze in front of them.
8. Encourage breathing in through the nose and out through the nose or mouth.
9. Mantra: "I am brave, like a warrior."
10. Repeat on the other side.
11. Check in and have them notice how their body feels after doing Warrior I Pose.
12. Option: Do a chair variation if the child struggles with standing or balancing.

### Warrior II (back foot at wall, back body at wall)

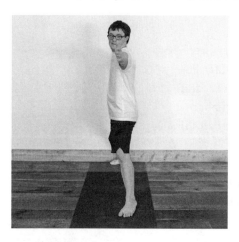 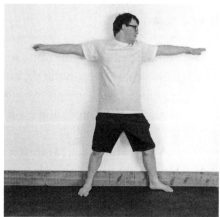

**Instructions:**

1. Tell the child they are going to do Warrior II Pose. Warriors are brave and courageous.
2. It can be helpful to practice this pose using the wall for stability.
3. Have the child place the edge of their right foot against the wall.
4. Have them step their left foot out wide (not too wide).
5. Have them tap their left leg and point their left toes out to the side.
6. Have them bend their left knee, making sure their knee is just above or slightly behind their ankle.

7. Encourage them to press the edge of their right foot against the wall as they push their left foot firmly to the floor.
8. Invite them to reach their arms out wide like a warrior shield, palms facing down. Their right hand is pressing to the wall for support.
9. Have them gaze towards their left fingers.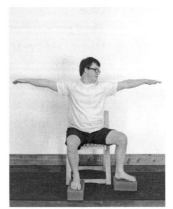
10. Encourage breathing in through the nose and out through the nose or mouth.
11. Mantra: "I am courageous, like a warrior."
12. Repeat on the other side.
13. Check in and have them notice how their body feels after doing Warrior II Pose.
14. Option: Practice this pose with their back body at the wall for more support.
15. Option: Do a chair variation if the child struggles with standing or balancing.

**Star (against wall)**
**Instructions:**

1. Tell the child they are going to do Star Pose. Stars shine bright in the sky and every star is unique. There are no two stars that are alike. Just as we are unique and we can shine bright like a star.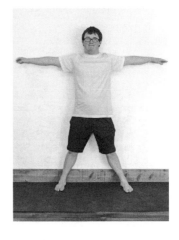
2. Have the child stand against a wall.
3. Have them spread their legs apart and open their arms out wide, their palms facing forward.
4. Encourage them to press their feet into the floor and press their arms against the wall to engage the muscles in the legs, shoulders and arms.
5. Option: Place a bean bag on their head and tell them to press their head into the bean bag to support lengthening the spine and upright posture.
6. Have them gaze forward.
7. Encourage breathing in through the nose and out through the nose or mouth.
8. Mantra: "I am a bright, shining star!"
9. As they say their mantra, they can spread their fingers wide, then

squeeze them shut a few times to mimic twinkling stars and to bring in more body awareness.

10. Check in and have them notice how their body feels after doing Star Pose.
11. Option: Practice this pose away from the wall.
12. Option: Do a chair variation if the child struggles with standing or balancing.

### Eagle (toe on floor, block under foot, eagle hug)

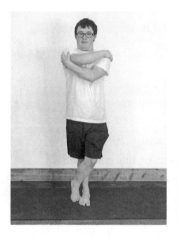 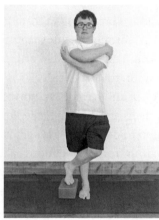

**Instructions:**

1. Tell the child they are going to do Eagle Pose. Eagles are strong and focused.
2. Have them stand with feet closer together, toes pointing forward.
3. Have them look down at their feet and check that their toes are pointing forward.
4. Encourage them to bring awareness to their feet, pressing their feet to the floor.
5. Tell them to tap their right leg and cross their right leg over their left with their right toes on the ground like a kickstand.
6. Option: Place blocks on both sides of their feet and have them place their toes on the block instead of the floor for extra challenge.
7. Encourage them to engage the muscles in their standing leg.
8. Invite them to open their arms wide, like an eagle spreading its wings.
9. Tell them to wiggle their left fingers and cross their left arm over their right arm.

10. Have them bring their hands to opposite shoulders and give themselves an eagle hug.
11. Option: They can bring the back of their palms together or bring their palms together, whatever variation is most accessible to them.
12. Encourage them to squeeze their thighs and their elbows together.
13. Option: Place a bean bag on their head and tell them to press their head into the bean bag to encourage upright posture and lengthening the spine.
14. Have them gaze forward (place a drishti image on the wall within their line of vision).
15. Encourage breathing in through the nose and out through the nose or mouth.
16. Mantra: "I am focused like an eagle."
17. Repeat on the other side.
18. Check in and have them notice how their body feels after doing Eagle Pose.
19. Option to do Eagle Pose against a wall, with a chair in front to facilitate balance, or seated in a chair if the child struggles with standing or balancing.

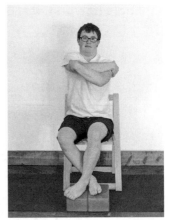

## Core Strengthening

These asanas promote core strength, spinal stability, self-confidence, focus and imagination.

**Precautions:** Be cautious with hypermobility.

### Standing and Balancing Poses

See above.

### Frog
**Instructions:**

1. Tell the child they are going to do Frog Pose. Frogs are curious and energetic.
2. Have them begin standing with their toes pointing out.
3. Tell them to crouch down with their knees wide like a frog.
4. Have them place their hands on the floor between their legs.
5. Encourage them to stay up on their toes rather than planting their feet

flat on the ground. This will facilitate more engagement in the muscles of the ankles and calves.

6. Option: Place a rolled blanket underneath their heels to provide more stability and grounding.

7. Encourage them to sit up tall, lengthening their spine and opening their front body like proud frogs.

8. Tell them to breathe in and lift their hips up slightly, then breathe out, stick out their tongue and say "ha!" as if they're hungry frogs catching a fly.

9. Mantra: "I am energetic like a frog."

10. Repeat 2–3 times.

11. Check in and have them notice how their body feels after doing Frog Pose.

### Butterfly (press feet together)
**Instructions:**

1. Tell the child they are going to do Butterfly Pose. Butterflies are graceful and free.

2. Have them sit on a folded blanket or two to facilitate a neutral pelvis and upright posture.

3. Tell them to bring the bottoms of their feet together, making wings with their legs.

4. Invite them to imagine and share what color they want their butterfly to be.

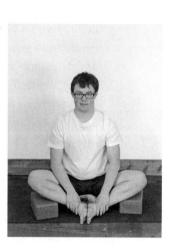

5. Encourage them to sit up tall, like a proud butterfly.

6. Have them place their hands on their shins or ankles.

7. Tell them to press their feet together to facilitate engagement of muscles.

8. As they press their feet together, encourage them to bring their knees up and down like a butterfly flapping their wings.

9. Mantra: "I am free like a butterfly."

10. Option: Place blocks under the knees to avoid overstretching.

11. Check in and have them notice how their body feels after doing Butterfly Pose.

### Bridge (squeeze block between thighs)

**Precautions:** Please avoid this pose if the child has atlantoaxial instability or a heart condition.

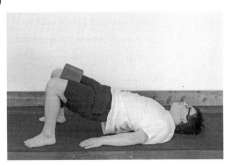

Using a block between the thighs can facilitate engagement of the adductors and keep the hips in a neutral position.

**Instructions:**

1. Tell the child they are going to do Bridge Pose. Bridges are sturdy and strong. Bridges have the shape of an arch. We can make our bodies into the shape of a bridge.
2. Have them lie down on their backs.
3. Ask them to bend their knees and place their feet on the floor.
4. Have them place their feet hips width apart with toes pointed forward.
5. Option: Place a block between the feet initially so the child can access the hips width cue.
6. Ask them to place their palms face down on the mat, next to their hips.
7. Have them place a block between their thighs.
8. Encourage them to squeeze the block so they begin to feel the engagement of their legs.
9. Tell them to breathe in, press their palms to the floor and lift their hips towards the ceiling while squeezing the block. Encourage them to image a bridge going up to let the boats through.
10. Tell them to breathe out, relax their leg muscles and bring their bottom to the floor.
11. Mantra: "I am sturdy like a bridge."
12. Repeat two more times.
13. Check in and have them notice how their body feels after doing Bridge Pose.

### Baby Cobra (block between thighs)

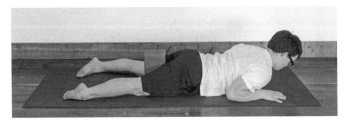

**Precautions:** Avoid hyperextension of the cervical spine.

**Instructions:**

1.  Tell the child they are going to do Cobra Pose. Cobra snakes are fearless.
2.  Have them lie on their bellies.
3.  Encourage them to point their toes back and place the tops of their feet on the mat.
4.  Option: Place a block between their thighs to squeeze in order to engage their adductors.
5.  Have them bring their palms underneath their shoulders, face down on the mat.
6.  Have them hug their elbows in toward their bodies.
7.  Tell them to breathe out, then breathe in, press their hands down and lift their shoulders up, gazing in front of them (this is to avoid hyperextension of the cervical spine).
8.  Option: Place a stuffed animal at the top of the mat for the child to gaze at to avoid hyperextension.
9.  Invite them to breathe out and make the "tsss" sound like a snake.
10. Mantra: "I am fearless like a snake."
11. Repeat two times.
12. Check in and have them notice how their body feels after doing Cobra Pose.

## Lightning Bolt Pose (against the wall with a block)
**Instructions:**

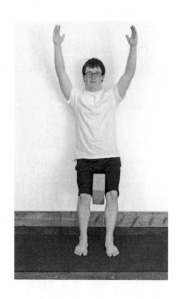

1.  Tell the child they are going to do Lightning Bolt Pose. Lightning bolts are energetic and powerful.
2.  Have the child stand against a wall with their feet hip-width apart and toes pointing forward.
3.  Option: Use a block as a tactile cue for standing hip-width with toes pointing forward.
4.  Have them press their back against the wall, then begin to walk their feet out until they come into a position as if they are seated in a chair.

5. Check that their knees are above the ankles or slightly behind them.
6. Have the child bring their attention to their belly and explain that their bellies are the energy center of their body.
7. Encourage them to squeeze their belly button in toward their spine so they can activate their lightning bolt energy.
8. Invite them to breathe in, then breathe out and shoot their arms up like a lightning bolt, making a "cheoooo" sound. This breath will facilitate engagement of the core muscles.
9. Have them hold that position for a count that is appropriate for their energy and stamina.
10. Mantra: "I am powerful like a lightning bolt."
11. Check in and have them notice how their body feels after doing Lightning Bolt Pose.

### Roller Coaster Twist (Seated Variations)

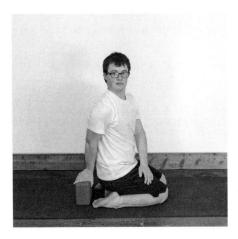 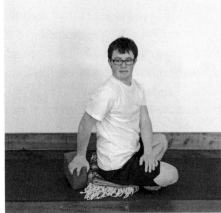

**Precautions:** Avoid extreme cervical rotation. Have the child do a supine twist if they are not able to have length in their spine for rotation.

**Instructions:**

1. Tell the child they are going to do Roller Coaster Twist. Our spines can twist like roller coasters!
2. Have the child sit in a criss-cross position or in Virasana (Hero's Pose). Option: If they are seated in a criss-cross position, have them sit on a blanket in order to help lengthen their spine.
3. Have them place a block behind them.

4.  Encourage them to sit up tall, then reach both their arms up as though they're riding a roller coaster.
5.  Breathing in.
6.  Have them wiggle their left fingers, then bring their left hand to the opposite thigh.
7.  Breathing out.
8.  Have them place their right hand on the block behind them.
9.  Invite them to look towards their right shoulder and say "hello" to their friends behind them on the roller coaster.
10. Repeat on the other side.
11. After doing the pose on both sides, consider the option to explore the "ch ch ch" sound as they move slowly into their twist (like the sound of a roller coaster when it's moving slowly on the track) in order to engage the core muscles during rotation.
12. Repeat 1–2 times slowly.
13. Check in and have them notice how their body feels after doing Roller Coaster Twist.

## Happy Baby
**Instructions:**

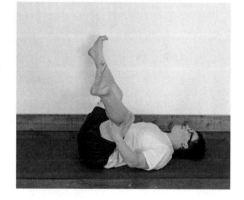

1.  Tell the child they are going to do Happy Baby. Babies like to lie on their backs and rock back and forth. We can be like happy babies.
2.  Have them lie on their back and bring their hands to their knees, shins, ankles or toes.
3.  Make sure the back of their head is on the mat.
4.  Invite them to rock back and forth gently like a happy baby.
5.  Ask what sounds a happy baby might make and explore those sounds with the child.
6.  Check in and have them notice how their body feels after doing Happy Baby.

## W-Sitting options
W-sitting is a sitting position in which children sit with knees bent and wide apart or close to touching and their feet out wide, with their bottoms on the

floor. If you were looking at the child from above, their legs would look like a W-shape. W-sitting is a typical sitting position in early child development. The reason for this is that W-sitting offers a wider base of support and does not require as much core strength. As children begin to develop their postural muscles, core strength and balance, they no longer need to W-sit; however, due to limited core strength, many children with Down syndrome may prefer to W-sit. Prolonged W-sitting can cause an increased posterior pelvic tilt, which can impact posture and breathing. This way of sitting also inhibits use of the core muscles that facilitate breathing, movement and coordination. W-sitting also does not require much weight shifting, which is essential for developing balance, integrating both sides of the body and development of fine motor skills. In order to support children with Down syndrome in accessing their core and postural muscles, we can offer variations of sitting positions.

*Hero Pose with Knees Together (option to sit on a block)*

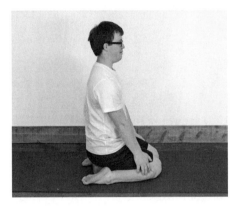

*Cross-Legged (option to sit on a blanket)*

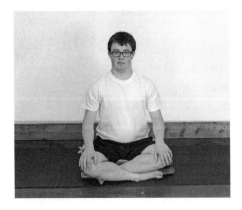

*Long Sit (option to sit on a blanket or have a rolled blanket under knees)*

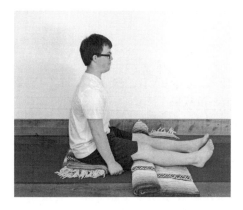

## Sitting in a Chair

Another way to encourage core awareness and activation, enhance attention, build self-confidence and provide opportunity for self-expression is through breathing practices, sound and chanting.

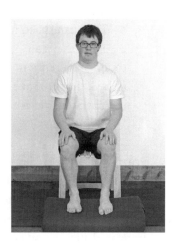

## Boxer Breath

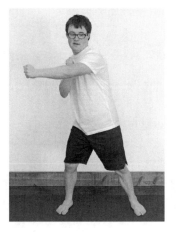 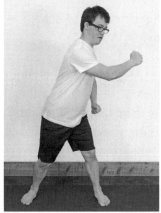

Boxer Breath is a great breath to energize the body and engage the core. The "huh" sound facilitates the belly button drawing in towards the spine for core activation.

**Instructions:**

1. Tell the child they are going to be a boxer and do Boxer Breath. Boxers have strong core muscles!
2. Invite them to put on their boxing gloves.
3. Encourage them to stand with legs wide apart and knees bent.
4. Invite them to imagine punching a boxing bag.
5. Have them punch with their right and say, "huh!"
6. Have them punch with their left and say, "huh!"
7. Ask them: "Can you feel your belly button coming in towards your spine when you make that sound?"
8. They can speed up their punching and breath.
9. Then they can slow down their punching and breath.
10. Encourage them to feel their feet on the earth.
11. Ask them to take their hands to their belly.
12. Check in and have them notice how their body feels after doing Boxer Breath.

## Sound Chanting

Sound chanting helps with accessing more diaphragmatic breathing. Speech initiates from the diaphragm; therefore, engaging the core muscles and connecting with the diaphragm can facilitate more awareness of the core and can support improved speech and communication.

We'll explore the sounds "shhh" and "ft."

### *Whisper Chant*
**Instructions:**

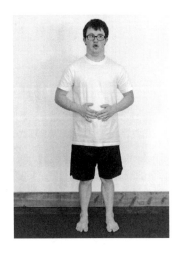

1. Have the child take their hands to the belly, just below the bottom of the rib cage.
2. Invite them to make the "shhh" sound until they empty their bellies of air.
3. Encourage them to notice how the belly button moves in towards the spine when they do the "shhh" sound.
4. Encourage them to take a natural breath.
5. Repeat 2–3 times.

6. Check in and have them notice how their body feels after doing Whisper Chant.

*Gila Monster Chant (pronounced hila)*

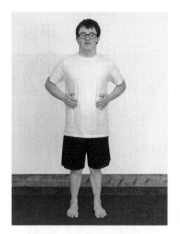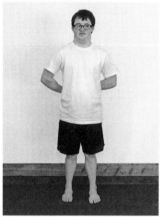

**Instructions:**

1. Have the child take their hands to the sides of the rib cage.
2. Invite them to combine the sounds "f" and "t" so it makes the "ft" sound, like a Gila Monster sticking out its tongue and hissing. Repeating the "ft" sound several times.
3. As they make the "ft" sound, have them notice how the rib cage hugs in tighter around the midline.
4. Have them extend the "f" sound—"ffff-t"—and notice the rib cage.
5. Have the child take their hands to their backs, right behind the belly button.
6. Invite them to make the "ft" sound and notice if they can feel the back muscles working when they do the Gila Monster Chant.
7. Have them extend the "f" sound—"ffff-t"—and notice the back body.
8. Check in and have them notice how their body feels after doing Gila Monster Chant.

## Crossing Midline
*Eagle*
See Chapter 4.

### Roller Coaster Twist
See earlier in the chapter.

### Apple Picking
See Chapter 7.

### Giraffe Toes
**Instructions:**

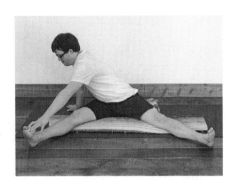

1. Have the child sit with their legs wide apart.
2. Encourage them to sit up tall, like a giraffe lengthening its neck.
3. Invite them to reach their arms up to the ceiling.
4. Have them wiggle their right fingers and bring their right hand across towards the opposite foot, reaching for their giraffe toes.
5. Repeat on the opposite side.
6. Option: Place a rolled blanket under the knees to avoid hyperextension of the knees.
7. Check in and have them notice how their body feels after doing Giraffe Toes.

## Weight-Bearing
Weight-bearing poses can be modified for children with Down syndrome in order to engage the correct muscles and avoid hyperextension and locking of the joints.

### Cat/Cow (chair)
Practicing Cat/Cow Pose in a chair offers the benefits of flexion and extension in the spine without putting unnecessary pressure on the elbow joints.

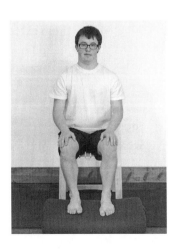

**Instructions:**

1. Tell the child they are going to move their spines like cats and cows.
2. Start with them seated upright in a chair with length in their spine.

3. Option: Place a bolster or blocks underneath their feet if their feet aren't touching the ground.
4. Have the child place their hands on their knees, then bring their belly and chest forward like a cow with a full belly.
5. Encourage them to look up with their eyes rather than lifting their chin in order to avoid hyperextension of the cervical spine.
6. Option: Have them moo like a cow.
7. Invite them to press their hands down on their thighs and look towards their belly button, arching their back like a cat.
8. Option: Have them hiss like a scared cat.
9. Repeat two more times.
10. Check in and have them notice how their body feels after doing Cat/Cow.

### Plank (elbows bent with block and on knees, wall plank)

There are several variations of Plank Pose that are accessible, encourage activation of the correct muscles and decrease risks of injury due to hypermobility. Below are three variations.

VARIATION 1

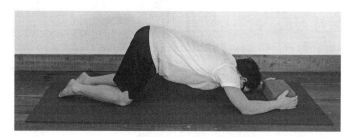

**What to emphasize:** Pressing the hands into the block and pushing the forearms to the floor to engage the muscles of the arms, shoulders and upper back.

VARIATION 2

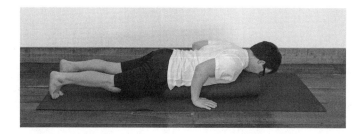

**What to emphasize:** Engaging the muscles in the legs, pressing the hands into the mat and keeping the elbows close to the body to engage the muscles of the arms, shoulders and upper back.

VARIATION 3

**What to emphasize:** Engaging the muscles in the legs, pressing the hands into the block and pressing forearms to the wall to engage the muscles of the arms, shoulders and upper back.

Mantra: "I am steady like a plank."

*Boat (hands behind, block between thighs, block under feet)*

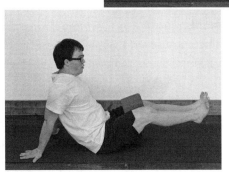

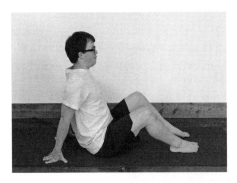

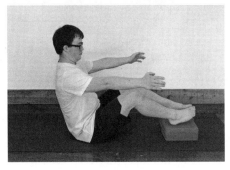

**Instructions:**

1. Tell the child they are going to do Boat Pose. Boats are strong and sturdy.
2. Have the child sit on the mat with their knees bent and feet on the floor.

3. Have them place their hands behind them to provide stability.
4. Invite them to stay right there, drawing their belly button towards their spine.
5. Encourage them to keep their spine long, with their chest upright.
6. Option: Lean back slightly and reach arms forward.
7. Option: Place a block underneath the feet and explore reaching the hands forward at the same time or keeping the hands down on the mat behind them.
8. Encourage breathing in and out while holding the pose for the count of "1, 2, 3."
9. Mantra: "I am sturdy like a boat."
10. Check in and have them notice how their body feels after doing Boat Pose.

### Upper-Body Strengtheners (chair)

These exercises can support engaging the muscles and building strength in the upper back, shoulders and arms.

#### *Pressing block between palms elbows bent*
**Instructions:**

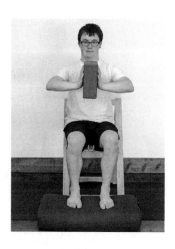

1. Have the child sit in a chair or on the floor, whatever is most optimal for them.
2. Give them a foam yoga block.
3. Encourage them to sit up tall.
4. Invite them to press their palms together on either side of the block (make sure the block is held with the long and wide side so the hands fit on the block), with their elbows out to the side.
5. Remind them to breathe.
6. Option: Count for the press, "1, 2, 3."
7. Then have them release and pause for a moment.
8. Repeat 3–4 times, depending on their stamina and energy level.

### Seated Mountain (block between hands)
**Instructions:**

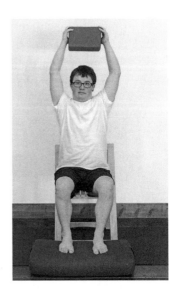

1. Have the child sit in a chair or on the floor, whatever is most optimal for them.
2. Give them a foam yoga block.
3. Encourage them to sit up tall.
4. Have them hold the yoga block so it's wide between their hands.
5. Have them inhale and draw the yoga block up overhead.
6. Encourage them to press their palms into the sides of the block as they reach the block upward.
7. Have them pause and exhale as they hold the yoga block up.
8. Option: Count, "1, 2, 3."
9. Have them release and pause for a moment.
10. Repeat 3–4 times depending on their stamina and energy level.

### Wooden Dowel Mountain
**Instructions:**

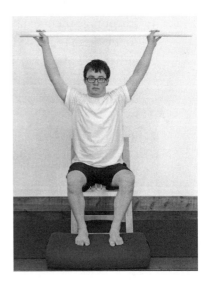

1. Have the child sit in a chair or on the floor, whatever is most optimal for them.
2. Give them a wooden dowel that is wide enough for them to have their hands more than shoulder-width apart.
3. Encourage them to sit up tall.
4. Have them hold the wooden dowel with palms facing down and a bit wider than shoulder-width (you can explore the width that is best for them).
5. Have them inhale and draw the wooden dowel up overhead, palms facing forward.
6. Encourage them to reach the dowel up towards the ceiling.

7. Have them pause and exhale as they hold the dowel up.
8. Option: Count, "1, 2, 3."
9. Have them release and pause for a moment.
10. Repeat 3–4 times depending on their stamina and energy level.
11. Option: Do this pose in Standing Mountain rather than seated.

### Weightlifter (bolster lift)

**Instructions:**

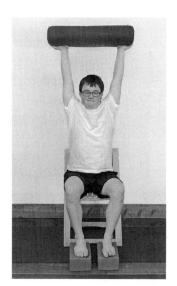

1. Have the child sit in a chair or on the floor, whatever is most optimal for them.
2. Give them a rectangular bolster.
3. Encourage them to sit up tall.
4. Have them imagine being a weightlifter who has to lift the bolster up like a weight.
5. Invite them to hold the bolster with palms face up, wrists in extension.
6. Have them inhale and press the bolster up towards the ceiling.
7. Have them pause and exhale as they hold the bolster up.
8. Option: Count—"1, 2, 3."
9. Have them release and pause for a moment.
10. Repeat 3–4 times, depending on their stamina and energy level.

## Yogic Eye Exercises

Children with Down syndrome are at increased risk for a variety of eye and vision disorders. Although early intervention including surgery and specialized optical supports are often necessary, eye exercises such as eye tracking and drishti (single point focus), can support strengthening the muscles around the eyes and increasing visual stability and focus.

*Eye Tracking*
**Instructions:**

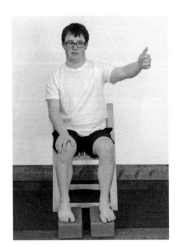

1.  Have the child sit in a chair or on the floor, whatever is most optimal for them.
2.  Invite them to hold their right thumb straight in front of them at eye level.
3.  Encourage them to move their thumb slowly to the right while following their thumb with their eyes, without moving their head.
4.  Encourage them to then slowly move their thumb back to the center while following their thumb with their eyes, without moving their head.
5.  Check in and have them notice how that felt for them.
6.  If it was a positive experience for them, repeat on the other side.

*Drishti Options*

-   A colored circle or favorite image posted on the wall at eye level
-   An object right in front of the child that is at eye level
-   Gazing at a soft light, glow stick or candle at eye level
-   Gazing at the thumb in a fixed point at eye level

## Mudras

Mudra practices for children with Down syndrome can support body awareness, focus, self-regulation and fine motor development. Each mudra has its own energetic effect on the nervous system, and some mudras are more accessible to children whose fine motor skills are impacted. We'll explore a few mudras that are accessible and supportive for children and teens with Down syndrome. As you explore mudras, you can also connect them to the chakras and specific areas of focus. Bear in mind, children with fine motor challenges may not present the gestures in a "perfect" manner. It is more about the intention and their own unique experience with each mudra. The recommended time to hold a gesture is 1–2 minutes, depending on the child's energy and attention.

### Gyan Mudra (Knowledge Mudra)

**Chakra:** Root

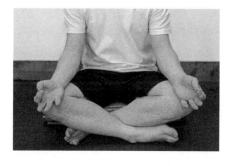

**Effects:** Reduces depression, anger, tension and agitation, improves concentration and sleep.

**Instructions:**

1. Begin seated in an upright position.
2. Bring the tips of your pointer fingers to the tips of your thumbs.
3. Keep the other fingers straight (as much as possible).
4. Rest your hands on your thighs with palms up.
5. Relax your shoulders.
6. Option: Close your eyes or keep them softly open.
7. Breathe naturally.
8. Mantra: "I am grounded and present."

### Dhyana Mudra (Concentration Mudra)

**Chakra:** Sacral

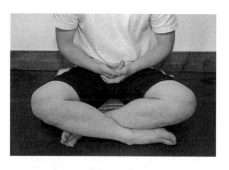

**Effects:** Releases tension, calms the mind, enhances creativity.

**Instructions:**

1. Begin seated in an upright position.
2. Rest your right hand in your lap, palm face up, with your elbow out to the side.
3. Place your left hand in your right palm, left palm facing up.
4. Touch the tips of the thumbs together lightly.
5. Relax your shoulders.
6. Option: Close your eyes or keep them softly open.
7. Breathe naturally.
8. Mantra: "I am supported."

### *Padma or Lotus Mudra (Heart Opening Mudra)*
**Chakra:** Heart

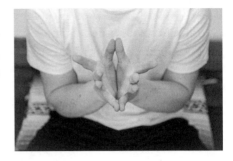

**Effects:** Inspires perseverance and compassion, brings awareness of inner beauty, supports cardio-respiratory and immune system health.

**Instructions:**

1. Begin seated in an upright position.
2. Bring your palms together at your heart center.
3. Keep the base of your palms, pinkies and thumbs pressing together.
4. Open your other fingers, making a blossoming flower.
5. Relax your shoulders.
6. Option: Close your eyes or keep them softly open.
7. Breathe naturally.
8. Mantra: "My heart is open and loving."

### *Ganesha Mudra (Energy Mudra)*
**Chakra:** Solar Plexus

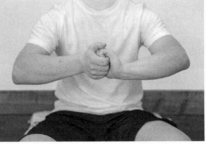

**Effects:** Lifts spirits, boosts confidence, relieves stress and tension, aids digestion, stimulates heart activity.

**Instructions:**

1. Begin seated in an upright position.
2. Hold your right hand in front of your chest with your thumb pointing down, palm facing out.
3. Bring your left palm in front of the right with the thumb facing up.
4. Clasp your fingers together and gently tug the fingers.
5. Bring your hands in front of the chest.
6. Option: Close eyes or keep them softly open.
7. Breathe naturally.
8. Switch the placement of your hands, clasping your fingers and gently tugging.
9. Breathe naturally.
10. Mantra: "I am confident and courageous."

### Angushtha Mudra (Communication Mudra)

**Chakra:** Throat

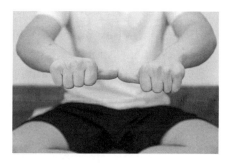

**Effects:** Enhances speaking, singing and communication, connects to intuition or inner knowing, supports thyroid health.

**Instructions:**

1. Begin seated in an upright position.
2. Curl all your fingers into your palm except your thumbs.
3. Bring your hands just above your belly button.
4. Bring the tips of your thumbs together.
5. Relax your shoulders.
6. Option: Close your eyes or keep them softly open.
7. Breathe naturally.
8. Mantra: "My voice is important."

### Trishula Mudra (Inner Wisdom Mudra)

**Chakra:** Third Eye

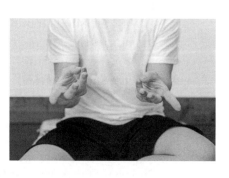

**Effects:** Enhances metal clarity and concentration, inner wisdom, supports health of nervous and endocrine systems.

**Instructions:**

1. Begin seated in an upright position.
2. Bring your pinky finger and thumb together to touch.
3. Straighten the other three fingers as much as you're able.
4. Rest your hands on the knees or keep them elevated with palms face up.
5. Relax your shoulders.
6. Option: Close your eyes or keep them softly open.
7. Breathe naturally.
8. Mantra: "I connect to my inner wisdom."

### *Hansi Mudra (Inner Smile Mudra)*

**Chakra:** Crown

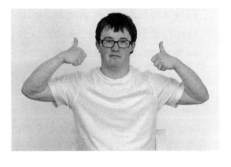

**Effects:** Invites positive feelings and contentment, supports improved mood, promotes increased circulation, enhances immunity.

**Instructions:**

1. Begin seated in an upright position.
2. Rest your hands on your thighs, palms facing up.
3. Bring the tip of your index finger, ring finger and middle finger to touch (on both hands).
4. Keep your pinky finger straight (as much as possible).
5. Relax your shoulders.
6. Option: Close your eyes or keep them softly open.
7. Breathe naturally.
8. Mantra: "I feel my inner joy."

### *Merudanda Mudra (Thumbs Up Mudra)*

**Effects:** Calms the mind, improves mental focus, supports respiration and circulation, supports improved posture, enhances self-confidence and self-esteem.

**Instructions:**

1. Begin seated in an upright position.
2. Curl your fingers in towards your palm.
3. Point your thumbs up.
4. Place your hands on your thighs or raise them up as a gesture of energy and positivity!
5. Mantra: "I got this!"

**Resources for future exploration of mudras:** *Mudra: The Sacred Secret (Arora, 2015), Mudras for Healing and Transformation* (Page et al, 2013).

## Social Communication and Connection

Building trust and connection with the child or teen will encourage openness and curiosity. This is the foundation of our work with children. Because many children with Down syndrome can struggle in areas of social communication, these practices can be building blocks in supporting them with social skills, communication and connection with others.

### Mirroring

This mirroring practice helps build connection and attunement with children and teens and also supports attention and imitation skills, areas in which children with Down syndrome can struggle.

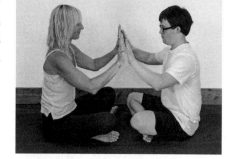

**Instructions:**

1. Sit face to face with the child or teen.
2. Hold your hands up, palms facing the child and say, "I'm going to move my hands and you can move your hands with my hands."
3. Have the child hold their hands up, palms facing your palms, close but not touching.
4. Move your hands slowly and encourage the child to move their hands with yours.
5. Hold the deep intention of connection and resonance as you do this practice together.
6. Switch and allow the child to move their hands and you mirror them (this supports autonomy, collaboration, building trust and connection).

## Partner Poses

Partner poses are a great way to build connection, enhance communication and teach collaboration and cooperation. As the adult practices partner poses with the child, they can also use their own bodies to assist and support the child with balance, body awareness and proprioceptive input. There is a beautiful felt sense of support and connection that can happen when practicing partner poses. This can also be a wonderful practice for the child to do with their caretakers, siblings, peers or other loved ones to build connection and enjoy yoga together.

**Note:** As with any practice where there is touch involved, it is important to get consent from the child first prior to doing partner poses.

*Tree Partner*

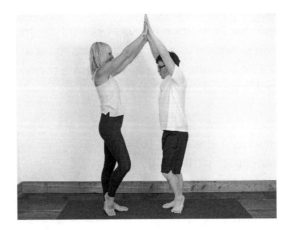

*Mountain Partner*

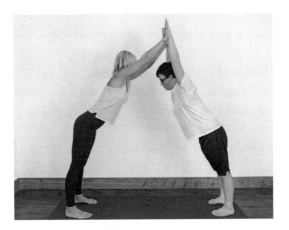

*Warrior II Partner*

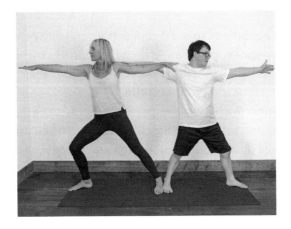

*Chair Partner*

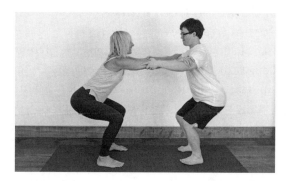

*Boat Partner*

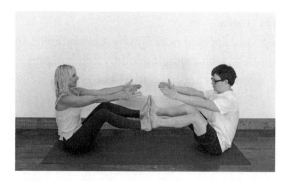

See sections on Chanting and Emotions breaths.

## Contraindications When Working with Children with Down Syndrome

- Avoid inversions if there is a heart condition or infantile glaucoma.
- Avoid extreme flexion, extension or compression of the cervical spine if the child has atlantoaxial instability or spinal issues or injuries. Avoid any extreme movement in general.
- **Epilepsy:** If a child has epilepsy, it is important to know the frequency, duration and seizure protocol as well as any specific triggers, precautions and contraindications. Medical approval to participate in yoga therapy and somatic movement sessions is recommended.
- See supports suggested in Chapter 3.

## CASE STUDY FOR THERAPEUTIC CONSIDERATION: SAM
## Information Gathered from Intake
## Form and Parent Interview

Sam is an 11-year-old boy with Down syndrome. He presents with moderate cognitive challenges and speech delays. He sees a speech therapist regularly. He processes information and communicates best when given visual and written supports and recognizes and uses some simple ASL signs. He struggles with attention and focus in the classroom and also has a diagnosis of ADHD. He experiences significant anxiety at times, mostly when unexpected situations occur or when he becomes frustrated with a challenging task. Parent stated that Sam likes to "be in charge." He can struggle with identifying and processing his emotions.

### SENSORY CHALLENGES

He is sensitive to unexpected noises in his environment and seeks out proprioceptive input through stomping loudly and banging into walls. He has a limited sense of body awareness and will often get into his peers' personal space, which causes some challenges with social relationships; however, he has many friends who he enjoys spending time with in school. Parent reports that Sam is not sensitive to touch and loves hugs and "rough play" with his older siblings.

### MEDICAL INFORMATION

Sam has hypothyroidism (low thyroid) and takes thyroid medication. He experiences frequent constipation. Parent states that he has a limited diet (mostly carbs) and is not great about drinking water throughout the day. Mom noted that he is not very active, which impacts his mood and energy levels. She stated that he can be quite stagnant and low-energy.

### STRENGTHS AND INTERESTS

Sam is loving and has a big heart. He loves to draw and do arts and crafts. He picks things up quickly, especially when it is something of interest to him. He loves dogs—all dogs—and likes to watch animal videos and read books about animals. He wants to be a veterinarian one day. He loves spending time in his room and enjoys being with his family. He loves listening to music, singing and dancing.

### Goals for Yoga Therapy Discussed by Sam and His Family — Shared by Sam

1. I want to learn how to tell people my feelings.
2. I want to feel less anxious.
3. I want to move my body and feel energy.
4. I want to learn animal poses.

### Initial Assessment

#### BEHAVIORAL OBSERVATIONS

Sam was able to follow 2–3-step directions with the use of visuals and direct and concrete instruction as well as modeling from the adult. He was easily distractible but was able to attend to a 45-minute session with redirection to the activity at hand. He seemed to enjoy the practice and smiled often throughout the session.

#### LEARNING PREFERENCES

Sam responded well to visual yoga cards and a "session schedule" with the poses and breathing strategies laid out visually for him to see what to expect. He helped turn the cards over after each one was finished and would sign "all done" using ASL. I did some signs along with the animal poses, which he seemed to be excited about, and signed the animal signs with me. He also responded well to taking turns in choosing the yoga poses and breathing practices to explore. When a card came up that he had chosen, he would say "mine" to remind me that the pose or breathing practice was "his choice."

#### PHYSICAL

**Posture and alignment:** Sam sits with a forward head, rounded shoulders and rounded back posture. He is able to sit in a criss-cross position, but it is apparent that his core is weak. He benefited from sitting up on a stack of folded blankets.

**Range of motion:** Sam presents with hypermobility as evident in hyperextension of his elbows and knees. He presents with low tone in his trunk, upper extremities and lower extremities.

**Balance and coordination:** Sam was able to sustain a single-leg stance for approximately 4 seconds on each side. He appears to struggle with body awareness and benefited from left/right visuals and tapping body parts.

**Bilateral movement and midline crossing:** Sam struggled with midline crossing but was able to do bilateral movements with relative ease. He does not know his left/right.

**Gait:** Sam walks with a wide base with limited trunk rotation. Gait presents as slouchy and uncoordinated.

**Breathing pattern:** Sam exhibited mouth breathing throughout the session as well as more collapsed breathing.

## Therapeutic Focus

1.  Stability and strength (core, postural muscles, prevent locking joints at elbows, knees).
2.  Balance.
3.  Therapeutic poses for thyroid.
4.  Increase energy, stamina and endurance.
5.  Diaphragmatic breathing.
6.  Improve focus and attention.
7.  Increase body awareness.
8.  Decrease anxiety.
9.  Support identification and expression of emotions.

Chapter 6

# Help for Teens with Scoliosis: The Yoga Therapy Approach

RACHEL KRENTZMAN PT AND
LIOR ZACKARIA HIKREY

Affecting 4 out of 100 teenagers, adolescent idiopathic scoliosis (AIS) is the most common form of scoliosis (Scoliosis Research Society, n.d.). "Idiopathic" means we don't know exactly why the curves happened, and often this diagnosis takes parents and adolescents by surprise—they may find themselves at a loss as to how to manage the condition. Regardless of whether there is pain, many are concerned about aesthetics, the need for bracing and the possibility of corrective surgery in the future.

Yoga therapy provides complementary solutions aimed at allowing the body to transform naturally. Because we look at the physical body as an integrated and organic structure, yoga therapists can offer tools that encourage a process of "letting go," along with functional realignment that is non-invasive and enjoyable.

A modern medical mindset can encourage us to look outside ourselves for solutions, forgetting that our own body and mind can be the most powerful healer. When teens learn ways to connect to their own bodies with both awareness and kindness, they can develop a program for self-care as an adjunct or even an alternative to bracing or surgery.

In a study examining the effects of yoga on scoliosis, doing one particular yoga pose called *Vasisthasana* (Side Plank) with appropriate cueing produced a 32 percent improvement in the Cobb Angle (degree of sideways curve) in a sample of 25 patients (Fishman, Groessl & Sherman, 2014). The Schroth approach, which focuses on patient education and breathing, has also been shown to be effective for teenagers with AIS (Burger *et al.*, 2019). Yoga therapy differs in that it addresses the individual on the physical, emotional and spiritual level, offering tools such as the asana (poses) mentioned here, as well as pranayama (breathwork), meditative and mindfulness practices and lifestyle changes. With yoga therapy, the focus is on the child, not on the curve, and therefore practices can be tailored to each individual's specific needs.

This chapter will outline 12 postures that can help teens with scoliosis, but working one on one with a yoga therapist can help tremendously in order to work on the broader issues of self-esteem, mood, embodiment and regulation of the nervous system as well as other postural issues. Yoga therapy is not a one-size-fits-all approach and therefore there are no strict protocols. A fluid and adaptive model is recommended for most teens, and therefore we recommend seeking an experienced yoga teacher or therapist who can offer more personal guidance and support.

## HOW DOES IT WORK?

Clients who have worn a brace in their teenage years often come with hypersensitivity to touch and decreased body awareness because of the constant pressure the brace placed on their curves. A brace may prevent progression of the scoliosis, but it can also create a great deal of muscular tension and rigidity. In addition, many of these young clients never received any guidance on physical exercises to help their condition, so they may have little connection to their body's needs and limited awareness of how their spine functions.

When offering yoga therapy for adolescents with AIS, we:

- normalize scoliosis and let them know that many others have the same condition
- maintain a light-hearted attitude and reassure them that they can participate in sports and activities with few restrictions
- teach them how to adapt yoga poses to help realign their specific curve(s)
- guide them to move breath into restricted areas in the chest and rib cage
- stick to a few key poses so they will succeed in practicing regularly (too many exercises can be overwhelming for anyone!)
- provide simple, clear instructions.

Adolescents need to develop a kind and loving relationship with their body—and with their scoliosis. We opt for an integrated approach that lengthens the shorter (concave) side of the curve while strengthening the weaker (convex) side; works toward alignment, symmetry and length on both sides of the waist; supports balanced posture and a strong core; increases breath awareness; and, most importantly, includes a practice of acceptance.

Yoga therapy can be a way for teens to develop a new relationship with their body and themselves, one that empowers them for the rest of their lives.

Yoga therapists will first need to teach teens how to adapt the yoga postures for their specific type of curve. It is then recommended to observe the students closely as they practice the following sequence and make appropriate adjustments and modifications as needed to normalize their curve. The therapist may choose to teach a few key postures for the student to practice at home or may offer the entire sequence to those with demonstrated body awareness. Helping students with verbal and manual cues will ensure more accuracy and proper alignment which, in turn, will lead to improved outcome measures.

The following text illustrates how to instruct your students with scoliosis:

## UNDERSTANDING YOUR UNIQUE CURVE

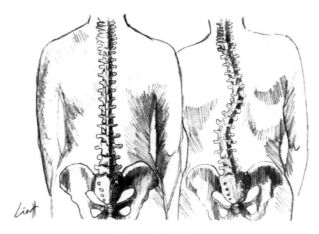

**Figure 6.1** Scoliosis

A scoliotic curve can be found in the upper or lower back and consists of a primary curve and often a secondary or compensatory curve as well (see Figure 6.1). The body, in its infinite wisdom and desire to achieve balance at all costs, finds a way to make sure that the head remains centered. In order to do this, the spine, like a delicate strand of pearls, adapts by curving in the opposite direction of the primary curve. This is a beautiful illustration of how the body is seeking balance at all times.

Another important consideration that is often overlooked is the rotational component of the spine with scoliosis. While most individuals understand the sideways bend of the curve, fewer realize that when a curve bends to one side, the vertebrae are actually rotated in the opposite direction. That is to say, if the curve is bent to the left, the vertebrae will be rotated to the right (see Figure 6.2a). Conversely, if the curve is bent to the right, the vertebrae will be rotated to the left (see Figure 6.2b).

The rotational component of the vertebrae is what gives rise to what we call a "rib hump" which is often visible on individuals when they move into a forward bend (see Figure 6.3).

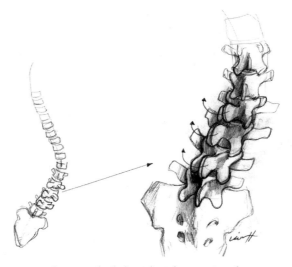

**Figure 6.2a** Curve bent to the left with right rotational component

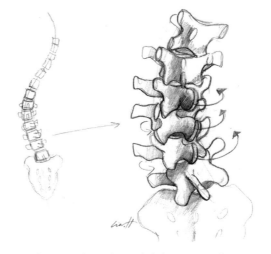

**Figure 6.2b** Curve bent to the right with left rotational component

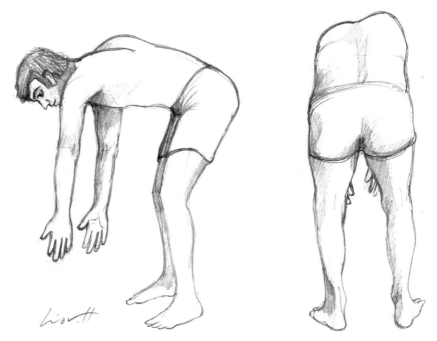

**Figure 6.3** Forward bend illustrating rib hump

In medical terminology, the curve is named for the convex side, or the side where there is a hump. For example, if your curve is side bent to the left, the convex side will be on the right and so will the hump. Therefore, this is called a right scoliosis. Similarly, if your curve is side bent to the right, the convex side will be on the left and so will the hump due to the vertebral rotation to the left side. This is called a left scoliosis. The curve may be in the thoracic spine, lumbar spine or both.

There are three main types of scoliosis (see Figure 6.4). Knowing which one of the three you have will help you move forward. It is good to visualize the different curvatures so you understand what each curve looks like. Your physician or physical therapist can help you determine which type of scoliosis you have.

- Thoracic curve: A C-curve that affects the upper back
- Lumbar: A C-curve that affects the lower back
- Double curve: A double major curve or S-curve in both the thoracic and lumbar spine, e.g. left thoracic, right lumbar or right thoracic, left lumbar curve

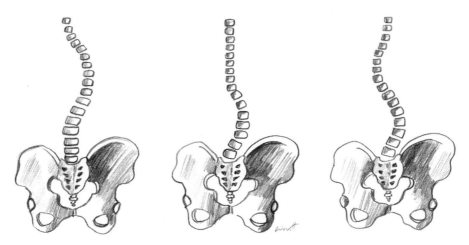

**Figure 6.4** Three main types of curves: C-curve—right thoracic (left image); C-curve—right lumbar (center image); S-curve—left thoracic, right lumbar (right image)

## HOW TO USE THIS PROGRAM

The following program is instructed for those with a right scoliosis (thoracic or lumbar). If you have a left scoliosis, reverse the instructions so that you emphasize lengthening the right side and strengthening the left side. If you have a double curve, work on the side that seems most prominent, your primary curve.

## YOGA SEQUENCE FOR SCOLIOSIS

The following sequence was designed for teens with scoliosis. It focuses on building body awareness and alignment with the need for only a few simple props including a strap or belt, chair, blanket and a wall. Students are encouraged to practice one or two postures a day until they feel confident to move on to the next pose. By the end, they have a repertoire of 12 postures they can practice daily or a couple of shorter sequences that they can do on alternate days. The key concept woven throughout the sequence is that, at all times, movement occurs in two opposing directions. In other words, there is always an "anchor" or grounding part of the body and another part that is reaching away. This contradiction that exists in each pose is what creates true length and change in structure.

You will need the following items for the practice:

- a yoga strap, belt or scarf that is looped or tied shoulder-width apart
- a strong, stable chair with rounded edges
- a blanket or towel
- two yoga blocks or books

- a wall
- a yoga mat.

Let's Begin!

## TWELVE KEY POSTURES FOR SCOLIOSIS
### 1. Yoga Mudrasana (Extended Child's Pose)
First Variation
**Instructions:**

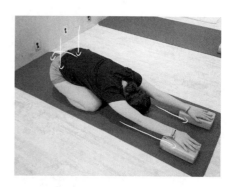

1.  Begin on your hands and knees with the knees wider than your shoulders and big toes touching.
2.  Sit back so that your buttocks touch your heels. (Note: If this is not possible, you may use a blanket, thinly folded and placed in the knee crease. If it is still difficult, you can sit back on a pillow placed between the thighs and calves. If the ankles or feet hurt, you can place a towel roll under the ankles for support.)
3.  Lift your chest and feel that you are lengthening your body forward as you walk your hands forward without letting the buttocks come away from your heels.
4.  Place your hands on two blocks or books.
5.  Keep your neck parallel to the floor by folding a blanket and putting support under your head. This prevents tension in the neck and collapsing of the spine.
6.  Make sure your hands are even so both sides of your trunk are long.
7.  Press your palms down onto the block and energize your arms so your elbows are straight.
8.  Inhale into your chest and lengthen more as you melt your upper back towards the floor.
9.  Lengthen both sides of your waist.
10. Hold for 15–30 seconds and come back to an upright seated position on your heels.

### Second Variation: Parsva Yoga Mudrasana (Child's Pose to the side)—for a right scoliosis

**Note:** For a left scoliosis, you would move to the left side twice as much as to the right. For a double curve, practice on both sides emphasizing the area you need to lengthen on each side.

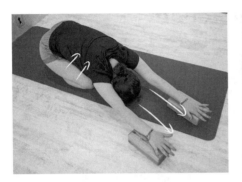
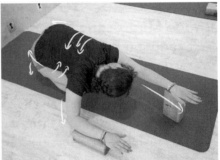

**Twist variation 1, with elbow bent**

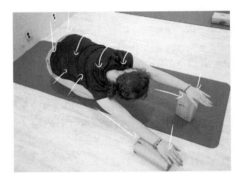

**Twist variation 2, with left arm straight**

**Instructions:**

1. Move the blocks and head support to the right side.
2. Lift the chest, inhale and lengthen the front body, then walk your hands to the right, pressing your left buttock back onto your left heel.
3. Put your hands on the blocks.
4. Reach your left hand forward, lengthening it more than the right side.
5. Hold for 15 seconds.
6. Then turn the left block up to a vertical position, so that your left side of the spine is higher than your right. Twist your spine to the left, gazing under your left arm. As you twist to the left, feel the right hump flattening out so that it becomes less prominent. It should feel as if you

are "absorbing" the rib hump into your body. This instruction will be important throughout the program.

7. Make sure your hips shift over to your left heel.
8. Breathe into the left side of your rib cage, inflating your left lung.
9. Hold for 30 seconds.
10. Repeat to the left for 15 seconds, lengthening evenly through both arms.
11. Go back to the right side and add the twist again. Hold for 15 seconds.
12. Come back to the center and hold for 15 seconds, lengthening both sides equally. Always end with general lengthening of both sides to create balance and come back to center.

## 2. Supta Urdhva Hastasana (Reclining Arms Overhead Posture)

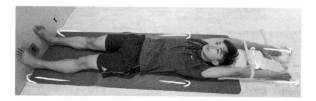

**Instructions:**

1. Lie on your back and place both feet against the wall with knees slightly bent.
2. Hold the sides of the mat and press the soles of your feet into the wall, sliding back along the mat (this helps to lengthen the spine).
3. Make sure your feet are parallel and hip-distance apart.
4. If your chin tilts back, place a blanket under your head (so your chin is facing your chest).
5. Bring your hands up to the ceiling and turn your palms to face each other. Then bring your arms overhead (make sure the blanket doesn't prevent your arms from reaching the floor).
6. Press your right heel into the wall and stretch your left arm, then press your left heel into the wall and stretch your right arm, then stretch both arms overhead while you press both feet into the wall.
7. There should be a little space between your lower back and the floor (don't overarch the spine).

### With a belt

1. Measure your belt so that it is shoulder-width apart.
2. Place the belt over your arms at your elbows.

3. Take your arms overhead with your palms facing the ceiling and reach as far back as you can with your fingertips while pressing both feet into the wall.

**To the side**

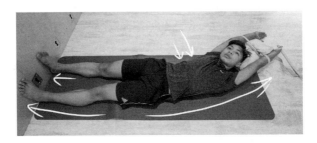

1. Keeping your feet against the wall and buttocks on the floor, move your upper body to the right side (press your elbows and lift your chest to do so).
2. Lift your arms up to the ceiling and resist into the belt, then take your arms overhead and reach out more through the left hand while you press your left heel into the wall to lengthen your left side body.
3. Go to the right, then left, then right again, then back to the center. Hold for 30 seconds in each position.

## 3. Urdhva eka hastasana (Side Body Lengthening Against the Wall)
**Instructions:**

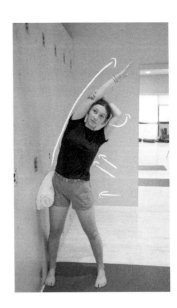

1. Stand with your left outer foot against the wall and a blanket roll between your left hip and the wall. Your feet should be parallel and a little wider than your hips.
2. Press your left hip towards the wall and lift your left arm overhead.
3. Hold your outer left elbow with your right hand and lengthen the side of your waist; lean to the right as you push your hip and heel into the wall.
4. Inhale, lengthen your spine and exhale as you move to the right side.
5. Hold for 5–7 seconds, lengthening your spine on every inhalation and leaning to the right side on every exhalation.

6. Do this twice to the right and once to the left.

## 4. Adho Mukha Svanasana (Downward Dog Variations on Chair)
**Instructions:**

1. Place a chair against the wall for support.
2. Hold the sides of the chair seat, look forward, bend your knees and walk backwards with your feet parallel and hip-distance apart.
3. Press your palms into the seat or hold the sides of the seat and lift the sides of your hips upward, lengthening your spine.

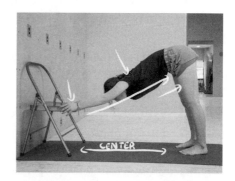

4. Lift your sitting bones up towards the ceiling, and press your thighs back.
5. Again, lift your pelvis up as you press your hands into the chair. Keep your head in line with your spine. Emphasize the lengthening of your spine away from the chair.
6. Bend your knees, walk forward and come up.

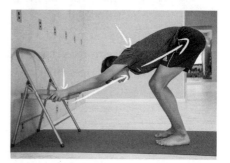

**Note:** if your hamstrings are tight, bend your knees. It is more important that your spine is straight. See the image above.

### With a twist

1. Put your palms on the chair seat, move backwards into Downward Dog and walk to the right, keeping your hands where they are.
2. Lift the left side of your pelvis back and press your left arm forward to lengthen the left side of your body.

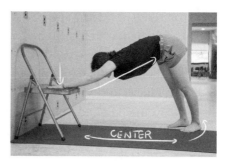

3. Bring your right rib cage towards the left.
4. Breathe into the left side of your rib cage.
5. Hold for 15 seconds.
6. Repeat on your left side, then your right side again.

**Bonus: Handstand with feet on the chair, to lengthen the spine and strengthen the upper back**

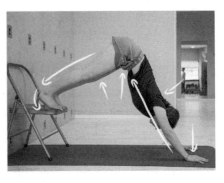

1. Bring your hands in front of the chair, press the ball of your foot onto the center of the chair seat with your knees bent and feet apart.
2. Lift your buttocks and straighten your legs.
3. Engage your quadriceps, using your thigh muscles as you lift your pelvis towards the ceiling.
4. Press your arms down into the earth, keeping your shoulders in joint.
5. Take your upper thighs back, and lengthen your outer hips up towards the ceiling.
6. Hold for 5–7 seconds.

## 5. Utthita Trikonasana (Triangle Pose)

This pose is practiced differently on the right and left side in order to balance out the curve. These instructions are for a right scoliosis. For a left scoliosis, reverse the instructions.

**Right leg forward**
**Instructions:**

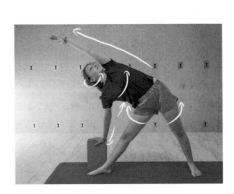

1. Stand in the center of the mat.
2. Take your feet at least four feet apart and stretch your arms out to the sides.
3. Press your feet into the ground, take your thighs back, inhale to your chest and lift it up, keeping your shoulders back and down.
4. Turn your right leg out to

90 degrees and make sure your heel is lined up with the center of your arch of your back foot.

5.  Engage your thigh muscles, lengthen the right side of your waist, and place the fingertips of your right hand on the block. Press your right hand into the block and move your right ribs into your body.

6.  Keep your left hand on your waist and roll your shoulder back.

7.  Keep your head in line with your spine (don't drop your head).

8.  Reach your left arm over your left ear and lengthen the left side of your trunk.

9.  Rotate your right rib cage forward.

10. Hold for 15–30 seconds and come up with your legs straight.

### Left leg forward

1.  Reach your left arm out and rest it on the top of the chair.

2.  Place your right hand at your waist and roll your right shoulder back.

3.  Lengthen the left side of your body by pressing the chair away from you. (It slides better if the chair is on a hard floor.)

4.  Absorb your right ribs into your body as you lengthen the left side of your trunk.

5.  Rotate your left rib cage forward.

6.  Hold for 15–30 seconds and come up with your legs straight.

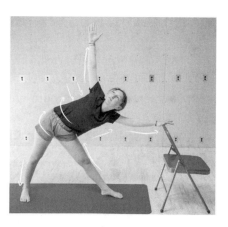

## 6. Utthita Parsvakonasana (Extended Side Angle Pose)

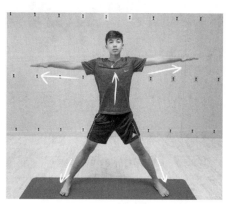 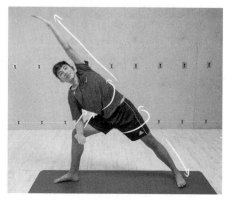

**Instructions:**

1. Take your legs a little wider than you did in the last pose. Turn your right leg out to 90 degrees and turn your back foot in to 30 degrees.
2. Take your arms out to your sides, keep your chest lifted, slowly bend your right leg, making sure your knee is in line with your hip and right ankle.
3. Make sure your knee doesn't cross in front of your ankle; if it does, widen your stance.
4. Press your back outer leg into the ground to stabilize.
5. Rest the back of your right forearm on your knee and lift your left arm up towards the sky.
6. Turn your palm towards your head and reach your arm over your left ear.
7. Rotate your chest towards the sky, moving your right rib cage forward and up.
8. Reach your left arm away from your back heel.
9. Hold for 15–30 seconds.
10. Repeat twice on your right side and once on your left.

## 7. Warrior I with Foot on Chair and Arm Variations
**Instructions:**

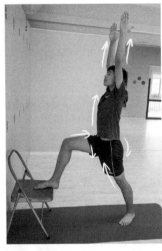

1. Place a chair against a wall for support.
2. Stand 3–4 feet away from the chair.
3. Stand with your feet slightly turned outward (about 30 degrees).
4. Place your right foot on the center of the seat, with the center of your heel on the front edge of the seat.
5. Keep your pelvis parallel to the wall.
6. Take your arms to the side, lift your chin and chest. Keep your chest lifted throughout the posture.
7. Bend your front leg forward so your knee is directly above your ankle.
8. Turn your palms up to the ceiling and take your arms overhead lengthening both sides of your waist.
9. Press your left thigh back so your back leg is straight.
10. Hold here for 15–30 seconds. Repeat on both sides.

11.  Be careful not to overarch your spine. You can avoid this by engaging your lower abdominal muscles. Draw your belly button back towards your spine on the exhalation.

### Second variation to balance the curve

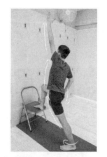

1.  Lift your left arm overhead to lengthen the shortened side of your curve.
2.  Place your right hand on your waist and pull the right side of your pelvis down.
3.  Do this twice on your left side and once on your right.

## 8. Prasarita Padottanasana (Standing Separate Leg Stretching Posture) with Hands on a Chair

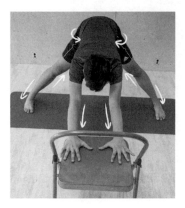
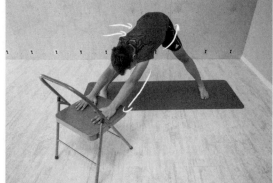

**Instructions:**

1.  Put your hands on your waist.
2.  Take your legs five feet apart, keeping them parallel.
3.  Engage your quadriceps (front thigh muscles) and lift your chest.
4.  Inhale, come forward, placing your hands on the chair seat and lift your chest again, drawing your shoulders away from your ears and bringing your chest forward.
5.  Push the chair forward and slowly bring your chest down towards the floor, moving your shoulder blades into your body.
6.  Keep your outer hips in line with your heels.
7.  Stretch forward and look towards the chair seat.
8.  Come back and take the chair to the right side.

9. Keep your left thigh back and lengthen your left palm a little more than the right.

10. Press your right rib cage into your chest.

11. Hold 15 seconds and repeat on the second side.

12. Go back for the last time to your right side.

13. Go to the center and then come back to standing with your hands on your waist.

14. Step your feet together.

## 9. Vajrasana with baddhanguliyasana (Sitting on Heels with Arms Overhead)

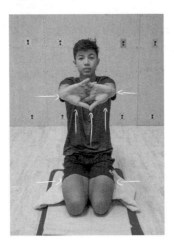 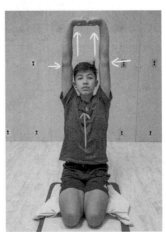

**Instructions:**

1. Come to a kneeling position with your feet and knees together and a blanket between your calf muscle and thigh. Pull the skin of the front of your knee up.

2. If you have pain in your ankles, roll a blanket and place it under the front of your ankles.

3. Sit for one minute, close your eyes, bring attention to your breath.

4. Keep your shoulders back, palms up on your thighs, chest lifted and gaze softly towards your heart.

5. Interlace your fingers, turn the palms away from your chest and press your palms forward.

6. Feel that you are sitting straight with your sitting bones pressing into the ground; lift your arms up overhead keeping your elbows straight.

7. Exhale, bring your arms down.

8. Change the interlock (switch pinky finger) and repeat.

9. If it is hard for you to bring your arms up with a straight elbow, take a belt (looped a little less than shoulder distance) and place your wrists inside the belt.

10. Then place your hands behind your back, interlace them, roll your shoulders back and open your chest.

11. Release your hands onto your lap.

12. Come forward into a Child's Pose, turn your toes in and sit on your heels for five seconds.

13. Then stretch your legs out in front of you, keeping your legs at the width of your pelvis.

## 10. Anantanasana (Side-Lying Pose)

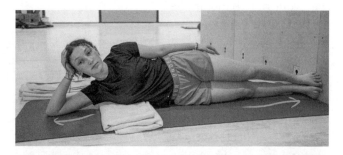

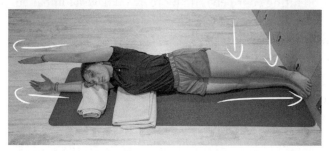

**Instructions:**

1. Take a blanket, fold it three times and place it under the convex side of your curve.

2. Keep your legs together and press both feet into a wall (if possible).

3. Make sure your whole body is in *one straight line*.

4. Stretch your right arm as far as possible away from the wall and place a small blanket or pillow under your head.

5. Inhaling, take your left arm overhead, pushing your feet in to the wall as you lengthen your hands away from the wall.

6. Inhale into the left side of your chest, filling up the concave side of your curve.

7. Hold for 30–45 seconds.

8. Only do this pose with the apex of the convex side of your curve resting on the blanket in order to balance out the scoliosis.

## 11. Vasisthasana (Side Plank Pose)
### Option 1: With hand on chair
**Instructions:**

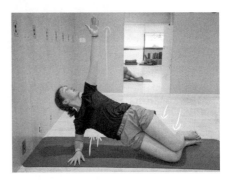

1. Place the chair against the wall.
2. Start with your right hand on the chair seat and walk your feet away from the chair.
3. Stack one foot on top of the other.
4. Straighten your left arm up.
5. Push your right palm down and focus on lifting your right rib cage up if you have a thoracic curve OR focus on lifting your pelvis up more if you have a lumbar curve.
6. Start to build strength by holding for 15–30 seconds, gradually building up to 90 seconds.
7. Repeat twice *on the convex side only*.

### Option 2: Modified Side Plank with Knees Supported
**Instructions:**

1. Rest your right forearm on the floor with your knees bent at a 45 degree angle. Keep the knees on the ground for the duration of the pose in this variation.
2. Repeat steps 5–7 above.

## 12. Bharadvajasana (Seated Spinal Twist) (on a Chair)

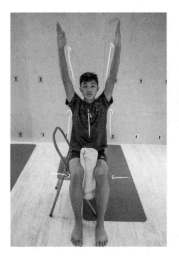 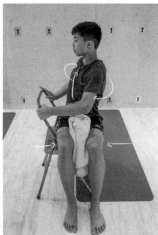

**Instructions:**

1. Sit sideways on a chair, keeping your knees together.
2. Place a block or blanket roll between your legs.
3. Press your feet into the ground and lift your arms overhead, lengthening the sides of your waist.
4. Turn towards the back of the chair; place your hands on the backrest, bending your elbows out to the sides.
5. Twist to the left side.
6. Press the right side of your rib cage into the body.
7. Pull with your left arm as you push with your right arm.
8. Hold for three breaths, inhaling as you lengthen, exhaling as you twist.
9. Keep your chin in line with the center of your chest throughout the pose.
10. Repeat on both sides.

Next version
**Instructions:**

1. Place your back hand on the chair seat.
2. Lift your chest and sides of your waist.
3. Roll your shoulders back as you twist evenly throughout the spine.
4. Hold for 15 seconds.
5. Lift both arms up come back to center.

6.  Repeat on both sides equally.

## Final Pose: Savasana — Relaxation

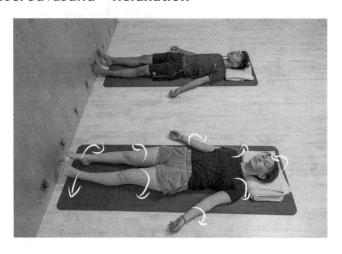

It is very important to take a few minutes to relax in a pose called savasana at the end of your yoga practice no matter how many poses you do. You may not realize it, but you are constantly being stimulated by messages from the outside whether it is through friends, school and, most often, technology and social media. Your feeds are blowing up with new videos and stories directing your attention away from yourself and your own inner feelings. Your yoga practice is a time for you to check back in and remember who you are and that you are okay at this moment. It is a precious opportunity to truly rest your body and mind from the stress of everyday life. Practicing savasana is also important so your body remembers and integrates all the stretching and strengthening into your nervous system. To prepare for savasana, make sure that you have a blanket under your head for support and that you roll your shoulders open so that your neck muscles are relaxed and your chest is open.

Begin by noticing the breath throughout your inhalations and exhalations. At first, you may notice that your belly rises as you inhale and falls as you exhale. As you progress, see if you can feel the rising of the chest as well on each inhalation, knowing that you are increasing and expanding your lung capacity. One of the effects of scoliosis is compression of the lungs, which can limit your ability to breathe deeply. We want to maximize lung capacity and expand the rib cage and surrounding muscles with each inhalation. On the exhalation, focus on letting go of any physical, mental or emotional tension. Stay in this position for five minutes before slowly rolling to the side and pressing up to a comfortable seated position.

Take your hands to the center of your heart and pause, giving thanks to yourself for taking the time to do something good for your body and your soul. You may use these few moments to set an intention for the day or to simply appreciate something or someone in your life. Bow your chin to your chest, honoring the wisdom that lies in your heart.

## CONCLUSION

Yoga is so much more than a physical practice and can be used therapeutically to help correct the curvature of the spine, maintain balance throughout a lifetime and create more peace and harmony in the mind. In addition, yoga can help teens accept and embrace and accept their bodies in its current state and cultivate a relationship that is loving and nurturing towards themselves. Scoliosis offers teens the opportunity to understand and work with their body at an earlier age than most, which can be viewed as a positive side effect, one that leads to healthier habits and lasting change.

If you look around in nature, things are rarely symmetrical. Most people have one leg longer than the other, or one shoulder higher than the other, or one foot smaller than the other. It is time to move away from the illusion of perfection and understand that imperfection and variation is inherent in being human. Yoga therapy is about being at peace with who we are, knowing that our essence is always perfect despite any inner or outer flaws.

It is truly our hope that teens learn to love their spines and themselves, knowing that with some mindful movement and attention, they can build a strong and stable foundation from which to blossom, move and grow.

## Chapter 7

# Anxiety and Depression in Adolescents and Teens

## PREVALENCE OF ANXIETY AND DEPRESSION IN CHILDREN AND TEENS

The incidence of mental health disorders in children and teens has been on the rise over the last few decades. According to a data analysis of a 2016 National Survey of Children's Health published online in *JAMA Pediatrics*, 1 in 6 U.S. children between the ages of 6 and 17 had a treatable mental health disorder such as depression, anxiety problems or ADHD (Whitney & Peterson, 2019). The data analysis also showed that the prevalence of children with mental health disorders who did not receive needed treatment or counseling from a mental health professional was 49.4 percent. It is clear that we have a mental health crisis on our hands when it comes to our children, and the numbers of children struggling with mental health disorders only continues to grow. A more recent study by *JAMA Pediatrics* reported a significant increase in the number of children diagnosed with a mental health condition. The study found that between 2016 and 2020, the number of children ages 3–17 years diagnosed with anxiety grew by 29 percent and those with depression by 27 percent (Assistant Secretary for Public Affairs (ASPA), 2022). This is an alarming increase in just four years.

## CAUSES

There are many factors that can contribute to mental health issues with children. The exact cause is not known, but research suggests that a combination of factors including heredity, biology, psychological, trauma and environmental stress might be involved (Brennan, 2006). Other factors such as disability, race, poverty and limited or no access to health care can also greatly impact a child's mental health (Centers for Disease Control and Prevention, 2022).

What we have seen change over the years that could be the reason for the growing number of children struggling with mental health challenges include:

- increase in use of technology and social media
- increase in exposure to violence and disturbing images/videos
- increase in mental health problems for the adults in the home
- increase in social and political tension
- the global pandemic
- decrease in opportunities for children to move throughout the day
- decrease in connection with nature
- decrease in personal or in-person contact with others.

## RESEARCH REVIEW: YOGA FOR ANXIETY AND DEPRESSION IN CHILDREN AND ADOLESCENTS

A systematic review of 16 yoga interventions for anxiety reduction among children and adolescents indicated, in nearly all of the studies, reduced anxiety after the yoga intervention (Weaver & Darragh, 2015).

An additional systematic review of yoga as an intervention for the symptoms of anxiety and depression in children and adolescents, including 27 studies involving youth with varying health statuses, showed overall improvements in 70 percent of all of the studies. For studies assessing anxiety and depression, 58 percent showed reductions in both symptoms, while 25 percent showed reductions in anxiety only. Additionally, 70 percent of studies assessing anxiety alone showed improvements and 40 percent of studies only assessing depression showed improvements. This review concludes that yoga generally leads to some reductions in anxiety and depression in youth regardless of health status and intervention characteristics (James-Palmer *et al.*, 2020).

## THE GUNAS AND MENTAL HEALTH
### Philosophical Foundation of Yoga

The philosophy of yoga teachings is that suffering arises from our relationship with, reaction to and misidentification with the body–mind environment (BME) (Miller, 2012; Stoler-Miller, 1998, 2004).

The aim with yoga practice is:

- self-awareness, to become aware of our thoughts, patterns of behavior and actions that cause us suffering
- to change our thoughts, patterns of behavior and actions in order to reduce suffering in our lives as well as the lives of others.

The process of inquiry and discernment to reduce suffering relates to recognizing the difference between prakriti and purusha, according to Samkhya philosophy (Jain, 2019):

- **Prakriti (Maya or illusion):** Prakriti includes everything that is changeable, not infinite. All that is illusion or unreal.
- **Purusha (reality):** Purusha is the only reality. The universe's only unchangeable element—the Self or soul.

Prakriti consist of three gunas or qualities of nature: sattva or balance, harmony and light; rajas or motion, passion and energy; and tamas or inertia. These qualities are present in everything: humans, food, animate and inanimate objects. Each of us consists of these three qualities in varying proportions according to our lifestyle and body types, and one quality is often more present than the others.

Only the soul—purusha—is eternal and unchanging, whereas prakriti is changeable and illusionary. Purusha refers to spirit and prakriti refers to matter. The aim in yogic practices is to learn to discriminate between the real and unreal. To see beyond illusion and see true reality, to connect with our Self or soul that is separate from the illusions.

## WHAT ARE THE GUNAS?

The Sanskrit word *guna* translates to "quality, peculiarity, attribute or tendency." According to yoga philosophy, everything is made up of the three gunas' qualities. The gunas are constantly in flux, but we as human beings can present as more dominant in one guna than the other. It is when there is excess of a specific guna that we experience mental and physical imbalance. Our thoughts, body states and behaviors set in motion the predominance or excess of a particular guna and vice versa. If we are in a balanced gunic state, each guna can serve as a positive force in our life. If there is excess of a guna, it can lead to mental/emotional and physical challenges.

### Sattva

Sattva is the guna of balance, harmony and light. In this state, we are present, connected, content and at ease. We are using our energy in sustainable ways and are able to set healthy boundaries with others. We are connected to our truth and are able to discern between illusion and reality. Our thoughts and actions are pure and free of fear, violence or malice. We are more connected to our sense of self and experience life mostly through a lens of harmony, joy and presence. We are able to live free of attachment to others' opinions or judgments (good or bad). We are free from judgment of ourselves.

## Rajas

Rajas is the guna of passion, energy and motion. When balanced and in harmony with tamas and sattva, rajas can help with motivation, mobilization, effort, right action and positive change. When imbalanced, too much Rajasic quality leads to impulsivity, anxious thinking, anger, greed, manipulation and too much energy/activation. Excess rajas can lead to perfectionism, overdoing, hyperactivity, being busy all of the time and exhaustion.

## Tamas

Tamas is the guna of impurity, dullness and ignorance but also has qualities of rest and stillness. When balanced and in harmony with rajas and sattva, tamas can help with grounding and stability. When imbalanced, too much Tamasic quality leads to laziness, lethargy, depression, foggy thinking and too little energy. Excess tamas can lead to lack of motivation, being stagnant, self-doubt, insecurity and fatigue.

Any imbalance or disease, according to ayurveda, the native Indian system of medicine and considered the sister science of yoga, is a manifestation of too much rajas or too much tamas; therefore, cultivating sattva is vital to our health and wellbeing.

The aim is not only to experience sattva but to have a balance and harmony of all three gunas.

Examples of ways to cultivate sattva are:

- physical/movement activities
- pranayama practices
- mindfulness and meditation practices (including chanting, mudras, mantras and gratitude practices)
- relationships/connection with other sattvic beings
- work/school/life balance (making time for experiences that spark joy and remind us of our authentic self as well as time for rest and restoration)
- nourishment/nutrition (sattvic diet)
- connection to nature.

## The Gunas and Polyvagal Theory

In their theoretical article "Yoga therapy and Polyvagal Theory: The convergence of traditional wisdom and contemporary neuroscience for self-regulation and resilience," the authors, comprised of yoga therapists and Stephen Porges, the neuroscientist who developed the polyvagal theory, explain the similarities and interrelationship between the gunas and the polyvagal theory (PVT) neural platforms. They state:

Both PVT and yoga provide frameworks for understanding how underlying neural platforms (PVT) and *gunas* (yoga) link the emergence and connectivity between physiological, psychological and behavioral attributes. By affecting the neural platform, or *guna* predominance, as well as one's relationship to the continual shifting of these neural platforms, or *gunas*, the individual learns skills for self-regulation and resilience. Moreover these frameworks share characteristics that parallel one another where the neural platform reflects the *guna* predominance and the *guna* predominance reflects the neural platform.

(Sullivan *et al.*, 2018)

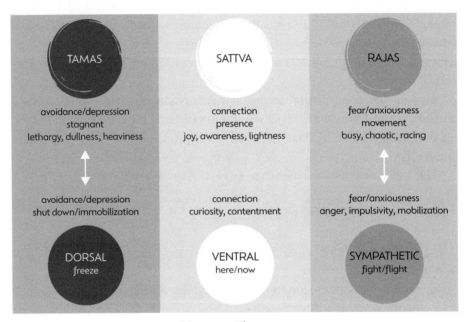

**Figure 7.1** The gunas

In the figure above, we can see the shared characteristics between the gunas and PVT related to the sympathetic nervous system (SNS), fight/flight and the branches of parasympathetic, ventral vagal and dorsal vagal:

- Fight/flight imbalance has similarities to the quality of too much rajas.
- Dorsal vagal imbalance or freeze has similarities to the quality of too much tamas.
- Ventral vagal is balanced dorsal vagal and SNS just as sattva is balanced rajas and tamas.

## ANXIETY AND DEPRESSION: SYMPTOMS AND SIMILARITIES

Both anxiety and depression present with specific symptoms as well as similarities (see Figure 7.2). Children and teens who are experiencing anxiety or depression may display observable emotional and behavioral signs such as anger, irritability, sadness, worry or lack of motivation, but there is often much more going on beneath the surface that can cue us into a child's or teen's mental/emotional state. Children, especially younger children, and even many teens who struggle with emotional awareness may not have the words to describe the emotions they are feeling. Instead, they may express that they have a "stomach ache" or a "headache." They may experience persistent or chronic physiological symptoms. They may have difficulty with sleep, show signs of persistent fatigue, experience chronic pain or struggle with attention and learning. The observable or "acting out" behaviors are the iceberg above the surface, but there is a wealth of information to attend to below the surface that can guide us in recognizing what nervous system state a child may be in and how we can best support them.

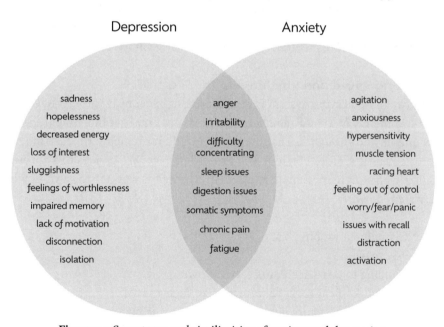

**Figure 7.2** Symptoms and similarities of anxiety and depression

The emphasis in working with anxiety and depression is to balance out the rajas and tamas in order to be in a more balanced, sattvic state.

We can work with rajas and tamas through the lens of nervous system states in order to bring the system back to homeostasis and a felt sense of safety, connection and self-empowerment.

## THERAPEUTIC APPROACHES FOR ANXIETY AND DEPRESSION

### Anxiety

#### Anxiety and Rajas

Anxiety shows up as excess rajas or too much activation in the nervous system. With persistent anxiety, there is a sense of hypervigilance. In this state, the SNS is on overdrive and the gas pedal is constantly on. The energy of the mind can be scattered, disorganized and focused on the future or what "could happen." This constant activation of the SNS can impact all aspects of a child's wellbeing.

#### Moving from more Dynamic Movement to More Slow/Subtle Movement

It's important to meet the child or teen where they are at. The intention with movement, breathing and meditation practices for anxiety is to meet their nervous system in that high activation state and support them in bringing their nervous systems to a more regulated, grounded and present state of being. Begin with more active and dynamic movement, then move towards more static and grounded practices. Once the nervous system is more regulated, the child will be able to access more meditative and contemplative practices.

#### Integrating Pause and Rhythm into the Practice

Often when the nervous system is in overdrive or constantly turned on, we will observe difficulty in a child's ability to pause. We may observe more rapid speech, movements and thoughts. The intention is to down-regulate the fast-moving energy towards a more efficient and grounded pace. We can do this through integrating pauses in movement and activities as well as working towards slowing the system down.

- Clapping or tapping fast to slow
- Freeze dance
- Dancing to fast-paced music then slowing it down
- Cheetah to Bear to Sloth (moving like each animal)
- Encouraging a pause between activities or during transitions
- Chanting, making animals noises or singing quickly, then slowing it down
- Using a metronome to pace movement

## Working with Grounding

Anxiety reflects excess rajas—airiness and movement. In working toward grounding the nervous system, we cultivate the opposite of airiness and movement—stability—in the mind and body.

## Practices to Bring More Focus or Organization to the Mind

In Patañjali's *Yoga Sutras*, *Yoga chitta vritti nirodha* is translated as "cessation of the fluctuations of the mind" (Graphics, 2020). When the nervous system is in a perpetual state of SNS activation or fight/flight, the mind can be scattered and disorganized, and the neuroception of danger can create a constant flow of anxious and worried thinking. Postures, breathing, mindfulness and meditation practices for children and teens that support focus and "taming the monkey mind" can bring more organization and clarity to the mind to support attention, mood, learning and a more grounded connection to the world around them.

## Moving from Anxious to Empowered

We often hear statements about "calming the anxiety." What if we were to take a different approach by teaching children that they can learn tools to channel their anxious energy into empowerment? Educating children and teens that in their anxious energy is a quality of mobilization that can be transformed into action, creativity, motivation and self-empowerment. Rather than asking them to just "calm" the anxiety, we teach them that they have the power to transform their anxiety and that active and mobilized energy in ways that can support them in their lives. Rather than teaching them to suppress the energy, we encourage them to acknowledge the mobilization and move the energy through and out. Children who experience anxiety often feel as though they have no control. Providing choice and taking a collaborative approach in their sessions will offer an experience of empowerment and agency.

## Therapeutic Approach

Integrate poses, breathing strategies, mantras, mudras and other activities to build self-esteem that support boundaries, self-agency and self-esteem.

## Self-Trust and Empowerment

A 16-year-old girl come to me at the start of the COVID-19 pandemic. She had been diagnosed with OCD, was experiencing significant anxiety, was having intrusive thoughts and was losing connection with her friends because she had begun to isolate from others. She had not experienced any of these issues prior to the onset of the pandemic. Her OCD behaviors involved obsessive hand washing and her intrusive thoughts were convincing her that she shouldn't be around other people because she might make them sick. She was also afraid to drive because she thought she might cause an accident and hurt or kill someone. There were many other fears, all centered around not trusting herself. She was seeing a therapist for her issues with a focus on cognitive behavioral therapy (CBT), which she was responding very well to. It is important to know our scope of practice. My role was not to be her mental health practitioner but to help her connect more with her body–mind environment and bring more of a bottom-up approach to her healing. Yoga therapy was an adjunct therapy to her CBT, and her therapist was quite supportive and excited about her exploring yoga as part of her mental health tool box.

The focus in her yoga therapy sessions involved:

- decreasing excess rajas
- building self-trust through empowered movement, breath, visualization and mantras
- increasing her interoceptive awareness
- building capacity to tolerate uncomfortable sensations in a titrated way
- developing healthy tools and coping skills to manage stress
- connecting to her authentic self.

### GABA, Anxiety and Yoga Research

There are numerous studies on the effects of yoga on the brain and levels of anxiety. A study published in *The Journal of Alternative and Complementary Medicine* found that certain types of yoga (a focus on yoga poses, as opposed to just breathing) increase gamma-aminobutyric acid (GABA) levels in the brain. Anxiety is associated with low GABA levels. GABA is the primary neurotransmitter known to counterbalance the excitatory neurotransmitter glutamate, which in the case of anxiety is overactive. The study found greater reductions in anxiety and greater improvements in mood compared with people who walked for exercise. These mood improvements and reductions in anxiety were correlated with changes in GABA levels. This study suggests that yoga, in particular, the asana practice combined with breathing, can be a promising approach to increasing GABA levels in the brain, thus decreasing anxiety (Streeter *et al.*, 2010).

## Depression

### Depression and Tamas

Depression shows up as excess tamas or stagnant energy in the nervous system. With depression, there is a sense of disempowerment or disconnection from self. In this state, the gas tank is empty, and the child or teen may feel as if they're running on fumes. With depression, there can still be activation beneath the surface as well as feelings of shame and worthlessness, which is why there is cross over between depression and anxiety.

## Moving from More Slow/Subtle Movement to More Dynamic/Active Movement

With depression, it's important to meet the child or teen where they are initially and build up energy from there. Many children and teens who experience depression may lack energy and fatigue easily. The intention is to begin the practice in a way that is attainable and allows the child to feel a sense of success in their practice. Beginning in a lying down or seated position, closer to the ground with slower, more static movement requires less energy and may feel "safer" for the child to explore; you can then build the energy up in a way that feels safe and attainable for the child. Integrate frequent opportunities to take breaks and rest between movements and activities.

## Integrating Rhythm and Patterning

Mirroring and entrainment are ways we can build connection as well as create a specific rhythmic patterning and energy. Begin with slow mirroring and rhythmic activities, then build up the pace and energy.

- Clapping or tapping slow to faster
- Dancing to slower music, then faster music
- Sloth to Bear to Cheetah (moving like each animal)
- Chanting, making animals noises or singing slowly or softly, then speeding up or increasing projection of voice
- Using a metronome to pace movement

## Working with Expansion

When we think of depression in the body, we see a rounded posture with the heart protected, head dropped and eyes looking down. The energy of the mind is often dull and constricted. The breath is often shallow and collapsed. Working with expansion of the body, breath and mind can support children and teens in building energy in the mind and body.

## Practices to Bring More Engagement and Expansion to the Mind

- Expressive arts
- Energizing breathing practices
- Stories
- Visualization

- Moving meditation
- Mudras
- Tapping into the five senses
- Novel experiences
- Music and sound

### Moving from Disempowered to Empowered

Often with depression there is a sense of disempowerment and feeling of a lack of choice or inability to make choices. Alternating choice with the child or teen can assist them in beginning to step into their power, while also feeling supported. Asking them to make too many choices at the start can feel overwhelming to them. An example of alternating choice would be for the adult to choose a pose, then give the child the option to choose a pose. Providing choice and taking a collaborative approach in their sessions will offer an experience of empowerment and agency.

### Therapeutic Focus

Integrate poses, breathing strategies, mantras, mudras and other activities to build self-esteem that support boundaries, self-agency and self-esteem.

### Brain Integration for Anxiety and Depression

Not only is crossing the midline an important developmental and functional skill, but it can also support reducing anxiety and depression by connecting both sides of the brain for whole-brain integration. Integration of both sides of the brain can help a child or teen move out of the "stuck" survival or emotional brain and access the more logical or thinking part of the brain. The corpus callosum is the connection between the two cerebral parts of the brain. Its function is to transmit neural messages between the right and left hemispheres of the brain. When the two sides of the brain are disconnected, it can impact a child's speech, language processing, motor coordination, learning, attention and emotional regulation. Movements that cross the midline, such as crossing an arm or leg across the body to the other side, stimulate the corpus callosum and support communication between the left and right hemispheres of the brain. A more integrated brain supports a more regulated and grounded child.

When children and teens experience anxiety and depression, they can become stuck in the emotional or reactive part of the brain. Activities that cross the midline can support in reducing anxiety and depression and moving children and teens out of "fixed" emotional states.

The ancient yogis carried this intuitive wisdom about the left and right brain relationship. We see the example of this represented in ida and pingala nadis.

According to the texts and teachings of yoga, prana flows through the subtle body within a network of channels, or *nadis* (Sullivan & Robertson, 2020). The sushumna nadi is the central channel, running along the spine. The left channel is ida nadi and runs along the left side of the body. The right hemisphere of the brain is in control of the left side of the body; therefore, Ida is right-brain dominant. The right channel is pingala nadi and runs along the right side of the body. The left hemisphere controls the right side of the body; therefore, pingala nadi is left brain dominant. Ida and pingala represent feminine and masculine, emotional and logical, the non-duality of our existence. The emphasis in yoga is balance. Brain integration practices can stimulate both sides of the brain, assist communication between the left and right sides of the brain, and bring balance to the mind, body and emotions.

### Crossing Midline Activities

These activities can be integrated to support emotional regulation, motor coordination, attention, focus and communication.

### *Cross March*
**Instructions:**

1. Begin standing.
2. Wiggle your right hand and cross it over to your left knee.
3. Release your right hand.
4. Wiggle your left hand and cross it over to your right knee.
5. Begin marching and crossing your hands to the opposite knee as you march.
6. Option: Add sound with the tapping.

### *Cross Tap*
**Instructions:**

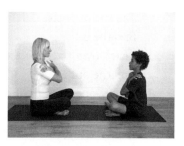

1. Begin seated.
2. Tap your left hand to your right shoulder.
3. Tap your right hand to your left shoulder.
4. Continue tapping these body parts with your opposite hand (hips, knees, ankles, feet).
5. Option: Name the body part being tapped.

*Bicycle*

**Instructions:**

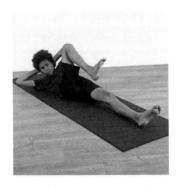

1. Lie on your back.
2. Bring your right knee towards your chest.
3. Cross your left elbow to your right knee.
4. Bring your left knee towards your chest.
5. Cross your right elbow to your left knee.
6. Repeat 4–5 times.

*Apple Picking*

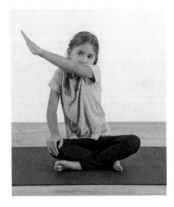
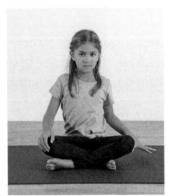

This pose not only supports midline crossing but also supports tapping into the senses.

**Instructions:**

1. Begin seated.
2. Imagine what color apple and what type of apple you are going to pick.
3. Wiggle the finger of your right hand.
4. Tap the opposite (left) shoulder.
5. Breathe in.
6. Reach over to the left as if you're reaching to pick an apple.
7. Breathe out.
8. Bring your hand back to the right side and drop your apple in the imaginary bucket.
9. Repeat 2 more times on that side.
10. Do 3 times on the opposite side.
11. Get an apple from the bucket.

12. Take a bite.
13. What color is your apple?
14. How does your apple taste? Sweet or sour?
15. Is your apple crunchy or mushy?

### Ear to Nose
**Instructions:**

1. Begin seated.
2. Touch your nose with your right pointer finger.
3. Reach your left hand to your right ear.
4. Give the earlobe a tug or squeeze.
5. Breathe in, breathe out.
6. Repeat on the opposite side.

### Pizza Dough Ear Stretch Crossed Arms
**Instructions:**

1. Cross your right arm over your left.
2. Take hold of your earlobes with your fingertips.
3. Gently tug on the earlobe and massage up and down the ear.
4. Breathe in, breathe out.
5. Repeat with the left arm over the right.

### Cross Row
**Instructions:**

1. Begin seated.
2. Extend your legs in front of you with your knees bent, feet on the floor.
3. Imagine you are rowing a boat on a lake.
4. Bring your hands together as if you're holding an oar.
5. Bring your hands over to the right.
6. Bring your hands over to the left.
7. Row back and forth several times.
8. Option: Sing "Row, Row, Row Your boat."

### Mix it Up
**Instructions:**

1. Reach your hands forward.

2. Keep your elbows straight, palms facing each other.
3. Turn your thumbs down towards the ground.
4. Face your palms out.
5. Wiggle your right finger and bring your right hand to your left palm.
6. Clasp your fingers together.
7. Reach your knuckles forward.
8. Breathe in, breathe out.
9. Repeat on the opposite side.

### Self-Hug
See Chapter 4.

### Ear Tug and Squat
**Instructions:**

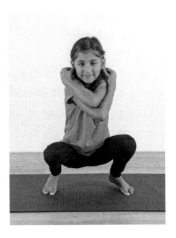

1. Begin standing with feet hips width apart.
2. Cross your right arm over your left.
3. Take hold of your earlobes with your fingers and give a gentle tug.
4. Breathe in.
5. Breathe out and come into a crouching position like a frog.
6. Stay for the count of 1-2-3, holding your earlobes.
7. Come back to standing hips width apart.
8. Cross your left arm over your right.
9. Take hold of your earlobes with your fingers and give a gentle tug.
10. Breathe in.
11. Breathe out and come into a crouching position like a frog.
12. Stay for the count of 1-2-3, holding your earlobes.
13. Come back to standing.

### Disco Dance
**Instructions:**

1. Begin standing.
2. Imagine you're doing a disco dance.
3. Point your right pointer finger.
4. Cross it over to the left.

5. Point your left pointer finger.
6. Cross it over to your right.
7. Option: Dance to or sing the song "Staying Alive."

### Figure Eight Breath
**Instructions:**

1. Begin standing.
2. We're going to draw the figure 8 in the air.
3. Extend the pointer finger of your right hand.
4. Breathe in.
5. Draw half of the 8 from the bottom to top.
6. Breathe out.
7. Draw the other half from the top to the bottom.
8. Repeat on the opposite side.
9. Do two more times on both sides.

### Cross Drumming
**Instructions:**

1. Begin seated.
2. Cross your right arm over your left.
3. Imagine you have drum sticks in your hands.
4. Begin drumming motion.
5. Repeat with the left arm over the right.

### Head Tap/Belly Rub
**Instructions:**

1. Place your right hand on your belly and your left hand on the top of your head.
2. Rub your belly in a circle with your right hand.
3. Tap the top of your head with your left hand.
4. Now try rubbing your belly and tapping your head at the same time.
5. Repeat with the opposite hands on belly and head.

### Seated Giraffe Toes
See Chapter 5.

## BREATHING

### Pranayama and Breathing Strategies

*Prana* is a Sanskrit word meaning "vital force" and *ayama* is another Sanskrit word meaning "expansion". *Pranayama* translates to "expansion of vital force."

Pranayama makes up the fourth limb of the eight limbs of yoga.

Prana is the life force which permeates both the individual and the universe. Prana, the breath, mind and body are linked to one another. Pranayama is the practice of breath control in yoga. It can be a practice of synchronizing the breath with movement in asana or a distinct breathing exercise on its own.

Pranayama typically follows asana, the third limb of yoga, because asana can open the body and allow more suppleness in the spine, rib cage and diaphragm for more diaphragmatic breathing; however, it can also be integrated as a practice on its own to support children with connection to their body and breath and as a tool for self-regulation.

Letting children and teens know their breath is their super power will encourage them to use their breath as a simple and accessible way to regulate their nervous systems.

Our breath is also the foundation for speech and communication. Speech initiates from the diaphragm and it is in the exhalation that we are able to express our thoughts and ideas, communicate and share and connect with others. Our breath is our voice, our unique "voice print" in the world, our tool with which to set boundaries, exhibit self-agency and express our authentic and unique selves.

Each pranayama breath practice has its own resonating effect on the nervous system. Because our nervous systems and constitutions are so diverse, there is no black and white in the effect each individual will experience with a particular breath.

There are certain breathing strategies that can be calming (cooling) and others that are more energizing (heating).

We integrate certain breathing strategies in a child's yoga protocol with the intention of giving them tools to up-regulate or down-regulate their nervous system, connect to their bodies/breath, express and release difficult emotions, support their asana practice, build self-confidence and self-esteem, calm the mind, prepare for self-exploration and meditation practices, and support physical, emotional and mental wellbeing.

### What is Diaphragmatic Breathing?

The diaphragm, a dome-shaped muscle located below the lungs, plays an important role in breathing. When you inhale, your diaphragm contracts (tightens) and moves downward. This creates more space in your chest cavity, allowing the lungs to expand. When you exhale, the opposite happens—your diaphragm relaxes and moves upward in the chest cavity. Many of us (due to posture, stress and dysfunctional breathing patterns), breathe relatively shallowly, relying on the secondary respiratory muscles rather than the primary respiratory muscles: the diaphragm, the rib cage muscles (intercostals) and the abdominal muscles. Diaphragmatic breathing is the optimal breathing for health and wellbeing in which we fully engage the diaphragm when breathing to increase the efficiency of our lungs and breath.

## Benefits of Proper Breathing

- Increases oxygenation to the systems in the body
- Activates the vagus nerve and brings the nervous system to a more relaxed state
- Supports up-regulating and down-regulating the nervous system
- Supports focus and attention
- Supports improved circulation
- Improves body awareness and connection to body
- Supports better sleep
- Supports improved communication

### MY DIAPHRAGM

*Did you know about the diaphragm?*
*A special muscle*
*That helps with breathing and respiration.*
*When I breathe in, my belly expands*
*Like a balloon that's big and grand.*
*When I breathe out, my belly contracts*
*Moves towards my spine and shrinks back.*
*I breathe in deep and my rib cage gets wide*
*I breathe out slowly and feel calmer inside.*
*This muscle does all it can*
*To help my lungs take in oxygen.*
*And then to let the toxins out*
*So I am healthy and can move about.*
*I love my amazing diaphragm.*
*My SUPER muscle.*
*My body's best friend.*

Shawnee Thornton Hardy

### Preparing the Body for Breath

#### Gorilla Breathing

Tapping the chest and integrating sound is a great way to prepare the body for breath. Gorilla Breathing can facilitate breaking up any mucus in the lungs, bringing energy to the lungs and supporting lymphatic functioning. This is a great breath for warming up the vocal cords, engaging the diaphragm and awakening the throat chakra.

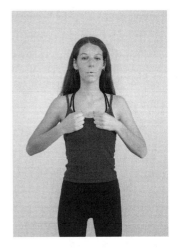

**Instructions:**

1.  Have the child stand or sit tall and upright.
2.  Have them begin to pound the chest gently.
3.  Have them begin to make the sound "ahhh."
4.  Encourage them to continue pounding their chest gently while making the "ahhh" sound.
5.  Repeat 3–4 times.
6.  Have the child check in and notice how they feel after doing Gorilla Breathing.

#### Lion's Breath

Lion's Breath or *Simha Pranayama* is a great way to stimulate the diaphragm and vocal cords, release tension in the face, jaw and eyes and enhance energy and vitality.

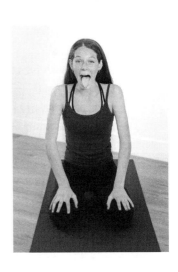

**Instructions:**

1.  Sit in Hero Pose or Criss-Cross Seat.
2.  Bring your hands onto your lap, straighten your arms and extend your fingers.
3.  Inhale through your nose.
4.  Exhale strongly through your mouth while sticking out your tongue and making a "ha" sound.
5.  Option: Have the child look up towards their third eye, gazing towards the tip of their nose with their eyes as they practice the breath.

## Preparing the Body for Breathing

Asana precedes pranayama in the eight limbs of yoga because the physical postures are intended to prepare the body for sitting in meditation and opening the body for more optimal breathing and flow of prana throughout the systems of the body. Pranayama is also a more subtle practice, beginning with connecting children and teens to their bodies (anamaya kosha), and will support them in *feeling* the breath in their bodies so they can notice how different breathing patterns and practices impact their nervous system states (pranamaya kosha). We can use visualization as well as tactile cues to bring more awareness to the body/breath connection.

Diaphragmatic breathing involves expansion of the front, sides and back of the rib cage. This can be explored through different seated postures that open the body for more optimal breathing.

### Front/Back/Side Breathing
#### *Seated Postures Opening the Front Body*
Option: Have the child or teen sit on a bolster or folded blanket in order to allow for more length in the spine and openness in the upper body.

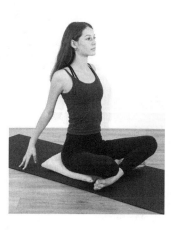 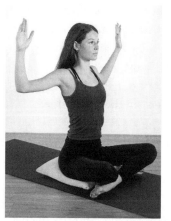

**Instructions:**

1. Begin seated in Sukhasana (Criss-Cross Seat).
2. Sit up tall, lengthening the spine.
3. Reach your arms back, bringing your fingertips to the floor or blanket/bolster.
4. Keep your ears in line with your shoulders.
5. Breathe your breath into the front of your body.

6. Breathe out slowly.
7. Bring your palms and elbows close together or touching.
8. Open your arms as if you're opening a book.
9. Keep your elbows in line with the shoulders.
10. Breathe your breath into the front of your body.
11. Breathe out slowly.

### *Seated Postures Opening the Side Body*
REACH FOR THE MOON

**Instructions:**

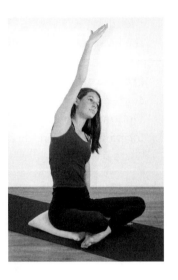

1. Begin seated in Sukhasana (Criss-Cross Seat).
2. Sit up tall, lengthening the spine.
3. Reach your right hand up, then over towards the left.
4. Keep your right hip on the floor.
5. Imagine bringing your breath into the right side of your body.
6. Option: Have the child take their left hand to the right side of their body to facilitate proprioception and awareness of the breath.
7. Breathe your breath into the right side of your body.
8. Breathe out slowly.
9. Repeat on the other side.

### *Seated Posture Opening the Back Body*
KOALA CUDDLE

**Instructions:**

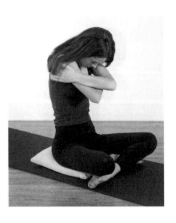

1. Begin seated in Sukhasana (Criss-Cross Seat).
2. Sit up tall, lengthening the spine.
3. Reach your arms out wide.
4. Cross your right arm over the left.
5. Tuck your chin slightly.
6. Feel your shoulder blades draw apart.
7. Breathe your breath into your back body.
8. Option: Gently place your hand between the shoulder blades to facilitate proprioception and awareness of the breath.

9. Breathe out slowly.
10. Repeat with the left arm over the right.

*Twists to Stretch the Intercostal Muscles and Bring More Mobility to the Trunk and Ribs to Facilitate Diaphragmatic Breathing*
SEATED TWIST
**Instructions:**

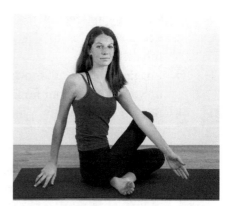

1. Begin seated in Sukhasana (Criss-Cross Seat) with the right leg on top.
2. Bring your right foot over towards your left hip.
3. Knee facing up.
4. Sit up tall, lengthening the spine.
5. Reach your left hand across to the right.
6. Bring your right hand behind you.
7. Inhale to lengthen.
8. Exhale, twist.
9. Repeat on the other side.

*Hip Openers to Release Tension and Support Diaphragmatic Breathing*
LOW LUNGE
**Instructions:**

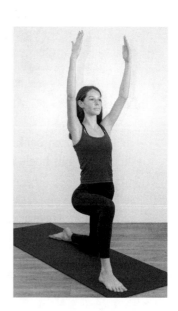

1. Begin kneeling on both knees.
2. Option: Have a folded blanket under knees.
3. Step your right foot forward.
4. Stack your front knee over your ankle.
5. Reach your arms up and find equal length on both sides of your upper body.
6. Bring awareness to the back hip and thigh.
7. Breathe your breath in.
8. Imagine your breath allowing your back hip and thigh to release tension.
9. Breath out.
10. Repeat on the other side.

## Neutral Spine/Alignment to Support Posture and Allow for Optimal Breathing

### Tall Mountain

**Instructions:**

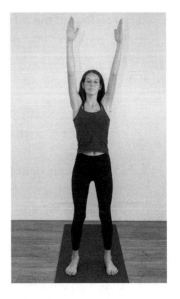

1. Stand with feet hip-width apart.
2. Option: Have your feet a bit wider if needed.
3. Point your toes forward.
4. Ground your feet down.
5. Reach your arms up.
6. Inhale.
7. Imagine your breath moving from your feet up your body to your fingertips.
8. Breathe out slowly.

### Core Activation

Allowing for a slight drawing in and up of the navel on the exhalation supports core awareness and activation.

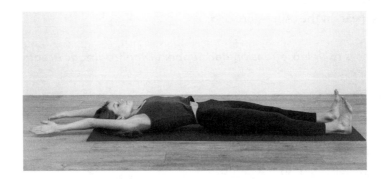

**Instructions:**

1. Lie on your back.
2. Press your heels away from your head and bring your toes towards your shins.
3. Stretch your arms back, palms facing up.
4. Option: Have a folded blanket or bolster under the arms to provide support.
5. Inhale.
6. Exhale, gently drawing the belly button in towards the spine.

## Typical Breathing Cue with Movement: Inhale on Expansion, Exhale on Contraction

The reason this is the typical cue when integrating breath with movement is that the body is more open and expansive to allow for the inhalation, and the inhalation brings more sympathetic energy to the nervous system. The exhalation occurs with the contraction because that is what is happening with the diaphragm. It recoils on the exhalation. The exhalation occurs with the contraction of the abdominal muscles, pressing the relaxed diaphragm against the lungs, causing air to be pushed out.

## Using Breath Practice to Regulate the Nervous System

Breathing practices can be integrated in a child's session to support up-regulation and/or down-regulation of the nervous system. It is important to observe and track a child's nervous system response to each breathing practice. Because of each child's unique body and nervous system, they will respond individually to the breathing practices. The focus with any breathing practice is bringing attention to the breath and noticing the resonating effect on their minds, bodies and nervous systems.

## Down-Regulating

### *Nyasa Finger Breathing*

Calms anxious energy, centers scattered mind, supports insomnia.

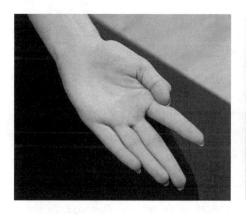 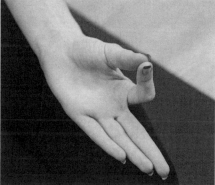

**Instructions:**

1. Sit up tall on the floor or in a chair.
2. Close your eyes or keep them softly open, gazing at your right hand.
3. Practice this breath slowly and mindfully.

4.  Bring your right thumb to the base of your pointer finger.
5.  Inhale, trace the thumb up your pointer finger.
6.  Exhale, trace the thumb down to the base of the middle finger.
7.  Inhale, trace the thumb up your middle finger.
8.  Exhale, trace the thumb down to the base of the ring finger.
9.  Inhale, trace the thumb up your ring finger.
10. Exhale, trace the thumb down to the base of the pinky finger.
11. Inhale, trace the thumb up your pinky finger.
12. Exhale, trace the thumb down to the other side of the pinky finger.
13. Check in and notice how you feel.
14. Repeat on the left hand.
15. Check in and notice how you feel.
16. Do both the right and left hand together.
17. Check in and notice how you feel.

### Taco Breath (Shitali Pranayama)

Shitali is a cooling breath which pacifies heat that builds in the body and balances out the nervous system.

**Instructions:**

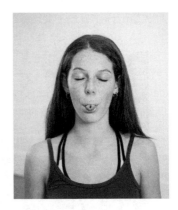

1.  Sit up tall on the floor or in a chair.
2.  Take a sip of cool water.
3.  Roll the outer edges of the tongue in to make a taco shape with your tongue.
4.  Draw the air in by sucking it through the rolled tongue.
5.  Natural breath out.
6.  Did you notice the cool air on your tongue?
7.  Repeat 2–4 times, taking sips of water as needed if the mouth becomes dry.
8.  Check in and notice how you feel.

### Moon Breath — Alternate Nostril Breathing (Nadi Shodhana Pranayama)

Nadi shodhana supports calming the nervous system and whole-brain integration. Breathing into the left side is more cooling and down-regulating.

**Finger position:** Pointer and middle finger bent.

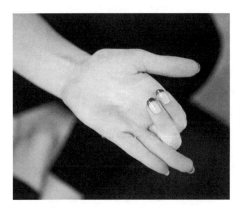 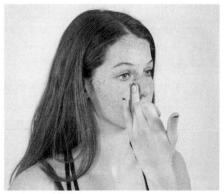

**Instructions:**

1. Sit up tall on the floor or in a chair.
2. Hold your right hand out in front of you, palm face up.
3. Bend your pointer and middle fingers in towards your palm.
4. Place your right thumb on right nostril.
5. Exhale through left nostril.
6. Inhale through left nostril.
7. Place your ring finger on left nostril and release your right nostril.
8. Exhale through right nostril.
9. Inhale through right nostril.
10. Place right thumb on right nostril.
11. Exhale through left nostril.
12. Repeat 3–4 times.

**Note:** Finger placement if the child is left-handed, ring finger on right nostril, breathe in through left.

### Wave Breath (Ujjayi Pranayama)
Calms the mind, eases anxiety and supports whole-brain integration.

When introducing this breath, you can use the movement of your hands to demonstrate the wave coming up with the inhale and going down with the exhale. When children do the movements with the breath, they cross the midline, which enhances whole-brain integration and focus.

**Instructions:**

1. Imagine a wave moving up and down.

2.  When you breathe in, the wave will come up.
3.  When you breathe out, the wave will come down.
4.  With this breath, you breathe in through your nose and out through your nose.
5.  You might even hear the sound of the ocean with your breath.
6.  Reach your right hand across your body.
7.  Breathe in through your nose as you bring your right hand up to bring the wave up.
8.  Breathe out as you bring your right hand down towards the right side to bring the wave down.
9.  Repeat two times on the right side.
10. Do three times on the left side.
11. Option: Alternate between right and left to enhance whole-brain integration.
12. Check in and notice how you feel.

### *Balloon Belly Breath*
**Instructions:**

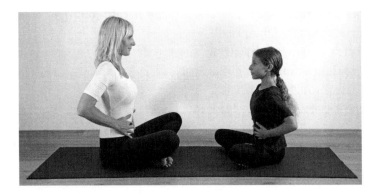

1.  Begin seated.
2.  Let's imagine your belly is a balloon.
3.  Think about what color you want your balloon to be.
4.  Place your hands on your belly.
5.  Sit up tall.
6.  Breathe in and fill your belly with air like a balloon.
7.  Breathe out slowly through your mouth, letting the air out of your balloon belly.
8.  Repeat 3–4 times.

### *Heart/Belly Breathing or Anchor Breath*
Grounding, supports connection to body, decreases anxiety.

## Instructions:

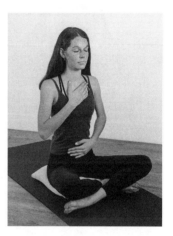

1. Sit up tall on the floor or in a chair.
2. Close your eyes or keep them softly open.
3. Place one hand on your belly.
4. Place the other hand on your chest or heart center.
5. Notice the self-contact of your hands on your body.
6. Breathe in through your nose.
7. Notice as your belly and chest expand out.
8. Breathe out slowly.
9. Notice as your belly and chest draw back in.
10. Bring your awareness to your hands and connect to your body as you breathe.
11. Think of your hands as an anchor, grounding you to the earth, connecting you to your body.
12. Repeat 3–4 times.
13. Check in and notice how you feel.

### *2-4 Breathing or Extended Exhalation*
Brings awareness to the breath, extends the exhalation which supports down-regulation of the nervous system. This breath is called 2-4 Breathing because the focus of the breath is to extend the exhalation twice as long as the inhalation.

## Instructions:

1. As you breathe in, count how long your inhalation is. This will be different for each child depending on their breath capacity. You can track their breathing and count how long their inhalation is, then guide them through the breath.
2. When you breathe out, extend your breath for twice as long as your inhalation.
3. For example: Breathe in 1-2, breathe out 1-2-3-4.
4. Repeat 3–4 times.
5. Check in and notice how you feel.

*Three-Part Breathing (Dirga Pranayama)*

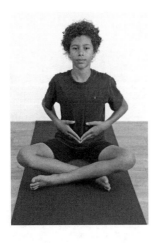 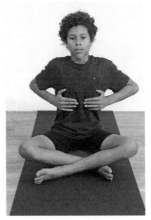 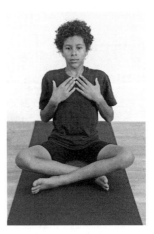

This breath brings awareness to the parts of the body where the breath should move and supports diaphragmatic breathing.

**Instructions:**

1. Bring your hands to your belly and tap your belly.
2. Bring your hands to your lower rib cage and tap your lower rib cage.
3. Bring your hands to your chest and tap your chest.
4. Belly, rib cage, chest.
5. We're going to breathe into these different parts of our body.
6. Place your hands on your belly.
7. Breathe in through your nose and fill it up like a balloon.
8. Breathe out slowly.
9. Bring your hands to your rib cage.
10. Breathe in through your nose and bring your breath into your rib cage, feeling it expand on the front, back and sides.
11. Breathe out slowly.
12. Bring your hands to your chest.
13. Breathe in through your nose and feel your lungs fill with air like balloons.
14. Breathe out slowly.
15. See if you can do one breath where it moves from the belly, to the rib cage, to the lungs.
16. Breathe in—feel belly, rib cage, lungs.
17. Breathe out slowly.
18. Repeat the full breath—feel belly, rib cage, lungs—3–4 times.

19. Check in and notice how you feel.

### Grounding Breath

Supports grounding and down-regulating the nervous system in the moment when the child or teen is experiencing a stressful event and is becoming overwhelmed or panicky. It is best to practice this during smaller, less overwhelming situations so the child has integrated the practice in their nervous system and can more easily access the Grounding Breath when they begin to feel overwhelmed or heightened levels of anxiety.

**Instructions:**

1. Feel my feet (have child bring their awareness to their feet).
2. Hands on my belly (have child bring their hands to their belly).
3. Breathe in 1-2 (have child breathe in to the count of 2).
4. Breathe out 1-2-3-4 (have child breathe out to the count of 4).

### Magic Carpet Breath

Magic Carpet Breath encourages diaphragmatic breathing. The use of a stuffed animal and a small bit of weight from a bean bag on the belly encourages body awareness and offers a cause and effect experience for the inhalation and exhalation.

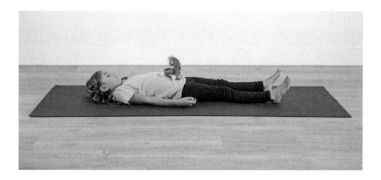

**Instructions:**

1. Let's go on a magic carpet ride using your breath!
2. Lie on your back.
3. Place a small bean bag on your belly button.
4. Place your stuffed animal on the bean bag so it's facing you.
5. The bean bag is your stuffed animal's magic carpet. Your mat is your magic carpet.
6. You can watch your stuffed animal go up and down on the magic carpet with your breath.
7. Breathe into your belly so your stuffed animal rises up towards the ceiling.
8. Breathe out and slowly let the air out of your belly as you watch your stuffed animal go back down.
9. Repeat 3–4 times.

### Sound Breathing

Sound breathing can be done through reciting vowel sounds, chakra sounds or animal sounds as well as when singing or chanting. Sound breathing supports extended exhalation and expression of voice and can also stimulate the vagus nerve in order to support up-regulation or down-regulation of the nervous system.

### Up-Regulating

It is important to consider the child's nervous system state when integrating up-regulating breathing practices. Rapid breathing, breath retention and breath holding are not recommended for children with significant anxiety. Such breathing practices could also be contraindicated for high blood pressure, epilepsy and heart, lung, eye and ear problems. It is important to know a child's medical information and any contraindications for breathing practices prior to beginning yoga therapy with them.

#### *Hum Breath or Bee Breath (Bhramari Pranayama)*

Hum Breath can be both down-regulating and up-regulating. Its vibrational sound provides stimulation to the vagus nerve which supports down-regulation, and it can also enhance feelings of joy, energy and vitality in both the mind and body. Offering different variations of the breath can offer different effects.

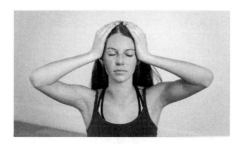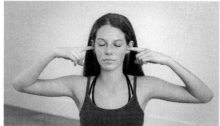
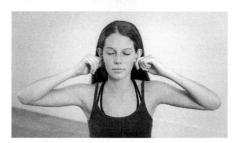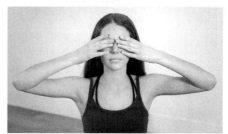

**Instructions:**

1. Think about the sound a beehive makes. It makes a humming sound.
2. We're going to hum just like a bee.
3. When we do Hum Breath, notice if you feel vibration in your body and where you feel it.
4. Sit up tall with your eyes closed or softly open.
5. Breathe in through your nose.
6. Close your lips with your teeth slightly apart.
7. Hum as long as you can until you feel you need to take a breath in.
8. Take a natural breath in and out.
9. Repeat 3–4 times or try different variations.
10. Notice if you feel differently with the different variations.

- Variation 1: Hands cupped over ears
- Variation 2: Pointer fingers pressing cartilage of ears to block sound
- Variation 3: Holding the earlobes and gently stretching them down
- Variation 4: Thumbs pressing cartilage of ears and fingers gently covering the eyes

### Elevator Breath

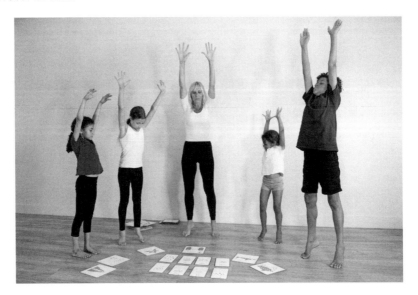

I created this breath for a child who loved elevators. The breath integrates breath retention on the inhalation, which is more energizing and up-regulating, as well as equal duration of the inhalation and exhalation. This breath also involves movement, so it can be more energizing.

**Instructions:**

1. Imagine being in an elevator, going up and down.
2. We're going to go to floor 3 on the elevator.
3. Squat down.
4. Breathe in through your nose, 1-2-3.
5. Come to standing and reach arms up.
6. Hold.
7. Breathe out through your mouth, 3-2-1.
8. Come back to a squatting position.
9. Repeat 3–4 times.
10. Check in and notice how you feel.
11. Option: Decrease or increase the number of floors you go to in order to meet the child's breathing capacity.

*Reach/Pull Breath*

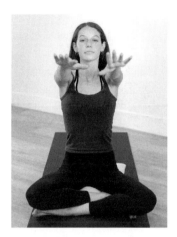 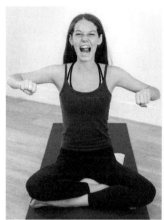

I call this Reach/Pull Breath. The intention of the breath is to extend the inhalation on the reach and exhale the breath quickly and forcefully on the pull. Because there is an extended inhalation and a forceful exhalation, this breath can be more alerting, energizing and empowering.

## Instructions:

1. This breath can be done seated on the floor, in a chair or standing.
2. Breathe in slowly through the nose as you reach your arms forward.
3. Breathe out quickly with an open mouth and make the sound "huh" sound as you pull your arms back.
4. The inhalation and reach should be slow and the exhalation and pull should be quick.
5. Repeat 3–4 times.
6. Check in and notice how you feel.

### Sun Breath — Alternate Nostril Breathing (Nadi Shodhana)

Ancient yogis ascertained that each nostril is connected to a *nadi*, which in Sanskrit translates to "river" or "flow." Each nostril corresponds to dominant activity that takes place in the opposite hemisphere of the brain. The left nostril is known as ida nadi, the lunar or moon channel. The moon is cooling and calming, which is why breathing into the left nostril is more down-regulating. The right nostril is known as pingala nadi, the solar or sun channel. The sun is heating and energizing, which is why breathing into the right nostril can be more up-regulating. Because each side correlates with the opposite hemisphere of the brain, nadi shodhana can support whole-brain integration.

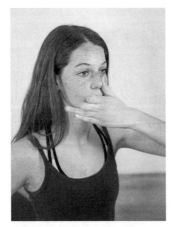 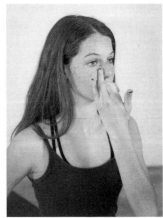

**Instructions:**

1. Sit up tall on the floor or in a chair.
2. Hold your right hand out in front of you, palm face up.
3. Bend your pointer and middle fingers in towards palm.
4. Place your ring finger on left nostril.
5. Exhale through right nostril.
6. Inhale through right nostril.
7. Place your thumb on right nostril and release your left nostril.
8. Exhale through left nostril.
9. Inhale through left nostril.
10. Place your ring finger on left nostril.
11. Exhale through right nostril.
12. Repeat 3–4 times.
13. Check in and notice how you feel.

Finger placement if the child is left-handed—left thumb on left nostril, breathe in through right.

*Lion's Breath (Simhasana)*
See Chapter 4.

## Breath of Joy
See Chapter 4.

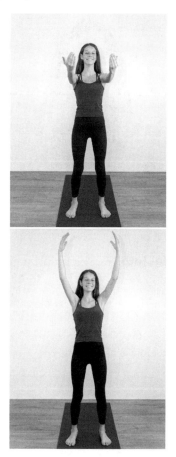
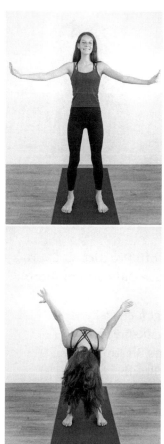
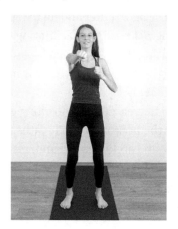
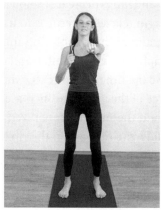

## Boxer Breath
See Chapters 4 and 5.

*Engine Breath: Voo and Waking the Bear Breath: Voo-Rarr*
See Chapter 8.

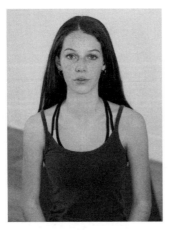 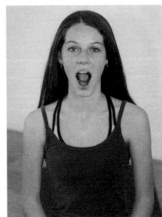

## Using Breath Practice to Express, Regulate and Release Difficult Emotions

- Dragon Breath
- Volcano Breath
- Lion's Breath
- Cat Breath
- Snake Breath
- Let it Go Breath
- I Don't Know, Let it Go Breath

### Mechanics of Breathing

The normal breathing process starts with the diaphragm. When the diaphragm, a dome-shaped muscle under the lungs, moves downward, the pressure in the thoracic cavity and lungs decreases, allowing the air to enter and fill the space. When the diaphragm relaxes, it returns to its original position, facilitating exhalation.

The amount of the air entering and exiting the body depends partially on the range of diaphragm movement. By relaxing and expanding the belly muscles, you can increase the range and breathe more deeply.

The force of the air can be increased or decreased by controlling the speed of breathing and the muscles mobilized for the breath. If you breathe in abruptly and forcefully, the muscles in the rib cage and abdomen expand, increasing the force of the breath.

Conversely, if you breathe out slowly and gently, the muscles in the airway, intercostal and abdominal regions relax, eliciting a calming effect on the mind and nervous system.

## Breathing Mechanics and Nervous System

The question is: What comes first, the chicken or the egg? Is it the breathing pattern that impacts the nervous system or the nervous system that impacts the breathing pattern? The answer to that question is *both*. Our nervous system states impact our musculature, breathing, sensory experience, emotion, thinking and behavior. If we are in a state of fight/flight, the musculature of our face, neck, shoulders and core becomes tense and hypervigilant. The rate of our heartbeat and breathing increases to prepare us to fight or flee. This in turn impacts our ability to breathe with ease. If we are in a state of freeze or immobilization, our respiration slows and becomes heavy and shallow, and our musculature can become more hypotonic and collapsed. If we are breathing rapidly, holding our breath or breathing in a more collapsed manner, this can directly impact our nervous system state. They both impact one another, so we work with regulating the child's nervous system states *and* changing abnormal breathing patterns.

## Abnormal Breathing Patterns and Practices

Irregular breathing patterns can be common in children with hypertonia and hypotonia, chronic progressive diseases, muscular dystrophies, spinal injuries, compromised spinal postures, asthma, anxiety disorders, sensory integration challenges, autism, ADHD and trauma histories.

## Reverse Breathing or Paradoxical Breathing

Paradoxical or reverse breathing is exactly what it sounds like. With correct diaphragmatic breathing, during the inhalation, the lungs expand and the diaphragm pushes down. This downward pressure causes the abdomen to expand outward. During the exhalation, the diaphragm compresses or moves up, which helps move air out of the lungs. When we breathe in, our belly should move out like a balloon filling with air, and when we breathe out, our belly should move in, with our belly button drawing closer to the spine. With reverse breathing, the belly moves in on the inhalation and out on the exhalation. The movement of the pelvic diaphragm is also reversed so the movement of the pelvic floor closes on the inhalation and opens on the exhalation (Farhi, 1996). This reversal of breathing can create confusion and tension in the mind and nervous system, eliciting an anxious or agitated response. Consider how tension in the body creates tension in the nervous system and the mind. Reverse breathers can also experience chronic tension in their neck, shoulders and upper back, muscles that become activated during sympathetic arousal. This can impact a child's sleep, energy level and ability to move with ease, often experiencing increased anxiety, fatigue and insomnia. Reverse breathing can also cause digestive issues such as indigestion, heartburn, bloating and flatulence (Farhi, 1996).

### Breath Practices

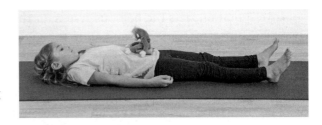

- Magic Carpet Breath
- Balloon Belly Breath
- Three-Part Breathing

## Chest Breathing or Constricted Breathing

Chest breathing is when we use the accessory muscles for breathing rather than the primary muscles of respiration. Chest breathing can elicit a fight/flight or sympathetic response in the nervous system which, when habitual, can impact our physical, mental and emotional wellbeing. Increased anxiety, hyperventilation and panic attacks correlate with habitual chest breathing.

### Breath Practices

- Three-Part Breathing
- Balloon Belly Breath
- Wave Breath

## Collapsed Breathing

Imagine a slouched and depressed posture with shoulders rolling forward in a protective manner, the chest drawn forward, forward head posture, the belly projecting outward, and low tone in the core and lower limbs. With collapsed breathing, there is more of a depressive breath, small puffs of air in and out with the chest and shoulders moving up and down in a stagnant manner. Collapsed breathers may sigh and gasp for air often in an attempt to get more oxygen. Collapsed breathing can be connected to more of a "freeze" response or disassociation from the body. This is also a breath that you might observe when someone is experiencing grief and loss. Collapsed breathing can also be connected to a child or teen's lack of confidence or trust in themselves, which can be a result of trauma or ongoing experiences of being bullied, ostracized or feeling that they don't "fit in." It can also be a common breath you might see with children or teens who are more low tone and whose posture tends to be more "floppy" and less engaged.

### Asana and Breath Practices

- Rooting and rising breath practices (grounding feet down and rising up with the breath)
- Asana in which you ground down and move the energy upward—Mountain Peak (Hasta Tadasana)
- Heart/Belly Breathing
- Elevator Breath
- Grounding Breath

## Hyperventilation

Hyperventilation can be subtle and chronic. With habitual hyperventilation, we breathe rapidly with short, constricted breaths. With hyperventilation, the diaphragm does not descend completely, which reduces the space in the chest and lungs for the breath to expand into. This creates a chain response of breathing more breaths, more rapidly, due to lack of oxygen intake. This in turn causes us to lose too much carbon dioxide, which shifts our metabolism from acid to alkaline and can have a significant impact on our physiological functions. Hyperventilation also causes a fight/flight response in the nervous system and, when habitual, can have significant effects on the mind, body and emotions.

### Breath Practices

#### Pursed Lip or Cool the Soup Breathing

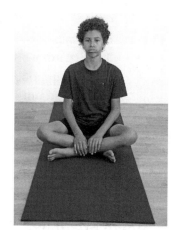

Pursed Lip Breathing focuses on slowing the breath down and making the breath longer and more intentional. When the breath is slow and elongated, it reduces the work of breathing by keeping the airways open longer. This makes it easier for the lungs to function and improves the exchange of oxygen and carbon dioxide (Gotter, 2018). Pursed Lip Breathing can be helpful for alleviating symptoms of asthma, anxiety and insomnia.

**Instructions:**

1. Sit up tall.
2. Breathe in through the nose for a count of 2.
3. Fill your belly with air.
4. Purse your lips as if you're blowing on hot soup to cool it down.
5. Breathe out slowly through pursed lips for the count of 4.
6. Repeat 2–3 times.

- Balloon Belly Breath
- 2-4 Breath or Extended Exhalation
- Heart/Belly Breathing

## Breath Holding

Breath holding is common in our society. We often hold our breath when anticipating something exciting, when we are nervous, afraid or startled, or as a habitual breathing pattern when the nervous system is stuck in a hypervigilant state. This pattern of breathing can continue the sympathetic feedback loop and keep our nervous system in a state of high alert. This can be a common pattern when a child has experienced significant trauma. There will often be signs of bracing and rigidity in the upper torso, shoulders drawing up and increased tone in musculature of the neck and face.

### Breath Practices

#### Open Mouth Breath or Cleansing Breath

Cleansing Breath can be a great breath practice to release built-up tension or stress in the body and down-regulate the nervous system. In fact, when we sigh or do an open mouth breath unconsciously, this can be a sign of down-regulation of the nervous system. So when we do an open mouth or cleansing breath, it can be a message to the brain that everything is okay right now.

### Instructions:

1. Sit up tall.
2. Take a natural breath in.
3. Open your mouth and go "haaa," extending the exhalation.
4. Breathe out until you feel the impulse to breathe in.
5. Repeat 3–4 times.

- Wave Breath
- Balloon Belly Breath
- 2-4 Breath or Extended Exhalation

## Mouth Breathing

Mouth breathing is a pattern of breathing in through the mouth and out through the mouth. Breathing in through the nose allows us to take fuller, deeper breaths into the lower lungs which stimulates the parasympathetic branch of the nervous system, whereas mouth breathing is more in the upper chest area, which elicits more of a sympathetic or fight/flight response and can lead to hyperactivity and restlessness. Mouth breathing can impact our sleep and body's ability to feel rested and is often associated with sleep apnea. Breathing through the nose also filters the air before it enters the body of allergens, bacteria and viruses, which supports a stronger and more protected immune system.

### Breath Practices
#### Flower/Wind Breath
This breath supports children with learning how to breathe in through the nose. This is a breath that I often use to first introduce children to proper breathing because there is a cause-and-effect experience they have with the breath practice.

**Instructions:**

1. Sit up tall.
2. Take the tips of your fingers together in one hand and imagine your hand is a flower.
3. Bring your hand to your nose and breathe in like you're sniffing the flower.
4. Open your hand and face your palm towards you.
5. Breathe out like you're blowing wind on your hand.
6. Did you feel the wind on your hand?
7. Repeat 3–4 times.

- Alternate Nostril Breathing
- Wave Breath
- Open Mouth Breath

#### Mindful Breathing
The power of mindful breathing should not be underestimated. Just bringing attention to the breath can shift a child's nervous system state out of fight/flight and into a more regulated state. Some children or teens may respond more intensely to certain breath practices for up-regulating and down-regulating—in particular, children who have experienced significant trauma and/or who have become accustomed to a specific breathing pattern. Mindful breathing might be the best place to start, just to bring awareness to their breath rather than expecting them to change their breathing. Encouraging a child to do mindful breathing can give them more insight into their patterns of breathing and can also help you to track their patterns of breathing so you know what types of breathing practices would be most supportive to them. Our breath can be a helpful internal resource, especially when we pay attention to the changes in our breath as our nervous system settles.

We can also track our nervous system state by becoming aware of moments when our breath becomes more restricted or rapid. Mindful breathing can also support interoceptive awareness and mind–body connection. Often, just bringing awareness to our breath can support one-point focus and more meditative practices. Mindful breathing can be practiced lying down or seated.

**Instructions:**

1. Sit up tall.
2. Close your eyes or keep them softly open.
3. Take a moment to notice your breath.
4. Just breathe naturally.
5. Notice when you are breathing in.
6. Notice when you are breathing out.
7. When you breathe in, are your lips closed or open?
8. When you breathe out, are your lips closed or open?
9. Where do you feel your breath in your body when you breathe in?
10. What do you notice about your breathing?
11. How does it feel to you to bring attention to your breath?

---

**PAUSE AND REFLECT**

Experience the mindful breathing practice for yourself. Notice your breath without the need to fix or change. Bring awareness and attention to your breath, then inquire about your own breathing patterns with compassion and curiosity.

What did you notice?

Option to journal about your experience.

---

# Chapter 8

# Trauma, Nature and Resilience

It wasn't until my 40s that I truly gained an understanding of just how much early traumatic events and experiences had impacted my emotional, mental and physical wellbeing throughout adolescence and into adulthood. As I learned more about the parts of our nervous system and how they respond to trauma, particularly in our early formative years, I was able to link my lifelong struggle with anxiety, my disconnection from my body and my experience with autoimmune issues since childhood. As I began to understand all of the ways in which my brain and body had worked so hard to help me survive, I felt less shame and more compassion for myself. It was in my own ability to show up for my younger self with tenderness, empathy, curiosity and care that true repair and healing has taken place.

## TRAUMA DEFINED

Because of its complexity, it can be difficult to identify one singular definition of trauma.

We often think of trauma as a specific event, but, in fact, trauma is not the actual event, rather our nervous system's response to an overwhelming event or a series of events.

According to Peter Levine:

Traumatic symptoms are not caused by the event itself. They arise when residual energy from the experience is not discharged from the body. The energy remains trapped in the nervous system where it can wreak havoc on our bodies and our minds.

(Levine, n.d.a)

Essentially, trauma occurs when a person's system goes into overwhelm and they have not been able to complete the defensive responses necessary in order to come back to equilibrium. The body and nervous system can become stuck in a fight/flight or freeze state and it can be difficult for the person to connect with the physiological sensations in the body and regulate states of arousal.

According to Peter Levine:

> Trauma happens when the organism is strained beyond its adaptational capacity to regulate states of arousal. The (traumatized) nervous system disorganizes, breaks down and cannot reset itself. This manifests in a fundamental loss in the rhythmic capacity to self-regulate arousal, to orient, to be in the present and to flow in life.
>
> (Levine, n.d.a)

Trauma is the antithesis of choice and empowerment. An individual's response to trauma can often result in feelings of helplessness, hopelessness, lack of choice and disconnection from their authentic self. Many traumatized people have difficulty experiencing pleasure and joy or in experiencing sensation or emotion altogether. They may struggle with boundaries, relationships with others and knowing themselves on a deeper level.

According to Bessel van der Kolk, trauma is something that happens to us that overwhelms us and causes us to feel unsafe. It is not the actual event, but how we respond to the event. He emphasizes that the largest mitigating factor against becoming traumatized is "who is there for you in that moment" and "what is your experience of the foundation of safety" (van der Kolk, 2021).

This perspective not only takes into account how our bodies and nervous systems respond to overwhelming events, but also emphasizes the relational and environmental factors to whether or not we become traumatized.

He highlights the importance of feeling safety in our bodies and experiencing safety with others.

Therein lies the question: How do we help people to live in bodies that feel fundamentally safe?

## Types of Trauma

Trauma has recently gained a lot of attention in the mental health field as well as in education and child development. As adults who work with children and teens, it is crucial that we have an understanding of trauma and how it impacts children's physiology, mood, behavior and overall wellbeing. When we understand trauma, we may understand ourselves a bit more and we can be better prepared to support children and teens from a trauma-informed and trauma-sensitive lens. It can be helpful to understand the different types or categories of trauma.

**Shock trauma:** A sudden or unexpected event that occurs very quickly and without warning, which overwhelms the system. With shock trauma, the event is too hard, too fast, sudden and unexpected. Some examples of shock trauma include:

- car or bicycle accident
- sudden loss or death of a loved one
- violent or sexual assault
- an unexpected medical diagnosis
- hospitalization or medical surgery or procedure
- witnessing or experiencing a frightening or horrific event
- experiencing a fall, serious injury or illness
- experiencing or witnessing a life-threatening event
- a frightening or near-death experience for the mother or baby during childbirth.

**Developmental trauma:** The impact of early, repeated trauma and loss which happens within the child's important relationships. Examples of developmental trauma include:

- neglect and abandonment
- physical or emotional abuse
- sexual abuse
- witnessing physical violence in the home
- growing up around caretakers with mental illness or substance abuse
- overly strict upbringing
- losing a parent due to divorce, abandonment, incarceration or death
- death of a close family member (parent, sibling)
- not having basic needs met (food, clothing, shelter)
- growing up in an unsafe home or community.

**Intergenerational trauma**: A concept developed to help explain generational challenges within families. The transmission (or sending down to younger generations) of the oppressive or traumatic effects of historical events within the family generations (APA Dictionary of Psychology, n.d.).

To simplify, a parent or grandparent may have experienced trauma that they were never able to resolve or heal from, so the effects of the trauma are passed down through the generations to the child.

**Collective trauma:** A traumatic event or history of events that is shared by a group of people.

**Societal trauma:** The trauma a person or group of people can experience from being ostracized, bullied, belittled or made to think they are "less than" according to society's idea of who is valuable/invaluable or "normal"/not normal. Examples of collective or societal trauma include:

- exposure to community violence
- global traumas such as pandemics, natural disasters and war
- mass shootings
- being a target of racism, homophobia, sexism and/or ableism
- being bullied
- living in a society where you are treated "less than" others.

### Impact of Trauma and Approaches to Healing

**PTSD** is included in the DSM-5, in the category of Trauma and Stressor Related Disorders. According to the DSM-5, there are specific criteria that must be met in order to receive a PTSD diagnosis. All areas of the criteria must be met. These criteria are specific to adults, adolescents and children over the age of 6.

Some of the symptoms of PTSD in children might include:

- nightmares and difficulty with sleep
- reliving the event over in their thoughts or through play
- intrusive thoughts
- hypervigilance
- avoidance of anything that is a reminder of the trauma
- lost interest in things that they once enjoyed
- difficulty with focus and learning
- intense and ongoing fear or sadness
- anxiety or depression
- dissociation
- increased neuroception of danger
- irritability and angry outbursts
- withdrawal from others
- regression such as bed-wetting, thumbsucking
- increased worry about death and dying
- physical symptoms such as headaches, stomachaches.

(McLaughlin, 2022)

Because PTSD can be expressed differently according to a child's developmental age, the DSM-5 now includes a developmental subtype of PTSD called "Post Traumatic Stress Disorder in preschool children." Because younger children have emerging abstract, cognitive and verbal expression capacities, the change in criteria is more behaviorally anchored and developmentally sensitive to detect PTSD in preschool-age children (U.S. Department of Veterans Affairs, n.d.).

It is important to note that we each respond to traumatic events differently, depending on our past experiences, upbringing, available support systems, unique sensory and nervous systems, and our capacity to respond to unexpected or prolonged stressors or events. An event could cause a traumatic response for one person and that same or similar experience or event may not cause a traumatic response for another person. There is an ongoing debate about whether or not one's capacity to bounce back more easily from traumatic events or prolonged stress is related to nature or nurture—nature being the unique personality and characteristics we are born with and nurture being our experiences at an early age with our primary caregiver/s.

Either way, it is apparent that trauma impacts not only our perception of ourselves and the world around us and how we engage with the world, but also our physiology and how we *feel* in the world. Recent research has shown the importance of bottom-up and somatic-based approaches in addressing trauma (Kuhfuß *et al.*, 2021). There is a saying, "We have to feel it to heal it." This makes sense when we consider the hierarchy of the brain and how and when we are able to access the "thinking and reasoning" part of the brain versus our survival brain. We experienced sensations long before we developed the language to communicate what we were feeling. Only through bottom-up approaches can we address the physiological impact of trauma and stress on the body and nervous system.

Bruce Perry (2020) discusses this in his sequence of engagement. According to Dr. Perry, this concept is based on two major principles:

1.  The initial sequence of processing of all experience from lower to higher networks in the brain (bottom-up).
2.  State-dependent functioning of the brain.

Perry asserts that if the lower brain is not regulated and well organized, the higher brain regions, such as the cortex, cannot function efficiently. Perry emphasizes this hierarchy of processing in the brain to parents and educators. Our education system often fails to support children and teens by over-emphasizing top-down processes in learning with standardized testing, outdated grading systems and top-down scaffolding rather than focusing on helping children to feel regulated and engaged in their environment prior to expecting them to think, reason and learn (see Figure 8.1).

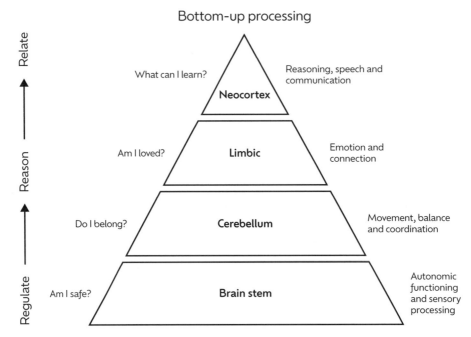

**Figure 8.1** Bottom-up processing
*Source: Adapted from Bruce Perry's Neurosequential Model*

My vision and dream is that every school takes a bottom-up approach to education by supporting our children's social-emotional health and helping them build emotional intelligence as a foundation for learning. Integrating yoga and mindfulness practices in schools is a step in the right direction. In fact, growing research suggests that yoga and mindfulness in the school setting is a viable and potentially efficacious strategy for improving child and adolescent health (Khalsa & Butzer, 2016).

Educating children and adolescents about how their brains work and the impact of unmanaged stress on their emotional, physical and mental wellbeing, while empowering them with tools to manage stress and regulate their emotions, can only benefit the children, educators, the education system and community as a whole. More empowered, embodied, compassionate and regulated youth = more empowered, embodied, compassionate and regulated community members and leaders.

It can be helpful for children and teens to understand the functions and roles of the different parts of their brain. Knowledge of the brain and its functions not only provides insight to why we may feel big emotions and experience dysregulation, but it can also reduce shame and empower us in learning tools for how to shift our states of regulation.

**MY BRAIN**

*My brain is an amazing organ*
*With so many parts that help it function*
*My amygdala is my alarm system*
*That tells me if there's danger I'm in*
*My hippocampus tells me how I'm feeling*
*My cortex helps me think and reason*
*Sometimes my amygdala is in charge*
*And makes me feel like small problems are large*
*When it takes over I can lose control*
*My heart starts to race and my mind starts to roll*
*All of my reasoning goes out the door*
*I might kick or stomp the floor*
*I can bring my cortex back online*
*Let my amygdala know everything is fine*
*I can take a breath in and breathe out slow*
*Move my body to and fro*
*Feel my emotions I'm feeling inside*
*Then let them out with a sigh*
*Remind my amygdala that its OK*
*Let my body rock and sway*
*Feel my feet on the ground*
*Use my eyes to look around*
*Let my amygdala take a rest*
*So my cortex can do its best*
*To help me learn and think and grow*
*So I feel more in the flow*

Shawnee Thornton Hardy

## WHAT IS ACES?

ACES stands for Adverse Childhood Experiences. In 1998, the *American Journal of Preventative Medicine* published a groundbreaking study that investigated the impact of ACEs on physical and mental health problems in over 17,000 adults. During the study, the adults were given a survey asking about ten different types of ACEs and if they had experienced them prior to the age of 18. The study showed a direct correlation between ACEs and future health complications (Felliti *et al.*, 1998).

The ten different types of ACEs are :

- physical abuse
- emotional abuse
- sexual abuse
- physical neglect
- emotional neglect
- mental illness of a parent/caregiver
- incarcerated parent/caregiver
- domestic violence in the home
- substance abuse by parent/caregiver
- divorce or loss of a parent/caregiver.

The higher the ACE score, the higher the risk for physical illness, mental illness and addiction in adulthood.

Physically, childhood trauma has been associated with autoimmune disease, cardiovascular disease, gastrointestinal symptoms, type 2 diabetes, poor dental health and obesity (Jiang *et al.*, 2019).

Childhood trauma has also been associated with many mental disorders including PTSD, anxiety, depression, insomnia, bipolar disorder, borderline personality disorder, disruptive behaviors, risky behaviors, antisocial behavior, substance abuse and eating disorders (Jiang *et al.*, 2019).

In 2012 and 2013, members came together to develop the Philadelphia Expanded ACE study to understand the impact of community-level adversities. The expanded ACE study includes:

- bullying
- experienced discrimination
- community violence
- living in foster care
- neighborhood safety.

The demographic of the initial ACE's study and the Philadelphia Expanded ACE study differed in that the majority of the participants in the original study were white, college educated and middle-income whereas in the Philadelphia study, roughly a quarter of the residents live in poverty.

The results of the study showed that 40 percent of Philadelphians had scored 4 or more on the ACE score (The Philadelphia ACE Project, n.d.).

It is clear that a child's wellbeing is impacted not only by their home environment but by their experiences in their community and society as a whole. We know that an individual's nervous system state is impacted by whether or not they feel a sense of safety and belonging in the world. We may not be able to change a child's circumstances at home or in the systems in which they navigate the world, but we can do our best to create an environment of safety and inclusion and be the supportive adult figure that the child or teen may not have or have had in their past experiences.

A high ACE score *does not* mean we will not be able to thrive in life.

Healing can come at any age and stage in life. That being said, early prevention and intervention can make a significant difference in whether or not a child is able to thrive. We may not be able to prevent trauma from happening, but we can do our best to give children and teens the tools and support to manage stress so their window of tolerance is bigger and they are able to come back to homeostasis or what Stephen Porges (2021b) refers to as health, growth and restoration.

## PAUSE AND REFLECT

Take a moment to check in and notice how the information about ACEs is landing in your own body. As you were reading about adverse childhood experiences, you may have been reflecting on your own experience as a child. You may have come to the realization that you tick off some or many of the adverse experiences listed. What do you notice in your body as you reflect on that? Now, picture your younger self in your mind, place your hands on your heart and say these words: "I'm sorry you went through what you did. You were just a child and you should have been protected. I am here now to acknowledge what you went through and to love and support you. We are a team. We can heal together."

What do you notice in your body when you say these words to yourself?

Invitation to write about your reflection and experience in your journal.

The emphasis with ACEs in early childhood is to:

- prevent trauma from occurring
- address trauma as soon as possible when it has occurred
- help build capacity and resilience in youth to increase their window of tolerance and manage life's stressors and any future trauma.

An essential factor in working with children who have experienced trauma is being a safe and consistent base of support. I liken this to being a flotation device for the child to go to for safety or the island in the middle of the ocean that can provide a sense of stability, predictability and safety. Peter Levine states that "trauma is not what happens to us, but what we hold inside in the absence of an empathetic witness" (Levine, n.d.b). We all have the need to feel seen, heard and understood. When we can show up for the children and teens we work with and bear witness to their pain and suffering, with compassion and empathy, we let their nervous system know that they are safe, they are supported and that someone is there to witness their struggles and celebrate their triumphs.

In John Bowlby's research on attachment, he uses the terms "safe haven" and "secure base" to refer to a child's felt sense of safety in their environment and with their primary caregiver (Kain & Terrel, 2018). More often than not, when a child has experienced trauma, particularly developmental trauma, there is an absence of safety with the adults in their life or within their environment. We can be that secure base and create a safe haven for them to experience safety and connection.

## CONNECTION

Developing a connection with the child or teen is the foundation for working therapeutically with them. When children feel a felt sense of connection, trust and safety, they are more likely to engage, explore and open their world to you. Think of connection as the foundation of a building. You have to lay the foundation before building the structure. Many children who have experienced developmental trauma may present as guarded, protected, distrusting and cautious of other adults. Going back to the metaphor of sticks and snakes, their neuroception of the world may be that every adult in their life is a snake. Patience, compassion and understanding are necessary ingredients in building connection, trust and a felt sense of safety with the child. We can build connection through attunement, tracking, mirroring, collaboration, co-regulation, love and play.

### Attunement

Attunement is the reactiveness we have to another person. It is the process by which we form relationships. According to Daniel Siegel, Madeleine Siegel and Suzanne Parker:

> When we attune with others we allow our own nervous system states to shift, to become resonant with the inner world of another. This resonance is at the heart of the important sense of "feeling felt" that emerges in close relationships.

(Siegel, Siegel, & Parker, 2016)

Children need attunement to feel secure and to develop well. We need attunement from and with others throughout our lives to feel close and connected. With developmental trauma, there is often lack of attunement from the primary caregiver. There is quite a bit of reparative work we can do just in attuning to the child and their needs.

## Behind Every Behavior Is a Need

I'll share a story with an example of attunement and identifying the need behind a behavior. I had a young girl in my program, age 12, who had experienced significant abuse and neglect early on. She had been in and out of group homes and foster homes her whole life. She had some learning delays, but her primary challenge was her dysregulation and acting-out behaviors, in both her school and home environments. I knew building a relationship of trust and creating an environment of compassion and safety were critical to her success in school, as well as her stability and placement in her current foster home. We worked a lot on self-regulation, communication, healthy boundaries and self-agency. This is a child who had the survival need to be in control, because, more often than not, she did not have control over decisions in her life, such as how she would be treated by others, where she would live and so on. She also did not have a choice when she was younger and experienced extreme abuse and neglect.

One day, I came into the classroom and she was yelling at an assistant, threatening to stab them with a pencil. My response was "You seem really upset. I want to help you. What is upsetting you?" She yelled, "She took my pencil away from me!" The assistant quietly let me know that she had taken her own pencil out of her pencil box and was upset that the assistant had taken the pencil away from her.

One of the rules in our classroom was that you had to use the classroom pencils, due to escalated behaviors when students brought and used their own pencils. On one hand, I wanted to maintain the rule or expectation of no personal pencils in the classroom. On the other hand, I recognized that when the assistant took the pencil away from her, it sent her into a fight response, an understandable survival response coming from a young girl who only had a few possessions and throughout her life had been bounced from one place to another. This pencil was a representation of safety to her. It was "her" pencil and she was fighting for what was hers.

My response to the young girl was "I know that pencil is really important to you. I want it to be in a safe place so you don't lose it and you know where you can find it when you get home. Where would you like to put your pencil, in the front pocket of your backpack or the middle pocket?" She quickly began to de-escalate and responded, "In the front pocket."

Her experience of being seen and understood by me and being given the choice of where to put her pencil took her out of her survival response into an experience of connection and empowerment, and I was still able to hold a boundary with her about the classroom rules. Later in the day, she came up to me, gave me a hug and said, "I love you, Ms. Thornton."

A simple moment of attunement and looking for the need behind the behavior helped to strengthen her feelings of trust and safety with me. I've remembered the importance of this moment years later.

## Tracking

Tracking means the ability for us to recognize and follow our own nervous system states as well as track the nervous systems of the children we work with. This comes with attention, awareness and practice. Our own consistent practices of mindfulness and self-reflection can support us in developing greater intuition and attunement to a child's nervous system. Often, children who have experienced trauma may not have the capacity to use words to express what they are feeling. If we are working with children who struggle with language and communication, we need to have the ability to track their nervous systems so we can be attuned to their needs. As we track, we notice moments of arousal, activation, shutting down or settling. This provides important information that can guide us in our sessions.

### What to Observe and Notice

- Facial expressions
- Rapid eye movement, fixated eyes or a "checked-out" gaze
- Change in skin tone
- Bracing in musculature
- Rigidity in the joints
- Breathing patterns
- Movement impulses
- Verbal sounds or expressions
- Signs of down-regulation or settling (diaphragmatic breathing, softening of musculature, relaxed face or smiling, signs of digestion (e.g. stomach gurgling, burping), normal skin tone, yawns or sighs, relaxed eyes, more mobility in the joints, more cohesive movement in the body)

**PAUSE AND REFLECT**

Take a moment to track your nervous system. Notice the musculature, breathing and internal sensations in your body. Notice your heartbeat, the temperature of your skin and any other sensations that are present. Allow a bit of time to be curious and notice without the need to judge, fix or change. As you observe, notice if there are any shifts in your nervous system as you bring your attention to your experience. Explore with non-judgment and curiosity.

Invitation to write about your experience in your journal.

### Mirroring

Mirroring is the behavior in which one person imitates the gesture, movement, speech pattern or behaviors of others. Mirroring supports connection, attunement and development of imitation skills. Imitation is a skill that infants develop early on through mirroring their primary caregivers' facial expressions, sounds and behaviors. Mirror neurons are neurons that fire both when an action is performed and when you see someone do the same action. Mirror neurons also cause us to feel emotion when we see another person experiencing the emotion. This neuronal firing is what enables babies to imitate, learn new skills, connect with others and develop empathy for others. Children learn how to engage in the world through "imitating" or mirroring their caregivers and peers. If there is a lack of attunement early on, the child may not have had the opportunity to develop imitation skills. If a child has struggled with attention, sensory processing and learning, their ability to imitate can also be impacted. The ability to imitate is necessary in learning new skills. This is particularly important in working with neurodivergent children and children who have experienced developmental trauma. When we do mirroring activities with the child, we meet them where they are at and we let them know that we are there to walk alongside them on their journey rather than walking ahead of them. We also help them to build attention, connection and empathy.

### Collaboration

Collaboration is a key element in building trust and healthy connection. Working together towards a common goal creates a sense of connection, support and interdependence with another.

## Co-regulation

Co-regulation is defined as warm and responsive interactions that provide the support, coaching, modeling and nervous system regulation needed to understand, express and modulate thoughts, feelings and behaviors. When babies are first developing, they rely on their primary caregiver to be their co-regulator, to attune and attend to their needs whenever they express a need. Gradually, as they continue to develop, they begin to learn ways to self-regulate (if they have a caregiver who consistently attends to their needs and supports them with co-regulation). As adults working with children and teens, we are the co-regulators. Our own capacity and ability to self-regulate will impact our ability to be effective co-regulators for the children. As we lend our own regulated systems to the children and teens we work with, they can then begin to learn tools to self-regulate on their own.

### Activities to Support Connection

#### Mirroring
**Instructions:**

1. Sit face-to-face with the child.
2. Hold your palms up facing the child and invite them to place their palms in front of yours, close but not touching.
3. Tell them you are going to move your hands and they can do the same movements as you.
4. Do simple and slow movements, so the child can follow and imitate.
5. As you do the mirroring activity, track your nervous system and the child's nervous system.
6. Tell the child that they now get a turn to lead and you will follow their movements.
7. Mirror their movements.
8. Continue to track and notice any shifts in their nervous system.

#### Scarves in the Wind
**Materials:** A colored scarf.

**Instructions:**

1. Sit face-to-face with the child.
2. Hold a colored scarf in your hand.
3. Tell the child you are going to play Scarves in the Wind.

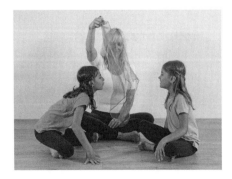

4. Demonstrate breathing in, then blowing on the scarf gently so it moves towards the child.
5. Tell the child it's their turn to blow the scarf towards you.
6. Continue blowing the scarf back and forth.
7. Track and notice both your nervous system and the child's as you do the activity together.

### Move the Ball

**Materials:** A light ball that can fit in the palm of the child's hand.

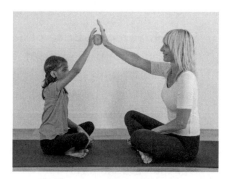

**Option:** Use a smooth ball or a ball that has some texture to it.

**Instructions:**

1. Sit facing the child.
2. Tell them you are going to work together to move the ball.
3. Bring the ball to the palm of your hand and invite the child to press their palm to the ball so you are both holding the ball between your palms.
4. Tell them you need to work together to move the ball without dropping it.
5. Begin to move your hand and encourage the child to move with you. Keep the ball between your palms.
6. Allow the child to initiate the movement and you follow their lead. Keep the ball between your palms.
7. Track and notice both your nervous system and the child's as you do the activity together.

### Back-to-Back Breathing
**Instructions:**

1. Tell the child you are going to do back-to-back breathing.
2. Sit in a criss-cross position with your back against the child's back.
3. Tell the child you are going to breathe together.
4. You can use verbal instruction initially, saying "breathe in, breathe out" to the child as you breathe in and out.
5. Invite the child to see if they can feel your breath and breathe in and out with you.

6. Tell the child it's their turn to breathe in and out and you will follow their breath.

7. Track and notice both your nervous system and the child's as you do the activity together.

### Partner Poses

Partner poses are a wonderful way to build connection and encourage collaboration, working together to support one another in the poses! See Chapter 5.

## Safe Haven and Base of Support
### Creating a Container of Safety

The second most essential element of working with children and teens who have experienced trauma is to create a container of safety or a "safe haven." This includes the environment in which the child is working with you as well as the relationship they have with you as a teacher or therapist. Creating a felt sense of connection, predictability and safety should be at the forefront of everything else. Our approach should always be trauma-informed and trauma-sensitive regardless of whether we are aware of a history of trauma or not.

## WHAT DOES IT MEAN TO BE TRAUMA-SENSITIVE AND TEACH FROM A TRAUMA-SENSITIVE LENS?
### Recognizing Diverse Learning Styles

When teaching yoga, somatic movement and mindfulness to children and teens, it's important to recognize that all children learn in different ways. Some are visual learners, some tactile learners, some auditory learners, some kinesthetic learners and many are a combination of several or all. Get to know what learning style each child has and honor the many ways in which children learn by teaching through multiple modalities:

- integrate all of the senses
- model
- use visual supports
- use tactile supports
- use auditory supports
- let them experience kinesthetically, through a hands-on approach
- have the necessary supports available for children with diverse communication needs
- repetition.

## Inclusive and Accessible Language

Words have so much power. We can use words to support and uplift or we can use words that may cause harm or disempower children. Consider the language you use as a teacher and the impact certain words can have on a child's nervous system and perception of self.

Words to avoid include:

- "Can't"—instead, say, "You can try...or you can try...whatever feels best to you."
- "I want you to"—instead, give direct and concrete language such as "Reach your hands up, bring your hands down" or use invitational language such as "You might want to..."
- Try not to imply that all children live with their parents or have a mom and dad. Many children live in single-parent homes, with aunts, uncles, grandparents, etc. and families are all different. Avoid, for example, saying do this with "your parents." Instead, say, "Practice these poses with your family or with your loved ones."
- Be intentional with your use of language. Instead of saying "Great job," be specific: "You are working so hard on balancing on one leg!"
- Offer choices through language to support self-agency and empowerment.

## Teaching from a Cultural Lens

Children come with many cultural backgrounds, races and ethnicities. Being inclusive of children's race, culture and ethnic background is important in creating a space for children to feel seen, heard, loved and equally valued. There are several ways to create an open, accepting and inclusive space for children of diverse backgrounds:

- Use diverse stories and books that represent a diverse community.
- Have children share about themselves and their culture with you. Integrate what the child shares in your sessions.
- Use visuals and images that represent a diverse community.
- Have an awareness of language that could be oppressive or create separateness.

## Trauma-Sensitive Teaching

When teaching yoga to children, it is always important to come from a trauma-sensitive lens. We often may not know the stories or histories of trauma with the children we work with, but we can have the intention of creating a safe space for children where they feel supported and connected.

- Connection, attunement and co-regulation
- Front-load information (write schedule, use visuals)
- Front-load expectations
- Create a predictable environment and routine
- Use invitational language
- Offer choices
- Be cautious with touch (always ask for consent)
- Be cautious with using sound and scents
- Recognize if certain poses, breathing strategies or activities are triggering to a child
- Encourage healthy expression of emotion
- Work with self-empowerment and self-agency
- Support them with boundaries (theirs and others)
- Teach to their skills

### Lens of Compassion

When we come from a lens of compassion and do our best in creating a space where children feel seen, heard, loved and equally valued, they will have more of a felt sense of safety and connection, their social engagement systems (ventral vagal) will be more online, and they will be willing to explore their worlds with curiosity, develop healthy relationships with others and experience more optimal mental, emotional and physical health and wellbeing.

## WHAT IS SOMATIC EXPERIENCING?

Somatic Experiencing® (SE), developed by Peter Levine, is a body-centered approach to treating trauma. The primary goal of SE is to modify the trauma-related stress response through bottom-up processing. It offers a framework to assess where a person is "stuck" in the fight, flight or freeze response and provides tools to help resolve fixated physiological states. The SE approach facilitates the completion of self-protective motor responses and the release of thwarted survival energy bound in the body (Somatic Experiencing® International, n.d.). The client's attention is directed toward internal sensations (interoception, proprioception and kinesthesia), rather than solely focusing on cognitive or emotional experiences.

Some key elements of SE are:

- resourcing
- orienting
- grounding
- self-contact

- tracking
- pendulation
- titration.

## Resourcing

Resourcing refers to ways we strengthen our sense of stability and safety in the world, connecting to safety and wholeness. We can have both internal and external resources. Resourcing can be an effective strategy to use at the start of a session with a child as well as a suggested practice outside of sessions.

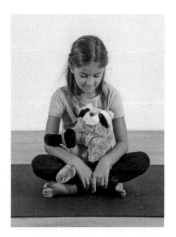

It can be helpful to have the child or teen list external and internal resources to refer to during their sessions or in their home/school/community environment.

### External

- Safe/peaceful place
- Nurturing memory, image or color
- Toys, stuffed animals or other objects that child or teen feels connected to
- Nurturing person or animal (parent, caregiver, grandparent, sibling, relative, friend, teacher, coach, pet)
- Protector figures (superheroes, angels, cartoon or book characters)
- Animal protectors

### Internal

- Pleasant or more neutral sensations
- Key intrinsic characteristics
- Qualities of personality or physical nature that the child or teen feels proud of or sees as positive qualities.

## Orienting

In the context of SE, the focus with orienting is developing more accurate neuroception in the present. According to Bessel van der Kolk (2015), trauma is fundamentally a disturbance in the ability to be in the here and now. He states that when something reminds traumatized people of the past, their brain reacts as if the traumatic event were happening in the present. With trauma, there is no sense of time. It can feel as if we are stuck in a perpetual state of danger and dysregulation. Orienting to safety and the present moment helps our survival brain know that we are safe in the here and now. This can help shift a child's neuroception of danger to a neuroception of safety. Orienting to the here and now can also bring a child out of fight/flight or freeze and into a more ventral vagal state.

It is important to note that visual orienting is not always an appropriate or accessible practice. For some children whose eyes have been so heightened and fixated towards danger and threat, visual orienting may not feel safe and can even feel dysregulating. Depending on a child's unique sensory system, other forms of orienting may not feel safe for them. Orienting can be experienced in many ways, through different senses. It is recommended that you explore orienting with each of the senses with the child in order to see which one is most comfortable for them. Once more safety and stabilization is established, then you may explore other ways of orienting that were not as accessible at the start.

### Orienting to Safety and the Present Moment

- Orienting visually to environment (what they see that is pleasant, soothing or neutral)
- Orienting to sensory experiences (what they see, smell, taste, feel, hear in the moment)
- Orienting to a person of safety (face, voice, image or memory)
- Orienting to an item of safety (e.g. favorite stuffed animal, pet, toy)

## Grounding

Grounding is the practice of feeling contact and connection with your seat, your feet, your body, the ground, the container that is supporting you and the earth. Grounding supports a feeling of embodiment. Often with anxiety and trauma, there can be an experience of not feeling connected to the ground or a feeling of not being in your body.

### Ways to facilitate grounding

- Weight on the body
- Self-contact
- Pressing feet and hands into a surface
- Lying down prone or supine
- Sitting or standing against a wall

- Somatic touch (therapist provides contact via touch to support with grounding the child's nervous system)

## Self-Contact

A recent study published *in Comprehensive Psychoneuroendocrinology* suggests that self-soothing touch such as placing a hand over one's heart offers similar stress-reducing benefits to being hugged by another person. The findings of the study have implications for people experiencing isolation, when touch from others is unavailable or when touch from others does not feel comfortable; that "self-soothing touch provides an alternative way to re-activate memories of support and compassion in the face of stress" (Dreisoerner *et al.*, 2021). In fact, we subconsciously use self-touch and self-contact all of the time. There can be a natural impulse to want to self-soothe and offer oneself compassion and support in the face of stress. Self-contact also provides proprioceptive input and can bring attention to areas of the body needing tending.

### Brain Stem/Frontal Lobe
*Calm the Cortex*
**Instructions:**

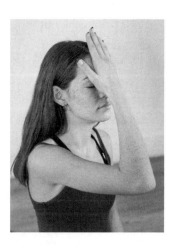

1. Begin seated.
2. Bring your palm to your forehead.
3. Allow your forehead to rest in your palm.
4. Fee the contact and support of your hand on your forehead.
5. Notice what amount of pressure feels supportive to you.
6. Breathe in through the nose.
7. Breathe out slowly.
8. Allowing your mind to rest and restore.
9. Slowly bring your hand down.
10. Notice how you feel.

### Amygdala/Cortex Communication

**Anchor the Amygdala**

**Instructions:**

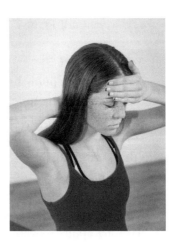

1. Begin seated.
2. Bring one palm to the back of the head, resting on the occipital ridge.
3. Bring the other palm to your forehead.
4. Press both palms evenly into the forehead and brainstem.
5. Feel the contact and support of your palms on your forehead and back of your skull.
6. As you explore the breath, repeat these mantras in your mind.
7. Breathe in through the nose.
8. "I am…"
9. Breathe out.
10. "Okay."
11. Breathe in through the nose.
12. "I am…"
13. Breathe out.
14. "Here."
15. Breathe in through the nose.
16. "1, 2."
17. Breathe out.
18. "1, 2, 3, 4."
19. Slowly bring your hands down.
20. Notice how you feel.

*Anchor Breath*

**Instructions:**

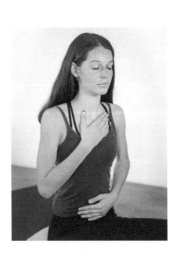

1. Begin seated.
2. Bring one hand to your belly, one hand to your heart center.
3. Feel the contact of your hand on your belly and your chest.
4. Notice how your belly feels.
5. Notice how your heart feels.
6. Notice your breath as you breathe in.

7.  Notice how your breath moves in your body on your inhalation.
8.  Notice your breath when you breathe out.
9.  Notice how your breath moves in your body on the exhalation.
10. As you breathe in, repeat in your mind, "I am breathing in."
11. As you breathe out, repeat in your mind, "I am breathing out."
12. Repeat these mantras with your breath two more times.

## Tracking Sensation

Tracking sensation brings awareness to body sensations. Inviting children to notice sensations they feel on the inside and track the changes in sensation facilitates increased interoceptive awareness as well as emotional awareness and is foundational for self-awareness and self-regulation. That being said, if a child has experienced trauma, they may not have established the necessary neural platforms to experience and track sensation. If they have been in a perpetual state of freeze or dissociation or it has not felt safe to *feel* or be in their bodies, they will struggle with experiencing and tracking sensation. This expectation could lead them to feeling as if they are doing something wrong or something is wrong with them if they are unable to access sensation in their body. In this case, it can be best to work from the outside in, scaffolding their experience with body connection and sensation in a titrated and safe manner.

Examples of ways to work from the outside in are:

- tapping
- self-contact
- exploring poses and movement with proprioceptive input
- activities that support inquiry of sensation (e.g. jogging in place then noticing heartbeat, temperature of skin, rubbing hands together and noticing sensation, temperature)
- exploring the senses (see Chapter 4)
- somatic touch.

## Pendulation

Pendulation is the shifting of awareness of body sensations or emotions between unpleasant, uncomfortable and pleasant/neutral sensations. Pendulation helps build capacity. It is the ability to move back and forth between contraction and expansion rather than having a fixed attention on the unpleasant, uncomfortable or even frightening sensations. As children learn to shift between the polar experiences, they build capacity in their nervous systems to manage both the pleasant and unpleasant sensations.

### Titration

Titration is working with sensation in small amounts at a time, in a slow manner so as not to overwhelm one's nervous system. This is particularly important when working with children whose systems are in more of an immobilized, shut-down or freeze state.

## WORKING WITH FIGHT/FLIGHT ENERGY

See the section on anxiety in Chapter 7 for additional suggestions:

- Grounding/Weight Bearing
- Movement
- Fight/Flight Musculature Release
- Restoration
- Breathing practices for working with fight/flight energy.

Please also refer to Chapter 7 for additional down-regulating breathing practices:

- Boxer Breath (release fight energy)
- Waking the Bear Breath (release fight energy)
- Let it Go Breath (release flight energy)
- Taco Breath (cooling)
- Balloon Belly Breath (diaphragmatic breathing)
- Grounding Breath (grounding).

### Grounding/Weight Bearing

Weight-bearing poses engage the fight/flight musculature and the experience of pressing or pushing into the floor or wall offers a way to tap into and move fight/flight energy through. They also support in embodying strength and empowerment.

- Table Pose
- Down Dog
- Wall Pushes
- Pushing feet into wall or hands

### Handstand (Adho Mukha Vrksasana)

Handstand engages the fight/flight musculature—the shoulders, arms, hands, core and legs. It also engages the cerebellum that is responsible for balance. Handstand is an inversion, which offers an energizing and calming effect to the body and mind. It can also offer an experience of empowerment and seeing the world from a different perspective.

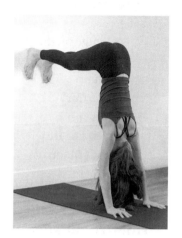

**Additional benefits:** Supports circulation, lymphatic functioning, bone density, focus and mental clarity.

**Contraindications:** See contraindications for inversions in Chapter 4.

**Instructions:**

1. Come into Down Dog with your heels against the wall.
2. Hands spread wide.
3. Begin to walk your feet up the wall until your hips are over your shoulders.
4. Press your hands into the mat and feel all of your muscles engaging.
5. Look back at the wall and keep your neck long.

## Movement

Movement can facilitate releasing stuck energy or activation in the body, completion of fight/flight impulses and bringing more mobility to the system which may be restricted, rigid or braced from being in a perpetual state of fight/flight or freeze. The movements suggested below can also facilitate more communication and integration of the left and right hemispheres of the brain which supports bringing more coherence to the system.

- Shifting weight
- Movement of spine
- Flow practice
- Crossing midline
- Follow impulse (how does your body want to move?)

## Balancing/Focus Poses

- Lunge modified
- Tree with proprioception
- Chair
- Warrior I
- Warrior II
- Warrior III
- Half Moon
- Eagle
- Triangle

## Fight/Flight Musculature Release

- Upper-body stretches
- Jaw massage
- Hamstring stretches
- Quad stretches

### Restoration

Being in a perpetual state of nervous system dysregulation takes a tremendous amount of energy and can result in adrenal fatigue and exhaustion. Encouraging children to take time to rest and restore is essential for their wellbeing. Restorative poses and practices can support with system restoration.

#### Supported Bridge to Legs up the Wall Variations

The third image provides support to the backs of the ankles to allow the child to feel supported and the legs to rest.

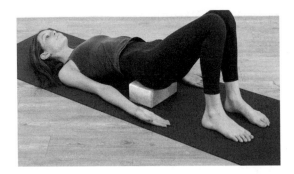

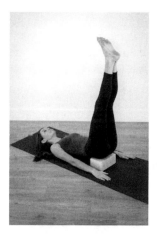
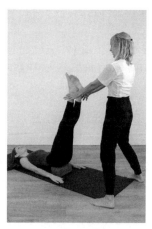
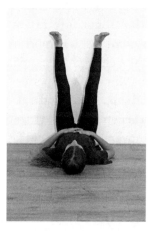
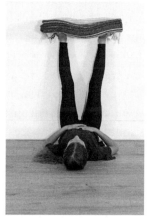

- Legs up the Wall variations
- Anchor Pose
- Koala Cuddle
- Facial Savasana


## WORKING WITH FREEZE ENERGY

See the section on depression in Chapter 7:

- Tapping
- Orienting with the senses
- Exploring sensation and pendulation
- Grounding
- Titration
- Somatic touch and self-contact

- Movement of joints.

Breathing practices for working with freeze energy (please also refer to Chapter 7 for additional up-regulating breathing practices):

- Bee Breath
- Engine Breath: Voo
- Boxer Breath
- Waking the Bear Breath: Voo-rarr
- Surprise or Startle Breath.

### Using Smovey Rings to Facilitate Embodiment

Because of the vibrational experience, smovey rings (www.smovey.info) can be a great tool to support body connection, whole-brain integration, interoceptive awareness and bringing mobilization to a system that is in more of a freeze state. When you introduce the smovey rings to the child or teen, invite them to get curious about the weight, the sound and the vibrational experience. Allow them to experiment in ways that are engaging and supportive for them. As you explore the movements with the child, encourage them to tune in to the vibration of the smovey rings. Explore different paces of movement (slow and fast), depending on the child's needs and comfort.

### Downhill Skier

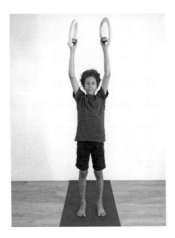 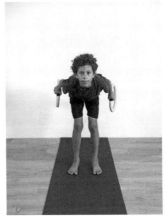

**Instructions:**

1. Hold the smovey rings in your hands with your arms by your side.
2. Reach your arms up.

3. Bend your knees and reach your arms back.
4. Imagine you're a downhill skier.
5. Option to explore a "hah" sound as they bend their knees and reach their arms back.
6. Repeat 4–5 times.
7. Check in and notice how your body feels.

## T-Shape

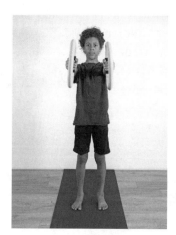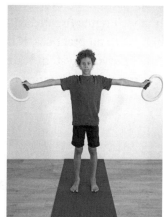

**Instructions:**

1. Hold the smovey rings in front of you with your arms straight.
2. Bring the smovey rings out to the side, making a T-shape with your arms.
3. Bring the rings back to the center.
4. Repeat 4–5 times.
5. Check in and notice how your body feels.

## Crossing Midline
**Instructions:**

1. Hold the smovey rings with arms out wide in a T-shape.
2. Cross the right arm over the left and reach arms across the body (crossing the midline).
3. Reach the arms out wide again.
4. Cross the left arm over the right and reach arms across the body.
5. Alternate both sides 4–5 times.
6. Check in and notice how your body feels.

### Engine Breath: Voo

Voo Breath was introduced by Peter Levine. Voo Breath stimulates the vagus nerve and supports coming out of a freeze response as well as accessing the rest and digest, parasympathetic nervous system. This breath reminded me of the sound of an engine hum and also has the effect of "starting the engine," so to speak, in coming out of a freeze state and getting the rest/digest response online. I interchange the terms "Voo Breath" and "Engine Breath" with the children I work with. As with all practices, it is important to track the child's nervous system response to determine whether the specific practice is supportive to them.

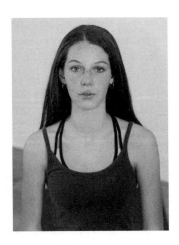

**Instructions:**

1. Take a full, natural breath in.
2. Make the extended sound "Voo" until the breath is emptied.
3. Breathe in again, filling the belly and lungs with air.
4. Make the "Voo" sound, coming from the belly.
5. Like the sound of an engine.
6. Repeat 3–5 times.
7. Notice how you feel after doing Engine Breath.

### Waking the Bear Breath: Voo-rarr

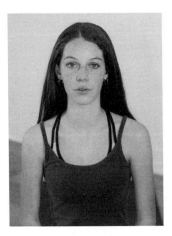
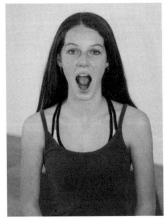

Voo-rarr is also a breath developed by Peter Levine. The intention of Voo-rarr is to stimulate the vagus nerve, access rest and digest (PNS) and experience self-empowerment and self-expression. I refer to Voo-rarr as Waking the Bear Breath. I imagine a sleeping bear, snoring, dormant and immobilized, then waking, mobilizing and expressing its fight energy. Moving from a frozen and disempowered state to a mobilized and empowered state. As with all practices, it is important to track the child's nervous system response to determine whether the specific practice is supportive to them.

**Instructions:**

1. Take a full, natural breath in.
2. Make the extended sound "Voo" until the breath is emptied.
3. Breathe in again, filling the belly and lungs with air.
4. Make the "Voo" sound, coming from the belly.
5. Begin adding the sound "rarr."
6. "Voo-rarr," extending the sound until the breath is emptied.
7. Like a bear waking from its sleep.
8. Repeat the "Voo-rarr" sound 3–5 times.
9. Explore exaggerating the movement of the mouth and the jaw as you make the "rarr" sound.
10. Notice how you feel after doing "Voo-rarr."

## Surprise or Startle Breath

When we experience unexpected or frightening events, our natural response is to startle. Exploring Startle Breath, where the child gets to experience the startle in a safe environment, can facilitate self-empowerment and a completion of a defensive response. When we take a surprise breath in, it brings a more sympathetic response or mobilization to the system; it can then initiate an exhalation. Extending the exhalation can support down-regulation.

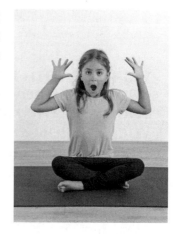

**Instructions:**

1. Imagine being at your surprise birthday party. You walk into the room and your friends and family jump up and yell, "SURPRISE!"
2. Bend your elbows and bring your hands up.

3. Take a surprise breath in and hold your breath for the count of "1, 2, 3."
4. Breathe out slowly.
5. Notice how you feel after taking a Surprise Breath.

Many children who are in a hypervigilant or shut down state may present with physical bracing in their bodies. Movement of the joints can support bringing more mobilization to their bodies and nervous system.

## Movement of Joints

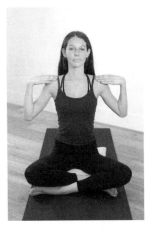 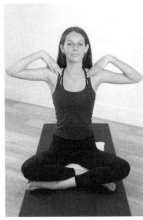 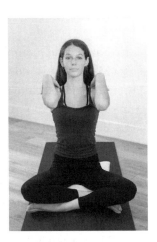

- Shoulders
- Wrists and ankles
- Hips

## WORKING WITH BOUNDARIES, SELF-AGENCY AND SELF-EMPOWERMENT THROUGH YOGA, SOMATIC MOVEMENT, BREATH, VOCALIZATION AND VISUALIZATION

The experience of trauma involves not having choice or control over what is happening to you or has happened to you. This can create feelings of hopelessness, helplessness, loss of sense of self and a greater need to be in control. An essential element in working with children and teens who have experienced trauma is to create experiences in which they are able to choose for themselves.

## Choice

- Choosing preferred poses, breathing strategies and activities
- Choosing preferred variation of pose or movement
- Choosing which side to begin with
- Choosing which mat to use
- Choosing where to sit
- Choosing colors
- Choosing preferred activity when session is complete
- Given an opportunity for choice as often as possible
- Invitational language

Another experience with trauma is that boundaries are ruptured. Oftentimes children who have experienced these boundary ruptures are less able to have healthy boundaries with others. Exploring healthy boundaries and choice through movement and play can support children in developing a greater sense of self-agency and healthy boundaries in relationships with others.

### Fawning and Healthy Self-Assertion/Self-Expression
A protective survival response that is not often considered or can be easily missed is fawning. If a child experienced or perceived danger or life threat, lacked attunement from a caregiver or lacked the felt sense of belonging, they may have developed adaptive strategies such as fawning or masking in order to "fit in," be accepted by others, gain others' approval or appease the people around them. With fawning, a child will perform prosocial behaviors regardless of the setting or their internal state. They may mask who they really are and mold themselves externally to who they think others want them to be. Fawning and masking requires a tremendous amount of suppression and "shutting off" or "tuning out" to one's emotions and internal sensations and connection to their authentic Self. Emphasizing choice, boundary, self-agency and self-empowerment are important in helping children and teens begin to develop healthy self-assertion, self-expression and connection to their authentic Self.

## Boundaries

- Give proximity choice (Where would you like me to sit? Would you like me to sit closer or further away?)
- Use visual tools as boundaries (e.g. hula hoop, yarn, mat)
- Request consent with touch and physical space

- Exploring boundaries with movement such as pushing forward, out, up, and down (where does my body end and the world begin?)

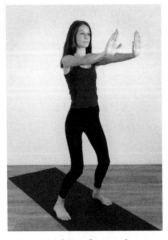

Pushing forward

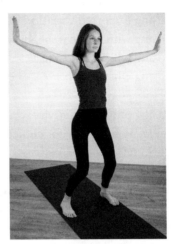

Pushing out

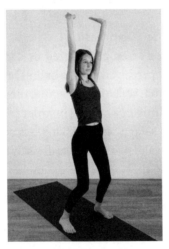

Pushing up

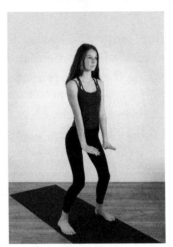

Pushing down

When children experience trauma, there can be a strong sense of disempowerment. They can develop belief systems that they have no voice, they have no choice, they are invisible, they aren't worthy of love, they are bad, they are broken, etc. Many children who experience developmental trauma may move through the world staying small, being afraid to take up space. Being afraid to be seen and heard. Practices that support children in embodying strength, agency, power and taking up space in the world can support them in engaging with the world with more confidence and self-esteem.

## Self-Empowerment
### Practices to Enhance Self-Empowerment

- Animal protectors
- Superheroes
- Asana and breathing practices (core strengthening, weight bearing, taking up space)
- Journaling (using writing prompts)
- Mantras

### Asanas
Exploring asanas with children in which they can embody strength, stability, power, courage, bravery and confidence can support them in connecting to those authentic qualities of themselves. Asanas or movements in which they are accessing their larger muscles, core and postural muscles can support them in accessing their fight/flight energy and embodying their inner strength and resilience.

### Standing and Balancing Poses
Goddess or Warrior series (embodying our inner warrior):

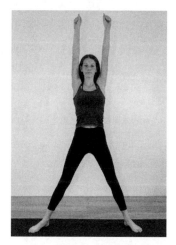

Stand strong with feet
wide apart, hands to fists,
breathe in, reach arms up

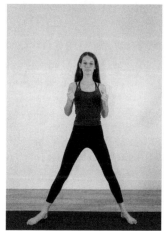

Bend elbows by side,
breathe out "haaa"

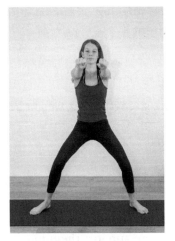
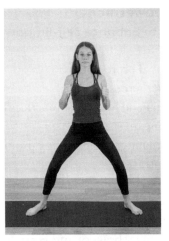

Bends knees, reach arms
forward, breathe in

Bend elbows, draw fists
in, breathe out "haaa"

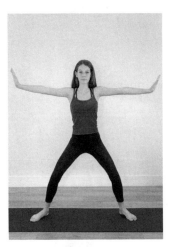
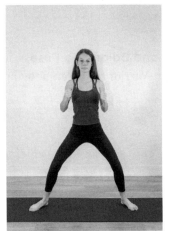

Reach arms out the
the side, breathe in

Bend elbows, draw fists
in, breathe out "haaa"

- Mountain (strength and stability)
- Tree (grounded and resilient)
- Warrior I (strength and confidence)
- Warrior II (courage and bravery)
- Star (energy and confidence)

## Core Poses

- Boat (strength and power)

- Plank (strength and perseverance)
- Chair (strength and stamina)

## Using Animals, Superheroes, Characters, etc. as Embodied Protectors

Children who have experienced trauma and have lost connection to their sense of self may struggle initially with being the "strong" ones. It may feel overwhelming for them to initially embody power as themselves. It can be helpful to use animals, superheroes or other characters that are of interest to the child to serve as "competent protectors" so they can explore these qualities initially outside of themselves, then work towards embodying these qualities as their own.

### Superheroes

BATMAN/WOMAN (AIRPLANE POSE)

**Characteristics:** Strength, intelligence, passion, curiosity.

SUPERMAN/WOMAN (SHARK POSE)

**Characteristics:** Strength, stamina, super speed, extrasensory powers.

CATWOMAN (CAT BREATH)

**Characteristics:** Clever, excellent balance, flexible, brave.

HULK (STAR POSE)

**Characteristics:** Super strength, emotional, expresses anger, protective.

CAPTAIN AMERICA (WARRIOR II POSE)

**Characteristics:** Strong, brave, noble, dependable.

WONDER WOMAN (WARRIOR II POSE)

**Characteristics:** Brave, strong, warrior heart, compassionate.

SPIDERMAN (FROG POSE)

**Characteristics:** Strong, fast, excellent balance, spider sense, intelligent.

WOLVERINE (MOUNTAIN POSE WITH TENSE-AND-RELAX HANDS)

**Characteristics:** Strong, fast, super stamina, agile, protective.

IRON MAN (WARRIOR I POSE)

**Characteristics:** Smart, strong, fast, super reflexes.

### Breathing Practices

- Waking the Bear Breath: Voo-rarr
- Empowered vocalizations
- Emotions Breaths
- Boxer Breath
- Lion's Breath

*Waking the Bear Breath: Voo-rarr with Movement*
*(self-empowerment and boundary)*
**Instructions:**

1. Take a full, natural breath in.
2. Make the extended sound "Voo" until the breath is emptied.
3. Breathe in again, filling the belly and lungs with air.
4. Make the "Voo" sound, coming from the belly.
5. Begin adding the sound "rarr."
6. Say, "Voo-rarr," extending the sound until the breath is emptied.
7. Option: Invitation to move your hands forward and out, making a boundary with your hands as you make the "Voo-rarr" sound.
8. Option: Invitation to move around your space as you make the "Voo-rarr" sound and move your hands.
9. When you feel the impulse to stop, stop and pause.
10. Notice how you feel after doing "Voo-rarr" with movement.

### Games

Games and stories can be a wonderful way to explore boundaries, self-empowerment, self-agency and choice. With trauma, children don't have the choice or the power. We want to give them the opportunity to lead, to be in the place of power and to have choice. Both the adult and child can become the leaders or the child can just be the leader, depending on the needs and specific focus with the child.

*Yogi Says*
**Instructions:**

1. Have the child give the commands, "Yogi says do (choice of pose, breath or movement)."
2. Example: "Yogi says do Tree Pose."
3. Adult does Tree Pose.
4. Repeat for several poses.

*Yogi Magician*
**Instructions:**

1. Give the child a magic wand (can use glow sticks).
2. The child says, "Magic wand, Magic wand turn _____ into a _____."
3. Example: Child says, "Magic Wand, Magic wand, turn Ms. Jessica into a frog."
4. Ms. Jessica goes into Frog Pose.
5. Repeat for several poses.

*Red Light/Green Light (working with boundaries)*
**Instructions:**

1. Child stands across from the adult.
2. Child can have a red sticker on one hand and a green sticker on the other hand.
3. Child holds up their hand with the green sticker and says, "Green light."
4. Adult moves towards the child slowly.
5. Child then holds up hand with the red sticker and says, "Red light" when they want the adult to stop.
6. The adult stops.
7. This continues until the adult reaches the child, then they choose a pose to do together.

*Yogi Freeze*
**Instructions:**

1. Child presses the button to start music and the adult dances to the music.
2. Child presses the button to stop music and the adult freezes in a pose.
3. The adult must wait for the child to start the music again to unfreeze.
4. Repeat several times.

## Stories
Make up empowered sequences with an empowered story that goes along with it.

### Embracing and Embodying our "Animal Nature"

#### Embodying our Animal Instincts

One of the things that gets thwarted when we have experienced trauma is connection to our natural instincts. In the animal world, there are both predators and prey. This is the same with our human experience. Embodying both their predator and prey nature can support children and teens in moving through important fight/flight responses that were inaccessible or suppressed. When this sympathetic energy is suppressed, children can remain in a constant state of activation or freeze.

Exploring and embodying the movements, shapes and sounds of predator/prey animals is a playful way to support children in accessing their "mobilization" or fight/flight energy. Our natural survival energy that supports healthy aggression, healthy escape and completion of defensive responses that were thwarted.

#### Predator: Fight Animals

Imagine being a bear. How would you move your body? How much space would a bear take up? What sound would an angry bear make? What do you notice in your body when you become a bear?

### I CAN BE A BEAR POEM

Explore movement and sound with the child as you recite the poem together.

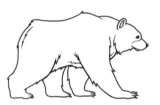

*I can be a bear*
*Strong and brave*
*Standing big and tall*
*Or sleeping in my cave*
*I can roar like a bear*
*Make a growling sound*
*Get on all fours*
*And walk around*

Shawnee Thornton Hardy

Other "fight" animals:

- Tiger
- Lion
- Snake

- Eagle
- Hyena
- Wolf
- Boar
- Shark
- Crocodile
- Leopard

## Prey: Flight Animals

Imagine being a rabbit escaping its prey. How would you move your body? Is your body moving fast or slow? What sounds does a rabbit make? What do you notice in your body when you become a rabbit?

### I CAN BE A RABBIT POEM

Explore movement and breath with the child as you recite the poem together.

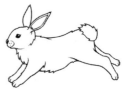

*I can be a rabbit*
*Running from its prey*
*Getting to safety*
*Hopping away*
*Breathing a bit faster*
*Then letting out a sigh*
*Far away from danger*
*Feeling so alive*

Shawnee Thornton Hardy

Other "flight" animals:

- Bird
- Bee
- Squirrel
- Fish
- Cat
- Lizard
- Coyote

### Protective Animals: Exploring Our Protective Animal Nature

Our survival instincts also include our protective responses. Think about when you poke a worm, caterpillar or a roly-poly insect. What do they do? Their natural instinct is to curl up and protect itself or to play "dead." If an opossum senses danger and can't escape, it will play "dead." This is the freeze or protective response. This is an important natural response to explore with children and teens, allowing them to fully experience their protective responses so they can begin to access their more defensive responses and connect with their fight/flight energy, moving into contraction before expansion.

Imagine being an opossum who is playing dead. How would your body move like an opossum playing dead? Can you let your body be really still? What do you notice in your body when you become an opossum?

### I CAN BE AN OPOSSUM POEM

Explore movement with the child as you recite the poem together.

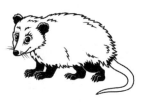

*I can be an opossum*
*When it plays dead*
*Keep my body frozen*
*Or curl up instead*
*Feel my body slowing down*
*Take a little pause*
*Moving when I'm ready*
*To show my teeth and claws*

Shawnee Thornton Hardy

Other "freeze" animals:

- Turtle
- Puppy
- Rolly Polly (Sponge Pose)
- Caterpillar
- Lizard

## Exploring Contraction to Expansion

*"Your hand opens and closes, opens and closes. If it were always a fist or always stretched open, you would be paralysed. Your deepest presence is in every small contracting and expanding, the two as balanced and coordinated as birds' wings."*

Rumi (Barks, 2004, p.174)

Exploring contraction and expansion with movement can facilitate pendulation and increased capacity and help children embody their inmate rhythm.

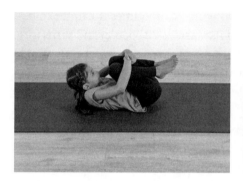 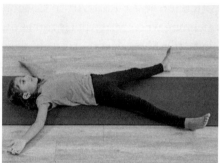

### Contraction Poses and Movements

- Forward bends
- Rounding the spine
- Tightening or squeezing body parts
- Making the shape of the body smaller
- Staying in one place

### Expansion Poses and Movements

- Backbends
- Opening the body
- Lengthening the spine
- Standing poses
- Warrior poses
- Making the shape of the body larger
- Moving around the space

*Butterfly to Cocoon*

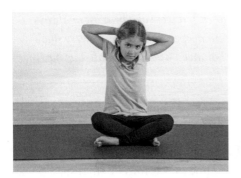 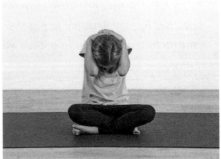

I often introduce Butterfly to Cocoon by saying: "Sometimes it can feel over-whelming when a caterpillar comes out of its warm, safe cocoon and turns into a butterfly. Some days it may want to go back into its cocoon when it feels afraid, worried or overwhelmed. Let's move our bodies in a way that we can go from butterflies back into our cozy cocoons."

**Instructions:**

1. Clasp your hands behind your head and spread your elbows wide like a butterfly out in the world.
2. Breathe in.
3. Breathe out and bring your elbows towards each other, curling back into your cozy cocoon. You get to decide how long you stay in your cocoon. Stay in your cocoon until you feel like spreading your wings and becoming a butterfly again.

**Option:** Have the child begin with their elbows together then decide when they want to become a butterfly. The intention is to let the child become a butterfly when they feel the impulse to expand and come out of their protective posture.

**BUTTERFLY TO COCOON POEM**

Explore movement with the child as you recite the poem together.

*Sometimes when I'm a butterfly*
*I get overwhelmed*
*By all the things around me*
*And all the noisy sounds*
*Some days I wish to be a caterpillar*
*Back in its cocoon*

*Feeling warm and cozy*
*Protected from the gloom*
*Other days I feel more open*
*Like a butterfly*
*Spreading its wings*
*Opening them wide*
*Either way, I get to choose*
*To shrink*
*Or expand*
*Whatever feels best to me*
*Is always the best plan*

Shawnee Thornton Hardy

## EMBODYING THE QUALITIES OF NATURE

Many of the yoga postures are named after what one would observe in nature, such as animals, mountains, trees, the sun, the moon and so on. Yoga is a practice of self-awareness as well as awareness of the world around us. Ancient yogis spent much of their time observing nature and their environment. In fact, Indian myths and mythology are rich with stories of sages, gods and deities and their experiences with and symbolism around animals and nature. Not only do the asanas in yoga have names of animals, but the essence of the postures is meant to embody the qualities of those animals. The ancient yogis knew there is much we can learn from animals and nature, and they also recognized that we are all a part of nature, interconnected and one with all living things. As we explore the shapes and even sounds and breath that represent nature, we can embody those qualities that are inherent in us. We can embody the stability of a mountain, the resilience of a tree, the awareness of an eagle, the fierceness of a lion, the inwardness of a turtle, etc.

Children or teens who have experienced trauma can feel disconnected from the world around them and may also lose connection to their own innate inner qualities that they share with animals and nature. Exploring movement by creating animal and nature shapes with their bodies and using movement, breath and sound can help them connect to their sense of power, curiosity, insightfulness, intuition and deepest essence of who they are.

Embodying an animal, a warrior or a bright shining star can also be less frightening than being "themselves." They may initially feel powerless as themselves and unable to show fierceness or bravery, or they may be fearful of taking up space in the world. By pretending to be an animal or something in nature, they can begin to explore what it feels like to tap into qualities of empowerment, boundaries, agency, healthy aggression, energy and vitality.

### Sun and Moon (Yin and Yang)
### The Energy of the Sun

Pingala: Extroverted, active, energizing, solar nadi

Right side of body, left side of brain

- Sun Salutations (Waking the Sun)
- Sunrise/Sunset Breath
- Solar Plexus Chakra
- Nadi Shodhana—Sun Breath
- Poses and movement practices that activate and strengthen the core and bring more energy and heat to the body

### The Cooling of the Moon

Ida: Introverted, regenerative, cooling, lunar nadi

Left side of body, right side of brain

- Moon Meditation
- Reach for the Moon
- Nadi Shodhana—Moon Breath
- Half Moon
- Sitali
- Poses and movement practices that allow for more introspection, going inward and bringing a cooling energy to the body.

### The Magic of the Stars
*Star Pose*
**Qualities:**

- Energetic
- Unique
- Vibrant
- Bright
- Warm

*Star Meditation*
"As you embody the shape of a star, feel the energy coming from the center of your body and moving out through your feet, your arms and the top of your head.

Like a five point star, shining bright. Imagine warmth filling your body and your body radiating warmth out into the world, sharing your unique and special light."

### The Stability of the Mountains
*Mountain Pose*
**Qualities:**

- Stable
- Strong
- Tall
- Immovable
- Powerful

*Mountain Meditation*
"As you embody the shape of a mountain, notice how your body is tall and stable. You are immovable. Connect with your inner power, knowing that you have a strength within yourself that will help you get through any of life's challenges."

### The Resilience of the Trees
*Tree Pose*
**Qualities:**

- Grounded
- Rooted
- Resilient
- Flexible
- Connected

*Tree Meditation*
"As you embody the shape of a tree, feel your feet connected to the earth, grounded and rooted. As you balance, allow your arms to sway back and forth, feeling how flexible you can be. If you fall, you can always get back up. You are resilient and can get through hard things."

### The Fluidity of the Rivers
*River Pose*
**Qualities:**

- Fluid
- Cool

- Graceful
- Refreshing
- Flowing

### River Meditation

"As you embody the shape of a river, notice how you move with grace. Your energy and emotions flowing through you with ease. Imagining how the cool water might feel on your skin. Refreshing and nourishing. Moving through the world with fluidity. Knowing that you can go with the flow."

## The Vastness of the Oceans

### Ocean Breath

**Qualities:**

- Deep
- Vast
- Life force
- Diverse
- Rhythmic

### Ocean Mediation

"As you embody the sound of the ocean with your breath, notice the rhythmic movement as you inhale and exhale, like the waves of an ocean. Noticing how your breath can begin to deepen as you breathe in and lengthen as you breathe out. Tuning into your life-force energy. Remembering the ocean is vast & diverse, just as we all are. You are not a drop in the ocean, you are part of the ocean."

## The Expansiveness of the Sky

### Floating on a Cloud (Savasana)

**Qualities:**

- Expansive
- Peaceful
- Brilliant
- Calm
- Soft

### Sky Meditation

"As you embody the sky and the clouds, allow yourself to feel into the expansiveness of your own breath. Allowing your muscles to soften. Inviting in, the peacefulness and calm of the clouds and the brilliance of the sky. Knowing that you carry your own inner peace and calm in your heart and brilliance in your mind."

## Nature as a Co-regulator

Nature can be a wonderful co-regulator. It can help generate feelings of calm, joy, groundedness, connection, vitality and creativity, and it can facilitate concentration. Connection to nature is associated with improved mental health and wellbeing (Weir, 2020). Connection to nature can be achieved through spending time in nature, experiencing nature through images, sounds and sensory experiences and integrating nature activities in a child's day.

### Activities to Support Connection with Nature

- Looking at nature images
- Watching nature videos or listening to nature sounds
- Nature art projects
- Visualizing being in nature
- Experience nature through nature yoga stories and adventures
- Weaving in colors of nature
- Embodying animals, plants, trees, mountains, etc. through posture and movement
- Planting and caring for plants
- Nature meditation walks
- Nature sensory box
- Nature stories
- Food as nature's medicine
- Spending time in nature
- Nature scavenger hunts
- Nature mandalas
- Gratitude practices (Sun Salutations, gratitude for nature)

### PAUSE AND REFLECT

Think of a resourcing experience you had recently in nature or when you were younger. What comes to mind? Where are you? What do you see? What do you hear? What do you smell? When you think back to your experience in nature, what do you notice in your body?

Invitation to journal your reflection.

# Chapter 9

# Trauma-Sensitive Therapeutic Uses of the Arts

## ANN DAVIS, EXPRESSIVE ARTS THERAPIST AND SOMATIC EXPERIENCING PRACTITIONER

### INTRODUCTION

Our bodies hold and tell the story of traumatic events and/or prolonged stress that words alone often cannot express. Peter Levine maintains that "our body communicates the memory of trauma through posture, movement, gesture, breath, sound and other somatic responses" (Malchiodi, 2019). Expressive arts are action oriented, that is, they utilize the sensory quality of movement, art making, touch and sound that involves active engagement of the body (Malchiodi, 2019).

The expressive arts, combined with yoga and somatic movement, are powerful tools that can develop one's capacity for self-regulation. For emotional regulation to occur, physical regulation must first be established. According to Dr. Bruce Perry, physical regulation begins to develop at eight weeks post-conception and is dependent upon touch, movement and rhythm, delivered as a patterned rhythmic activity. The pairing of expressive arts with yoga and somatic movement provides a bottom-up approach that not only supports physical regulation but also promotes a felt sense of safety, allowing the body to tell its story. Throughout this chapter, you will learn expressive arts tools and activities that are grounded in touch, movement and rhythm, aimed specifically at supporting children's and teens' capacity for physical regulation. In addition, I offer extension activities that integrate yoga, movement, mantras and connection to nature.

In my professional practice, I provide integrative experiences utilizing various arts forms—movement, art making, gesture, sound, breathing and silence—so that my clients can connect with multiple sensory experiences. For it is through our sensory experiences that we begin to explore and make meaning of our lives, and can, in the words of my first expressive arts mentor, Dr. Judith Greer Essex, "restore what might have been lost, missing or broken" (Archer, 2022). This restoration of the self happens in the space of a safe, supportive, loving and nurturing relationship no matter your scope of practice.

## WE ARE THE CO-REGULATORS

The best gift we can give children is our own regulated, grounded, attuned, loving, compassionate presence. I believe that it is our ethical responsibility as adults working with any child to do our own healing work so that we may be a contagion of calm. Some children we have the honor of working with may have never experienced a regulated adult, let alone what regulation feels like in their own body. They may need to, temporarily, borrow our regulation while we simultaneously support them in growing their own capacity for self-regulation. Trauma expert Deb Dana expresses that connection is a biological imperative. We come into *being* because of connection. She states that, "trauma compromises our ability to engage with others by replacing patterns of connection with patterns of protection" (Dana, 2021). How, in our work with children with complex needs, can we emanate a felt sense of safety that invites connection? We start with ourselves.

Our own healing work, according to my expressive arts mentor, Dr. Greer Essex expands our capacity for compassion for ourselves so that we may have it for others. When we co-create healing spaces with children that are grounded in love and openhearted curiosity, we are able to truly *see* what another is doing and extend ourselves from our heart to support their healing process (Archer, 2022). It is where we honor and celebrate similarities and differences in culture, race, religion, gender, values and beliefs. Healing occurs within a space of genuinely feeling seen, heard and known.

Throughout this chapter, I will offer moments to pause and reflect. Dr. Perry (2021) has found that our reflective moments are when we engage our cortex, when we are able to problem solve, generate new ideas, make connections and begin to lay down new neural pathways in our brains. We learn by doing. I invite you to read, and experience, this chapter from a space of openhearted curiosity.

**PAUSE AND REFLECT**

Before you continue reading this chapter take a moment to reflect on how you currently show up with children. What brought you to this work? Who, if anyone, was a source of regulation for you as a child? How has that impacted you both personally and professionally?

Invitation to draw, doodle, write, move and/or make sound in response to these questions.

## WHY USE THE ARTS FOR TRAUMA HEALING?

The arts support trauma recovery work because they are sensory by their very nature. Playing with the arts and various art materials provide visual, tactile, auditory, olfactory, vestibular and proprioceptive experiences. Malchiodi (2020) states that "they are believed to predominantly access the right brain and implicit memory because they include a variety of sensory based experiences including, images, sounds, tactile and movement experiences that are related to right hemisphere functions." Malchiodi (2020) goes on to reference Rothschild (2000) who posits that "trauma memories can be encoded as a form of sensory reality, underscoring the idea that expression and processing of implicit memories have an important role in successful trauma resolution." The arts *are* somatosensory. For example, visual arts are tactile, visual and sensorimotor. Music is auditory and visual. Dance and theater are visual, auditory, kinesthetic and tactile.

Dr. Perry (2020) proposes that one of the most important associations we ever make as infants in the womb occurs when somatosensory cues from the outside world meet in the brainstem. For example, the rhythmic vibratory rocking movement of the mother and the sound of the mother's heart beat along with touch cause our brains to associate patterned repetitive rhythmic activity with feeling safe, nurtured and regulated. The arts enlist both our brains and our bodies, offering an opportunity to give the brain precisely what it needs to feel safe. The arts—walking, listening to music, doodling, humming, dancing—by their very nature are patterned, rhythmic activities. The arts speak the language of safety and regulation. Malchiodi (2020, pp. 24–31) identifies the following key reasons to include the arts in trauma healing. The arts:

- provide a way for the senses to tell the story
- engage and self-soothe the body and the brain
- enhance non-verbal communication

- support experiences of mastery and empowerment which are essential to expanding resilience
- provide action-oriented and hands-on experiences where narratives can be rescripted through imagination and play
- support restoration of joy, vitality and life force, all embodied experiences that we cannot be talked into.

## WHAT DOES IT MEAN TO USE THE ARTS FOR TRAUMA HEALING?

The arts can be a vehicle for self-determination that facilitates the psychological, emotional and social development of not only children but all humans. Therapeutic uses of the arts explore all of the different forms of creativity and expression, such as visual arts, creative writing and poetry, music, sound and silence, creative enactment, movement and dancing, yoga, imagination and play, as well, as cooking, building and construction, nature and land art. What sets therapeutic uses of the arts apart from traditional arts education is that the focus is on the richness of the process, rather than the outcome or product. It is not about focusing on artistic skill or technique, creating the perfect museum-ready art piece, writing a publishable poem or a performance-ready monologue. Instead, the therapeutic use of the arts provides a safe and supportive space where a child can express their inner sensory experience through an outer image. This is especially important for children with diverse needs and abilities, and those who have experienced developmental trauma. Often with developmental trauma, language centers in the brain have not yet been developed. Asking a child to recount a preverbal experience through language may inadvertently re-traumatize them. When language is not available, the arts have the ability to communicate what has been lost, is missing or is broken.

We are sensory beings and comprehend our environment through our senses. You've likely experienced this with children. Some are visual, some are auditory, some are kinesthetic, and some may be a combination. It is through artistic play and imagination that our sensory experiences reveal new information and strengths, we find solutions to challenges, experience success and mastery, make meaning, rewrite our narratives and reshape our identities. Creativity, expression and art making each involve some level of play. Play exists across all cultures. Play is the most accessible way to the imagination. Play *is* the work of children. Play is our brain's favorite way of learning. We are hardwired to play.

> **PAUSE AND REFLECT**
> Check in with your body and ask how it might like to express itself in response to the following question: How do you bring a sense of play, curiosity, and wonder to your work with children and teens?
>
> Invitation to write, move, doodle and/or make sound in response to this question.

## HOW TO INCORPORATE THE ARTS INTO YOUR PROFESSIONAL PRACTICE: PILLARS AND ACTIVITIES

I consider myself a detective of sorts when working with children as I look and listen to what and how a child is responding, simultaneously tracking and noticing shifts in their physiology, staying attuned to what each child is showing me that they need. Children *will* show us exactly what they need if we slow down and take the time to interpret what their behavior is communicating. We must stay grounded in ourselves, and remember most of all to *play*. There are multiple ways "in" to the body.

As mentioned earlier, the most important tool you can bring to incorporating the arts into your professional practice is your own regulated, accepting, attuned and loving presence. I have adapted an article by artist Beth Herrild (2022), founder of Outside the Box Creation, to provide you with some tips to begin incorporating the arts into your practice.

- Follow the child's passion.
- Work within the child's window of tolerance, offering activities that are exciting and not overwhelming.
  - Focus on process over product. *Play* with different art materials and mediums, paying close attention to the child's sensory response.
  - Create small "doses" of time to create, tracking the child's physiology and offering breaks when necessary.
  - I rarely sit and watch children create art. I make art right alongside them. Not only does this provide attunement and co-regulation, but it allows them to learn by doing.
  - Provide structure and predictability. For many children, knowing what to expect can provide a sense of ease, relaxation and calm.
- Provide developmentally appropriate (developmental stage, not age) art offerings.

- Always ask permission, use invitational language and offer choices. In this way, we work with a "living consent" and provide opportunities to support a child's agency.
- Sensory comfort level. Before I begin working with any child, I ask the child (and, where appropriate, their caregiver) to complete a sensory survey. The sensory qualities of the arts can lend themselves to safety in some children and overstimulation in others. It is important to know the child's sensory seeking and sensory avoiding behaviors so you can develop activities that match their "just right" level of sensory input.

Addressing the needs of children who have either experienced trauma, lived in prolonged stress, or have diverse needs is not a one-size-fits-all. We must view each child through the lens of their lived experience, be it intrapersonal, interpersonal, religious, cultural, racial, social or environmental. Throughout my professional practice, I have had to wind around, bump up against and fumble my way to pillars that consistently guide and ground my work. They are: Safety, Relationships, Stabilization and Resources, and Empowerment. My guiding pillars are not linear. I am always doing my best to meet the needs of the child as they present themselves. What I provide here is not a recipe, but rather a menu. The activities do not focus on skill or technique, but on the sensory experience of working with, and through, the arts. My hope is that these activities will inspire you to incorporate the arts into your practice to enhance a child's sensory experience. I encourage you to make these activities your own—modify, re-create, re-purpose—to meet the children you are working with exactly where they are.

## Pillar I: Safety

Not all children have access to safety, embodiment, imagination and creativity. Children with trauma histories may not have the capacity to feel, experience, or sense their bodies. They may have learned to dampen the very thing that provides a sense of aliveness, that is our sensory experience, in service of survival. Sean McNiff (2011) reminds us: "Humans are aesthetic beings. We communicate, learn, make meaning through the experiences of our senses." The expressive arts use gesture, intonation, rhythm, visual, tactile, vestibular and proprioceptive experiences. They have the potential to help individuals both sense safety and feel more secure with others and their environments (Malchiodi, 2020). The arts, therefore, can be a portal back home.

**PAUSE AND REFLECT**
**What does safety mean to you?**
How do you present yourself as safe to the children/teens you work with? How do you create a safe environment for them?

Invitation to draw, doodle, write, move and/or make sound in response to these questions.

### Art Activities Related to Safety
*Journal*

Adapted from Dr. Judith Greer Essex's Expressive Arts Therapy program at The Expressive Arts Institute

**Art supplies:** 8 x 12 blank book of unlined paper, magazines for collage, scissors, glue.

**Instructions:** Journals come in all shapes and sizes. They can be visual and written diaries. Journals are a great place to document progress, "house" visual art projects created in your sessions, a place to write down "home-fun," responses to reflection questions, yoga sequences or tools to practice between sessions. I encourage children to work in their journals in between sessions to record their thoughts, feelings and experiences. You can reflect on the entries the child chooses to share during your session. I usually introduce journaling early on in our work together. The initial prompt is simple: Collage and decorate the journal cover to represent *you*, your likes and dislikes (see Figure 9.1).

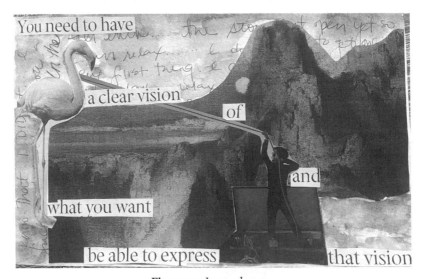

**Figure 9.1** Journal cover

### Competent Protector

Adapted from Levine, n.d.a

**Art supplies:** Paper and any mark-making materials (e.g. colored pencils, colored markers, pastels).

**Instructions:** When a child's sense of safety has been disrupted, or is even non-existent, they may not have experienced another human "having their back." We can support a child with this imagined experience of safety so they can develop a felt sense of what it would feel like to have someone protect them. Invite the child to imagine someone who they would like to "have their back", or to be their *competent protector.* This can be an actual person from their past, present or future. It can be a pet, or an animal, a character from a movie, TV show or book or anything they imagine. Invite the child to explore as much detail as possible. What qualities would they have? What would they look like? What would they say or do to protect you? What superpower might they have? Once they have a clear image, invite the child to draw, paint, sketch or doodle.

**Reflection questions:**

- How was your experience of bringing to life your competent protector? What did you notice or what surprised you?
- Is there a situation where you can imagine your competent protector defending you? Would they use words, sounds or a superpower?
- Is there anything else you need from your competent protector (e.g. kindness, comfort, reminder that you are worthy)?

**Accommodations:** If the child has difficulty imagining a competent protector, inquire about their interests. For example, I worked with a child who was chronically bullied and no one came to her aid. She lived and breathed Marvel superheroes. Her interests and passions were our launching point. Her competent protector became Iron Man.

See Chapter 8 for superhero embodiment practices.

**Extensions:**

- Create a 3D version of your competent Protector, utilizing clay, found objects around your home or items from nature.
- Write a story/poem or create a dance about your competent protector.
- Create a mantra and choose a yoga pose to represent your competent protector.

- Invite the child to choose an animal as their competent protector, then have them embody that animal. How would it protect them? How would it move? What protective sounds might it make? See Chapter 8 for embodied animal practices.
- What might be the competent protector's theme song? Create a power playlist.

### Body Mapping

Adapted from Malchiodi, 2020

**Art supplies:** Large roll of butcher paper, mark-making materials (e.g. colored pencils, colored markers, paint, stickers), collage materials (magazines, printed papers), scissors and glue, My Body Sensations cards, My Body outline (www. asanasforautismandspecialneeds.com/product-page/sensation-language-cards).

**Instructions:** Body maps are usually drawn as life-size and represent stories about oneself, specific body experiences or memories. With children, body mapping is an excellent activity to pair with psychoeducation and/or to support them in understanding how they experience emotions, tell the story of their emotions and reduce fear around uncomfortable sensations related to emotions. I like to use large rolls of butcher paper for this activity. Beginning this activity with movement or a yoga sequence is an excellent warm-up and a good way to awaken the child's sensory experience. Once you have completed a movement sequence, offer a choice to the child between working with a life-size body map or with the My Body outline (see art supplies ). If the child consents to having their body traced on the paper, you can invite them to lie down on their back on the paper and begin tracing. Once their body tracing is complete, invite them to decorate their body.

**Reflection questions:**

- How was the experience of having your body traced?
- What do you notice as you look at your life-size body?
- What did you learn about your body?

**Accommodations:** For children who may not be ready to have their body traced, you can use the My Body outline and create a smaller version, scaffolding to the 'life-size' body tracing if and when the child shows you they are ready. If the My Body outline is too overwhelming for the child, you can invite them to draw or collage their body. Creating "bodies" from pipe cleaners or clay is also an option. Always work within the child's window of tolerance.

**Extensions:**

- Build a sensation vocabulary. I use the My Body outline and My Body Sensations cards in almost every session with children. The brain loves repetition. The more we practice these tools in session with children, the more we support them in building a felt sense of their sensory experiences.
- Use My Body Sensations cards to begin to identify sensations the child experiences with different experiences/emotions. Invite the child to display their "body" somewhere in their house where it is visible. They can collaborate with their caregiver to "map" their sensations on their body.
- Trace the child's body on colored butcher paper, inviting the child to lie on the paper in their favorite yoga pose. Cut out and decorate. Create a mantra with the child for their body map. This mantra can be written inside their body map and hung in their home as a reminder.
- Create a symbol of the child's personal power or strength and include it on their body map. Invite the child to embody their power pose.

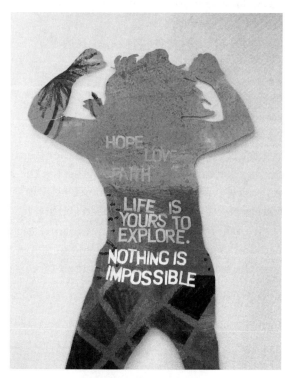

**Figure 9.2** Body Is Home

## Pillar II: Relationships

Therapeutic uses of the arts are guided by fostering a felt sense of safety with self, with others and within the environment (Malchiodi, 2020). Humans are relational creatures. We are wired for connection. We come into the world reliant on another human for every aspect of our survival. Connection and relationships, like food, water and sleep, are biological imperatives. Carl Rogers was a humanistic psychologist who developed person-centered psychotherapy (McLeod, 2014). Rogers asserted that the person-centered therapist learns to recognize and trust human potential, which can facilitate change, growth and restoration. For it is in trusting this potential that we can support our clients in learning to rely on their vast internal resources for change. The power to change resides within the client and is not a result of advice, direction or information the therapist offers (Landreth, 2002). Together, therapist and client co-create the conditions for healing.

Rogers outlines four essential ingredients for a successful therapeutic relationship which he believed facilitated such growth. They are empathy, positive regard, congruence and alliance (McLeod, 2014). Dr. Perry states, "Relationships are the agents of change and the most powerful therapy is human love" (Perry & Szalavitz, 2017, p.258). How does love show up in your practice?

### Art Activities Related to Relationships
*Relation to Self: Torn-Paper Portrait*

Adapted from Levine, 2015

**Art supplies:** Colored construction paper, glue.

**Instructions:** Invite the child to think of a time when they felt they were at their best, a time when they demonstrated their strengths. Let the child know that they will be creating a self-portrait at their best; it will be abstract, not representational. They will tear pieces of paper for the head and any facial features they would like to include (hair, eyes, nose, mouth, neck, shirt) and glue them onto another piece of colored paper. Encourage the child to get as abstract as they would like; for example, using the color green for their face or purple for their hair (see Figure 9.3).

**Reflection questions:**

- How was it to not use scissors?
- How were you able to overcome this challenge?
- What positive qualities do you see in yourself?

- Does your portrait have a message for you?

**Accommodations:** For some children, not using scissors can either be liberating or activating. Notice how the child responds to the activity. Support them as necessary so they remain within their window of tolerance. If the child is overwhelmed by this activity, co-create the portrait together.

**Extensions:**

- This is a great activity to do with caregivers to support them in thinking about their child in a positive way. Caregivers can share their completed art with their child, reflecting on the qualities they value in their child.
- I like to include a poetry component with this activity. Reflect with the child on their positive qualities. If they are able, invite them to write from one of the following prompts: "I Matter Because..." or "I am the one who..." You can also scribe while the child shares their story and then reflect their words back to them. The child can write phrases or words that resonated with them on their portrait.
- Create a yoga sequence or mantra that embodies the child's positive qualities.

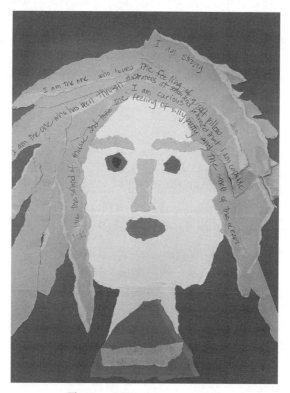

**Figure 9.3** Torn-paper portrait

### Inside/Outside Box

Adapted from Dr. Judith Greer Essex's Expressive Arts Therapy program at The Expressive Arts Institute

**Art supplies:** Shoe box or any craft box with a lid, magazines for collage, scissors, glue, paper.

**Instructions:** The focus of this activity is to help a child identify how they see themselves, as well as how they think others perceive them. This activity can support the child in considering the questions: "Who am I? Who do I want to become? What are the things about me that are loveable and of value?" Peruse age-appropriate magazines and support the child in finding images/words/colors/textures/designs that represent how they view themselves and images that represent how they believe others perceive them. They will then cut and glue images that represent themselves on the inside of the box and images that represent others' views on the outside of the box and lid (see Figure 9.4).

**Reflection questions:**

- Explore how others' perceptions may or may not be true, what the client thinks about and feels while looking at their "outside box."
- What do you notice as you look at the outside and the inside of the box?
- What would you change or add to the outside of your box, if anything?

**Accommodations:** Co-create the box with the child and their caregiver.

**Extensions:**

- Writing prompt: If you were to look at me on the outside you might notice _____ , but on the inside I am _____ .
- Scavenger hunt in nature: Find items in nature that are a resource and reminder for finding calm and ease, or that represent a favorite yoga posture or breath. Store the items in the box.

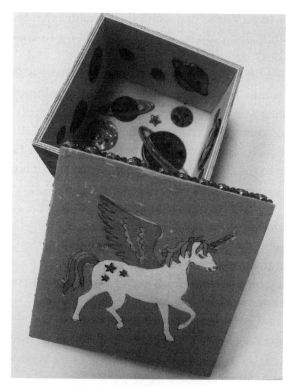

**Figure 9.4** Inside outside box

## Pillar III: Stabilization and Resources

Stress and trauma influence the way we think, feel and behave. The body is the container of all of our sensations and feelings. Our bodies are a boundary between us, our environment and others (Levine, 2008). This boundary often gets ruptured with trauma. In trauma work, we are guardians at the gates of overwhelm. We want to begin by providing opportunities and experiences to take in the good in a titrated way. That is, to stabilize the dysregulated nervous system *before* working with the trauma narrative.

### Art Activities Related to Stabilization and Resources
*Three Parts of Your Life*

Adapted from Rachelle Archer's Expressive Arts Therapy program at the Monarch School

**Art supplies:** 18 x 24 inch paper and any mark-making materials (e.g. colored pencils, colored markers, patels).

**Instructions:** I like to use this activity when I am first getting acquainted with a child. It allows me to get a sense of not only their resources but also the challenges in their life. Additionally, it can be a launching point for co-creating goals. This activity can also be done with their caregiver.

On a large piece of paper, invite the child to create three different sections in any way they would like. Ask the child to think of all of the things they love, things that are going well and people who support them. Instruct them to doodle, draw or write those things in their first section. In the next section, ask the child to think of and doodle, draw or write challenges they may be facing. In the last section, ask them to think of and doodle, draw or write their hopes for our time together.

**Reflection questions:**

- Was there anything that surprised you?
- Is there anything you notice when you look at your lists?
- How was it for you to create these lists?

**Accommodations:** For non-verbal children, stickers can be used to create their three sections.

**Extensions:**

- Use My Body Sensations cards and the My Body outline (two copies) to have the child identify sensations related to one of their resources and one of their challenges. Compare the two and reflect on their noticings, similarities and differences.
- Use cards from the CALMM toolkit (www.asanasforautismandspecial needs.com/product-page/c-a-l-m-m-yoga-tool-kit) to invite the child to find a yoga posture and/or breath to support them during one of their challenges.

### Resource Zine

Adapted from Levine & Kline, 2007

**Art supplies:** Paper and any mark-making materials (e.g. colored pencils, colored markers, pastels), My Body Sensations cards, CALMM toolkit.

**Instructions:** A resource is anything that nurtures and supports a sense of physical, emotional, mental and spiritual wellbeing. It can be anything that helps soothe and settle, provides a sense of goodness, is used to help anchor us to the here and now or prevents a downward spiral of thoughts, emotions or memories. A resource can be external, outside of yourself such as an object like a weighted pillow, a person, a pet, nature, an activity such as sports, dancing, music or art. A resource can also be internal or something that you feel inside of yourself without the help of an external resource such as a spiritual practice, your breath, grounding, orienting self-contact. Ask the child to think about their resources. What has supported or got them through challenging times? How did they cope? What has got them to the place they are now? What inner strengths did they enlist? Write down their resources. Ask the child to choose four resources (two internal and two external) that stand out and remind them of when they most feel like themselves. When they think of these resources, what sensation(s) do they experience in their body? Is there an image that comes to mind? A color, shape, texture? An emotion?

**Reflection questions:**

- Were there any surprises about your resources?
- How might your resources support you?
- Is there a time when you can practice using one of your resources?

**Accommodations:** This activity is geared toward older children but can easily be adapted for younger children. The word "resource" may be new or advanced for a child. Work with them, and their caregiver, to find a word for "resource" that makes sense to them. If the child is having difficulty thinking of resources, you can use the CALMM toolkit and find yoga poses together that are resourcing for them.

**Extensions:**

- Create a zine or booklet incorporating images of the child's resources.

---

**PAUSE AND REFLECT**

What types of things do you do to self-soothe? There are no right or wrong answers, only what supports you in feeling most like yourself.

Invitation to draw, doodle, write, move and/or make sound in response to this question. Perhaps create your own resource zine!

## Pillar IV: Strengths and Empowerment

Therapeutic uses of the arts in trauma healing are an empowerment model. The arts provide opportunities for children not only to explore self-image and find safety and ease, but to gain a stronger sense of who they are. Because working with the arts is an embodied experience, they naturally identify strengths and resources. The arts move us away from pathologizing behaviors and toward understanding that behaviors are management strategies for overwhelming sensory experiences. Children with diverse needs and abilities, as well as those who have been impacted by traumatic experiences, possess a wealth of strengths—often untapped or unnoticed. At every possible opportunity, we can seek ways to identify strengths and build upon and celebrate them with the ultimate goal of reestablishing a child's sense of mastery, success and agency.

### Art Activities Related to Strengths and Empowerment
*Boundaries Exercise*

Adapted from Levine, n.d.a

**Art supplies:** My Body outline, My Body Sensations cards, mark-making tools (e.g. colored pencils, colored markers, pastels, paint, stickers), different-colored yarn.

**Instructions:** It is important to support children in repairing boundary ruptures so they can feel safe and contained. Have the child choose a color of yarn. You can provide simple psychoeducation and briefly describe boundaries to the child in a developmentally appropriate way. Invite the child to imagine the yarn represents their boundary, asking them to create a shape on the ground with the yarn. Invite the child to walk around the inside of their boundary, noticing any sensations or images that may arise. The child may want to create a mantra or embody a yoga pose to represent their boundary. Once the child has become acquainted with their boundary, invite them to show you on the My Body outline and My Body Sensations cards what they experienced.

**Reflection questions:**

- What sensations do you notice inside of your boundary?
- Is there anyone you would like to imagine with you inside (or outside) of your boundary?
- What gesture or movement would represent your boundary?
- Share a situation where you might need your boundary?

**Accommodations:** This activity can be done without the yarn, if that feels too overstimulating for the child. Simply use the My Body outline for this experience. If the child needs even more distance from their body, use pipe cleaners or clay.

**Extensions:**

- The boundary exercise can be used to establish a felt sense of safety, an embodied "yes" and "no." The child could imagine what it might feel like to have someone who "has their back" or who "hasn't had their back" walk toward their boundary. How might their boundary change with or without this person? Ask the child to record their experience using My Body Sensations cards and the My Body outline.
- See Chapter 8 for embodied boundary practices.

### Bilateral movement

Adapted from Malchiodi, 2020

**Art supplies:** 18 x 24 inch paper and any mark-making materials (e.g. colored pencils, colored markers, pastels).

**Instructions:** Bilateral movement means using both sides of the body for dance/movement or drawing/painting. Malchiodi (2020) proposes that bilateral movements can support children in sensory integration. It can be a grounding activity, providing ease and calm to heightened stress responses. Mark making with both hands can move attention away from uncomfortable sensations to a more action-oriented, self-empowered focus (Malchiodi, 2020). Demonstrate creating large circles with both arms while simultaneously crossing the midline. Invite the child to move slowly, then fast, forward and then backwards. Ask the child which movement they preferred, then have them choose two different colors (one in each hand) and replicate these movements several times on a large sheet of paper, making marks as they move.

**Reflection questions:**

- How did you know which movement felt most pleasant in your body?
- What sensations in your body let you know the movement felt pleasant?

**Accommodations:** In addition to demonstrating the bilateral movements, you can also mirror the movements. Have the child first follow your movements and then follow theirs. This provides an opportunity for co-regulation, attunement and leadership.

**Extensions:**

- Invite the child to give a title to their image.
- Have the child create the bilateral movements while listening to their favorite song.
- Ask the child to name ten action words to describe the image that resulted from their bilateral movement. You can work with the child to reduce the words to a phrase and create their personal mantra.
- Pair the bilateral movement with a yoga breath from the CALMM toolkit.
- See Chapter 4 for bilateral brain integration practices.

## CONCLUSION

My aim with this chapter was to provide information, activities and experiences that support the arts' role in connecting us to different sensory forms of expression, visual, auditory, tactile, interoceptive, proprioceptive and vestibular. Trauma-sensitive uses of the arts can either be a bottom-up (brain stem to cortex) or a top-down (cortex to brain stem) experience, depending on the needs of the child. For example, with a bottom-up approach, we can begin with the body's sensory and kinesthetic experiences such as yoga, movement or breathing, which naturally relax the mind and begin to tap into a deeper level of implicit experience; then we can move to art making, a more limbic experience; and finally transition to language, meaning and integration, which is mediated by the cortex. Not every child will work through all brain "areas" in a session, or even several sessions. And some might be more comfortable beginning with the narrative piece. Ultimately, if a child can access all three areas of their brain (brain stem, limbic area and cortex), a harmony of embodied intelligence emerges and becomes the foundation of trauma reparation and integration via the arts (Malchiodi, 2020).

When working therapeutically with the arts, we are looking for expression of the human condition. Therefore, we do not interpret or translate art images. It's important to leave opinions, judgments or critiques out when speaking with children about their art. We must learn how to be quiet and listen. Follow the art. Lead with openhearted curiosity, encourage children to "say more" and adopt a "Yes! and" mindset. Art speaks differently to different bodies. What piques your interest about a child's art may not be what piques theirs. Always ask. Not only does asking respect the child and the therapeutic relationship you have developed, but it also models healthy boundaries, speaks to the living consent and communicates the value and worth of the child's form of expression. When providing feedback on a child's art, it is important to use "I" language and speak of how you are impacted by their art. For example, you can use statements such as "I see," "I feel," "I imagine." Be mindful to hold loving, attuned, non-judgmental space for the child's sensory experience to emerge.

Children are individual beings who possess a wealth of resources waiting to be mined. Children are not problems that need to be fixed. If we listen, if we witness, if we hold space, children show us exactly what they need to succeed. It is the responsibility of the adults in their life to guide them in finding—and cultivating—their strengths and resources. The arts provide a shift away from what is not working to focus instead on how to build upon their strengths and resources. The arts are a way of making sense of our lives, growing our capacity and resilience. The greatest teachers I have had are my own children and my students. Watch. Listen. Learn. Children will always guide the way. We simply need to lead with curiosity and love.

---

**PAUSE AND REFLECT**

How might your grounded, regulated, loving presence support you in working with children with complex needs?

Invitation to draw, doodle, write, move and/or make sound in response to this question.

# Chapter 10

# Assessment and Developing a Therapeutic Protocol

When assessing a child or teen and developing a therapeutic protocol specific to their needs, rather than looking at each system as separate or individualized, we want to see from an integrated lens. Assessing from the framework of the Kosha model ensures that we are looking at all of the layers of the child's being, rather than just their physical challenges or faulty breathing patterns. As mentioned earlier, integration is the communication and working together of different systems to support homeostasis. Each layer in the Kosha model communicates with and impacts the others. When one is out of balance, it impacts the functioning of the other layers. When we come from a lens of nervous system regulation rather than "fixing" a child, we can better support them in moving through the world with more confidence, connection and curiosity.

As evidenced in the original ACE study (Felliti, *et al.*, 1998), prolonged and unmanaged stress in childhood can impact children's physical and mental wellbeing later on in life. In order to prevent children and teens from developing health problems such as heart disease, autoimmune conditions, digestive disorders and risk of early death, as well as mental health issues that lead to addiction and other unhealthy adaptive behaviors, we want to support them in learning tools to help them cope with stress and build their capacity and resilience. Rather than focusing on one physical challenge or one mental health diagnosis, we approach them from a nervous system perspective, looking at the whole child with an intention of integration and coherence of all the layers.

In this chapter I'll share my process in developing a therapeutic protocol, from intake to therapeutic co-facilitation.

## INTAKE PROCESS

The intake process is necessary in order to gather information about the child or teen, so that I have the background information to ensure safety and individualized support to meet their unique needs.

### Intake Form

The first step in the yoga therapy process is to have the parent (and child if they are able) complete the intake form. Teens may be able to complete the intake form on their own with some parental guidance. This is where I gather important information about the child or teen. The intake form encompasses the five koshas, gathering information about their physical, mental, emotional, social and spiritual (connection to authentic Self and the world around them) experience in the world.

- Medical history
- Primary/secondary disability (if applicable)
- Trauma history
- History of anxiety/depression
- Sensory needs
- Energy level
- Diet and sleep
- Communication style
- Learning style
- Behaviors that impact their daily life
- Relationships with family, peers and other community members
- Challenges
- Strengths and interests

### Parent/Child Interview

Following the review of the intake form, I conduct a parent/child interview. The interview is an opportunity to ask more specific questions and discuss with the parent/child/teen what their goals are for yoga therapy. I like to involve the child or teen in the goal setting as much as possible, so they feel a sense of autonomy and collaboration in the process. When a child or teen feels their voice is heard and they get to have a "say" in their therapy, there is more buy-in and more accountability for them to engage in the therapeutic experience.

### Assessment

Depending on the child's needs, there are several assessments I may choose to do. If the child presents as having sensory challenges, I have the parent complete a sensory questionnaire. This gives me helpful and important information with regard to their sensory system. I will also observe the child's response to specific sensory input and use that information to guide me in developing a protocol specific to their sensory needs. I also do a complete asana assessment which gives me insight into their physical strengths and challenges. This helps to guide my choices of asanas, movement and any supports they may need. I also use the neurodevelopmental sequence to assess a child following the kosha model. As I am doing the physical and sensory assessments and reviewing the intake information, these are the questions I am gathering answers to.

### Annamaya Kosha

- How do they move?
- How much body awareness do they have?
- What is their nutrition like?
- How much water do they drink?
- How is their sleep?
- What are they ingesting (television, social media, video games) and how are they digesting what they take in?

### Pranamaya Kosha

- How do they breathe?
- How do they communicate with others?
- Where are they blocked in relation to their chakras (safety, creativity, self-confidence, compassion for themselves and others, ability to express themselves, intuition, connection to their authentic Self)?

### Manomaya Kosha

- How do they think?
- How does their sensory system function?
- What is their mental and emotional state?

### Vijnanamaya Kosha

- How do they feel about themselves?
- Do they have healthy or unhealthy boundaries?
- Are they able to identify what they feel inside?

Anandamaya Kosha

- Do they have connected and meaningful relationships with others?
- Do they have supportive resources?
- How often do they connect with nature?
- Do they do things that spark joy in their life?
- Are they connected to their authentic Self?

This process does not happen in one session. It takes several sessions to gather enough information to create an informed and individualized protocol. In fact, the assessment is ongoing. As I am doing sessions with the child or teen, I am continually gathering information that will help guide me in our future sessions.

## Ongoing Observation and Data Collection
Following each session, I write notes, including any information that was gathered in regard to challenges, responses to specific practices, what I observed in terms of their nervous system state, what they expressed that they liked/disliked, any improvements in goal areas and any other noteworthy information.

## Working Towards Independence
The goal in yoga therapy is always moving towards self-empowerment and independence. What will often happen with my yoga therapy clients is that we will begin with weekly sessions in order to develop connection, trust and an intuitive sense of what to integrate in their protocol. After several months or even a year, depending on their needs, we may begin tapering the sessions to bi-weekly, then eventually doing monthly check-ins. Part of the yoga therapy focus is helping the child or teen practice and develop tools they can use in their home, school and community environments to support their wellbeing. What I have found to be so rewarding is when a child begins with weekly sessions and is able to develop a consistent practice at home either with the support of their family members or independently so they are not in need of such frequent sessions.

One example in particular is a 14-year-old, autistic girl who came to me for weekly sessions. She experienced significant anxiety and wanted to learn how to manage her anxiety and emotional outbursts in her school and community setting. Her intense anxiety was impacting her ability to develop healthy relationships with her peers and her ability to have positive experiences in the community with her family. As part of her protocol, I created short 20-minute video practices for her to do at home that reinforced the work we were doing in our sessions together. We discussed her attainable goal for her home practice and she committed to doing her yoga practice two times a week. She loved doing the practice videos so much that she was practicing three or four times a week! We eventually moved from weekly sessions to monthly check-ins. This is self-empowerment. I'll never forget what she said to me after doing her first home video practice. When she came back the following week for a session, she said, "I love doing the videos with you. It feels like you're with me and we are doing yoga together!" Heart melt…this is what it's all about—the power of connection! This doesn't mean that all of a sudden her challenges were gone. It just means that she now has a consistent practice that will support her nervous system regulation and a better understanding of her brain and body, along with tools to support her needs.

# A Closing Note

## SELF-COMPASSION AND SELF-CARE AS THE FACILITATOR OF HEALING

I would be remiss not to include the importance of self-care and tending to our own growth, healing and wellbeing if we intend to be facilitators of healing with children and teens.

Perhaps you are a parent, a grandparent, a caregiver, an educator, a therapist, a yoga teacher, a Somatic Experiencing practitioner, an embodied movement facilitator or just simply a human being seeking more wisdom and knowledge in caring for our greatest hope for our future—our children.

The greatest gift we can offer to our children is our own commitment to healing.

When we tend to the needs of our own inner children and their little wounded hearts, we break the cycles of abuse, shame, anger and grief, and we build our capacity to hold space for others.

When we have greater capacity, we have the energy, strength, patience and resilience to do our heart's work.

There is no need to be perfect. We are all human, finding our way in this beautiful, messy and unpredictable world.

What children desire most from us is authenticity, love, understanding and connection.

May we do our best and may we offer ourselves grace and understanding when we mess up.

May we strive to help all children feel seen, heard, loved and equally valued.

May we find peace in ourselves so we can spread peace and love to the children and families we serve.

## PAUSE AND REFLECT

How do you show up for yourself when it comes to self-care and your own daily practice? Take a moment to reflect on each practice and ideas or intentions of how you can tend to the ones that need tending.

- Self-compassion
- Self-care
- Resourcing
- Rest
- Daily Sadhana
- Sangha

Option to write your intentions or reflections in your journal.

A parting poem...

### HEART TENDRILS

*The heart does not exist in isolation*
*It nests between the lungs*
*Receiving comfort with each breath*
*Its tendrils spiral out*
*Searching for a place to expand*
*Reaching for connection*
*It is only when it is touched*
*In a harsh way*
*That it shrinks back*
*A self-preservation*
*With each careless word*
*It clings*
*But with tenderness*
*It grows stronger*
*Wraps itself around*
*And moves through*
*And there*
*Cradled in a bed of warmth and love*
*The healing begins*

Shawnee Thornton Hardy

# Resources

## TEACHER TRAININGS AND COURSES WITH SHAWNEE

Use the QR code or the link below.

www.asanasforautismandspecialneeds.com

www.yogatherapyforyouth.com

## SHOP FOR THE CALMM YOGA PRODUCTS

- Visual Yoga Toolkit
- Body Sensations Curriculum
- Supplementary Products
- Books

www.asanasforautismandspecialneeds.com/shop

## YOGA FOR SCOLIOSIS

happybackyoga.com

## SOMATIC EXPERIENCING TRAININGS

https://traumahealing.org

## INTERNATIONAL ASSOCIATION OF YOGA THERAPISTS
www.IAYT.org

## YOGA THERAPY ACCREDITED TRAINING
Optimal State with Amy Wheeler

https://amywheeler.com

# Contributor Biographies

**Shawnee Thornton Hardy** has worked with children and teens with complex needs for nearly three decades. She holds a Master's in Special Education, is a certified yoga therapist through the International Association of Yoga Therapists and a Somatic Experiencing practitioner through the Trauma Institute. Shawnee is the founder of Asanas for Autism and Special Needs and the founder/director of Yoga Therapy for Youth. She is passionate about making mind–body practices inclusive and accessible to all brains, bodies and abilities. She leads trainings internationally and throughout the US and offers one-to-one sessions in mind–body practices to support children and teens with complex needs, to include: autism, ADHD, neurodiversity, developmental disability, sensory processing challenges, communication difficulties, anxiety/depression and trauma. She is also the author of *Asanas for Autism and Special Needs: Yoga to Help Children with their Emotions, Self-Regulation and Body Awareness*. She combines her unique experience as an educational/behavioral specialist and her knowledge and passion for yoga and somatic practices in her work and teachings. Her heart's longing is in facilitating healing in the world.

**Rachel Krentzman**, PT, C-IAYT, is a physical therapist and yoga therapist. She is the author of two books: *Yoga for a Happy Back* and *Scoliosis, Yoga Therapy and the Art of Letting Go*. Rachel is the co-director of Wisdom-body Yoga Therapy, an 850-hour certified yoga therapy training in Israel and is an active advocate for integrating yoga into healthcare.

**Lior Zakaria Hikrey** is a certified Iyengar yoga teacher Junior 1 level 2 and an artist. Iyengar yoga is a precise, alignment-based method used to treat various skeletal problems. He lives in Ramat Gan, Israel.

**Ann Davis** is a trauma trained expressive arts and Somatic Experiencing practitioner with 30 years' combined experience in public health and education. She has extensive experience working with youth and families living with chronic stress and trauma. For several years she was the expressive arts therapist at a school for unhoused youth. Currently, she is the expressive arts therapist at a center for mental health and wellness where she provides individual and group sessions. Ann has an active visual arts practice which deeply informs her personal and professional practice.

# Bibliography

Algoe, S.B., Kurtz, L.E. & Grewen, K. (2017) "Oxytocin and social bonds: The role of oxytocin in perceptions of romantic partners' bonding behavior." *Psychological Science 28*, 12, 1763–1772. doi:10.1177/0956797617716922

Ali, F.E., Al-Bustan, M.A., Al-Busairi, W.A., Al-Mulla, F.A. & Esbaita, E.Y. (2006) "Cervical spine abnormalities associated with Down syndrome." *International Orthopaedics 30*, 4, 284–289. doi:10.1007/s00264-005-0070-y

Alluri, V., Toiviainen, P., Jääskeläinen, I. P., Glerean, E., Sams, M. & Brattico, E. (2012) "Large-scale brain networks emerge from dynamic processing of musical timbre, key and rhythm." *NeuroImage 59*, 4, 3677–3689. doi:10.1016/j.neuroimage.2011.11.019

Ambitious About Autism. (n.d.) "Repetitive behaviours and stimming." Accessed on 12/19/2022 at www.ambitiousaboutautism.org.uk/information-about-autism/behaviour/repetitive-behaviours-and-stimming

American Psychiatric Association (2022) *Diagnostic and Statistical Manual of Mental Disorders, Fifth Edition Text Revision DSM-5-TR*. Washington, DS: APA.

APA Dictionary of Psychology (n.d.) "Intergenerational trauma." Accessed on 12/19/2022 at https://dictionary.apa.org/intergenerational-trauma

Archer, R. (Host) (2022, April 8) The importance of healing centered aesthetic education with Dr. Judith Greer Essex (No. 106) [Audio podcast episode]. In *The Artful Leader*. https://podcasts.apple.com/us/podcast/106-the-importance-of-healing-centered/id1615123011?i=1000556619840

Arora, l. (2015) *Mudra: The Sacred Secret*. Yogsadhna LLC.

Asala, S.A. & Bower, A.J. (1986) "An electron microscope study of vagus nerve composition in the ferret." *Anatomy and Embryology 175*, 247–253. doi:10.1007/bf00389602

Assistant Secretary for Public Affairs (ASPA) (2022, March 14) "New HHS Study in JAMA Pediatrics Shows Significant Increases in Children Diagnosed with Mental Health Conditions from 2016 to 2020." Accessed on 12/16//2022 at www.hhs.gov/about/news/2022/03/14/new-hhs-study-jama-pediatrics-shows-significant-increases-children-diagnosed-mental-health-conditions-2016-2020.html

Ayres, J.A. (1972) "Treatment of sensory integrative dysfunction." *Australian Occupational Therapy Journal 19*, 2, 88. doi:10.1111/j.1440-1630.1972.tb00547.x

Backes, E.P. & Bonnie, R.J. (Eds.) (2019) *The Promise of Adolescence: Realizing Opportunity for All Youth*. Washington, DC: National Academies Press. Accessed on 12/19/2022 at www.ncbi.nlm.nih.gov/books/NBK545476

Bailey, R. (2021, August 17) "The olfactory system and your sense of smell." ThoughtCo. Accessed on 12/19/2022 at www.thoughtco.com/olfactory-system-4066176

Barks, C. (2004) *The Essential Rumi: reissue*. San Francisco, CA: HarperOne.

Bart, O., Bar-Haim, Y., Weizman, E., Levin, M., Sadeh, A. & Mintz, M. (2009) "Balance treatment ameliorates anxiety and increases self-esteem in children with comorbid anxiety and balance disorder." *Research in Developmental Disabilities 30*, 3, 486–495. doi:10.1016/j. ridd.2008.07.008

Billman, G.E. (2020) "Homeostasis: The underappreciated and far too often ignored central organizing principle of physiology." *Frontiers in Physiology 11*. doi:10.3389/fphys.2020.00200

Blomberg, H. & Dempsey, M. (2011) *Movements that Heal: Rhythmic Movement Training and Primitive Reflex Integration*. Independently published.

Bordoni, B., Mankowski, N.L. & Daly, D.T. (2022) "Neuroanatomy, Cranial Nerve 8 (Vestibulocochlear)." StatPearls [Internet]. Treasure Island, FL: StatPearls Publishing. Accessed on 12/19/2022 at www.ncbi.nlm.nih.gov/books/NBK537359

Brennan, D. (2006, February 2) "Mental illness in children." WebMD. Accessed on 12/16/2022 at www.webmd.com/mental-health/mental-illness-children

Brewer, R., Murphy, J. & Bird, G. (2021) "Atypical interoception as a common risk factor for psychopathology: A review." *Neuroscience and Biobehavioral Reviews 130*, 470–508. doi:10.1016/j.neubiorev.2021.07.036

Bruni, M. (2016) *Fine Motor Skills in Children with Down Syndrome, Third Edition*. Bethesda, MD: Woodbine House.

Bundy, A.C. & Murray, A.E. (2002) "Sensory Integration: A. Jean Ayres' Theory Revisited." In A C. Bundy, S.J. Lane & E.A. Murray (Eds.) *Sensory Integration: Theory and Practice* (2nd ed., pp.3–33). Philadelphia, PA: F.A. Davis.

Burger, M., Coetzee, W., du Plessis, L.Z., Geldenhuys, L. *et al.* (2019) "The effectiveness of Schroth exercises in adolescents with idiopathic scoliosis: A systematic review and meta-analysis." *South African Journal of Physiotherapy 75*, 1, 904. doi:10.4102/sajp.v75i1.904

Cafasso, J. (2018, September 18) "What is synaptic pruning?" Healthline. Accessed on 12/19/2022 at www.healthline.com/health/synaptic-pruning

Carozza, S. & Leong, V. (2021) "The role of affectionate caregiver touch in early neurodevelopment and parent–infant interactional synchrony." *Frontiers in Neuroscience 14*. doi:10.3389/fnins.2020.613378

CASEL (2022, August 3) "What is the CASEL framework?" Accessed on 12/19/2022 at https:// casel.org/fundamentals-of-sel/what-is-the-casel-framework

Cedars Sinai (n.d.) "Childhood apraxia of speech." Accessed on 12/19/2022 at www.cedars-sinai. org/health-library/diseases-and-conditions---pediatrics/c/childhood-apraxia-of-speech. html

Centers for Disease Control and Prevention (2022, November 28) "Improving access to children's mental health care." Accessed on 12/16/2022 at www.cdc.gov/childrensmentalhealth/access. html

Cerebral Palsy Guide (2022, April 15) "Does high muscle tone always indicate cerebral palsy?" Accessed on 12/19/2022 at www.cerebralpalsyguide.com/blog/high-muscle-tone

Craig, A.D. (2009) *How Do You Feel? An Interoceptive Moment with Your Neurobiological Self*. Princeton, NJ: Princeton University Press.

Damasio, A. (2010) *Self Comes to Mind: Constructing the Conscious Brain*. New York, NY: William Heinemann.

Damasio, A.R. (1994) *Descartes' Error: Emotion, Reason, and the Human Brain*. New York, NY: Grosset/Putnam.

Damasio, A.R. (1996) "The somatic marker hypothesis and the possible functions of the prefrontal cortex." *Philosophical Transactions of the Royal Society of London: Series B, Biological Sciences 351*, 1346, 413–1420.

Dana, D. (2018) *The Polyvagal Theory in Therapy: Engaging the Rhythm of Regulation*. New York, NY: W.W. Norton & Company.

Dana, D. (2020) *Polyvagal Flip Chart: Understanding the Science of Safety*. New York, NY: W.W. Norton & Company.

Dana, D. (2021) *Anchored: How to Befriend Your Nervous System Using Polyvagal Theory*. Louisville, CO: Sounds True.

Desikachar, T.K.V. (1999) The Heart of Yoga: Developing a Personal Practice. Rochester, VT: Inner Traditions.

Dreisoerner. A., Junker, N.M., Schlotz, W., Heimrich, J. *et al.* (2021) "Self-soothing touch and being hugged reduce cortisol responses to stress: A randomized controlled trial on stress, physical touch, and social identity." *Comprehensive Psychoneuroendocrinology 8*, 100091. doi:10.1016/j.cpnec.2021.100091

Ekholm, B., Spulber, S. & Adler, M. (2020) "A randomized controlled study of weighted chain blankets for insomnia in psychiatric disorders." *Journal of Clinical Sleep Medicine 16*, 9, 1567–1577. doi:10.5664/jcsm.8636

Evan, S., Galantino, M.L., Lung, K. & Zeltzer, L. (2016) "Yoga Therapy for Pediatrics." In S.B.S Khalsa, L. Cohen, T. McCall & S. Telles (Eds.) *The Principles and Practices of Yoga in Healthcare*. Pencaitland: Handspring Publishing.

Farhi, D. (1996) *The Breathing Book: Good Health and Vitality Through Essential Breath Work*. New York, NY: St. Martin's Press.

Felliti, V.J., Anda, R.F., Nordenberg, D., Williamson, D.F. *et al.* (1998) "Relationship of childhood abuse and household dysfunction to many of the leading causes of death in adults. The Adverse Childhood Experiences (ACE) Study." *American Journal of Preventative Medicine 14*, 4, 245–258.

Field, T. (2010) "Touch for socioemotional and physical well-being: A review." *Developmental Review 30*, 4, 367–383. doi:10.1016/j.dr.2011.01.001

Fishman, L.M., Groessl, E.J. & Sherman, K.J. (2014) "Serial case reporting yoga for idiopathic and degenerative scoliosis." *Global Advances in Health and Medicine 3*, 5, 16–21. doi:10.7453/gahmj.2013.064

Foley, J.O. & DuBois, F.S. (1937) "Quantitative studies of the vagus nerve in the cat. I. The ratio of sensory to motor fibers." *The Journal of Comparative Neurology 67*, 1, 49–67. doi:10.1002/cne.900670104

Galantino, M.L., Galbavy, R. & Quinn, L. (2008) "Therapeutic effects of yoga for children: A systematic review of the literature." *Pediatric Physical Therapy 20*, 1, 66–80 doi:10.1097/PEP.0b013e31815f1208

Goldman, J. (2022) *Healing Sounds: The Power of Harmonics* (4th ed.). Healing Arts Press.

Gotter, A. (2018, March 23) "Pursed lip breathing." Healthline. Accessed on 12/19/2022 at www.healthline.com/health/pursed-lip-breathing

Govender, S. (2015, October 13) "Is crying good for you?" WebMD. Accessed on 12/19/2022 at www.webmd.com/balance/features/is-crying-good-for-you#:%7E:text=%22%5BCrying%5D%20activates%20the%20parasympathetic,to%20cultural%20or%20personal%20reasons

Graham. J. (2021, August 12) "Bulletin #4356, Children and brain development: What we know about how children learn." Cooperative Extension Publications, University of Maine. Accessed on 12/19/2022 at https://extension.umaine.edu/publications/4356e

Graphics, O. (2020) "The Yoga Sutras of Patanjali." Accessed on 04/11/2023 at https://worldyogainstitute.org/2020/05/17/the-yoga-sutras-of-patanjali/

Guglielmo, A., Tourville, J. & Potter, G. (2018) *How to Build a Hug: Temple Grandin and Her Amazing Squeeze Machine*. Atheneum Books for Young Readers.

Harvard School of Public Health (2018, June 22) "The importance of hydration." Accessed on 12/19/2022 at www.hsph.harvard.edu/news/hsph-in-the-news/the-importance-of-hydration/#:%7E:text=Drinking%20enough%20water%20each%20day,quality%2C%20cognition%2C%20and%20mood

Helbert, K. (2019) *The Chakras in Grief and Trauma: A Tantric Guide to Energetic Wholeness*. London: Singing Dragon.

Herrild, B. (2022) "Tips for Doing Art with Your Neuro-Divergent Child." Accessed on 1/26/2023 at https://outsidetheboxcreation.com/tips-for-doing-art-with-your-neuro-divergent-kiddo/

IAYT (n.d.) "Contemporary definitions of yoga therapy: IAYT definition." Accessed on 1/26/2023 at www.iayt.org/page/ContemporaryDefiniti

Jain, R. (2019) "A Complete Guide To The Three Gunas Of Nature." Arhanta Yoga Blog. Arhanta Yoga Ashrams. Accessed on 04/11/2023 at https://www.arhantayoga.org/blog/sattva-rajas-tamas-gunas

James-Palmer, A., Anderson, E.Z., Zucker, L., Kofman, Y. & Daneault, J.F. (2020) "Yoga as an intervention for the reduction of symptoms of anxiety and depression in children and adolescents: A systematic review." *Frontiers in Pediatrics 2020*, 8, 78. doi:10.3389%2Ffped.2020.00078

Jiang, S., Postovit, L., Cattaneo, A., Binder, E.B. & Aitchison, K.J. (2019) "Epigenetic modifications in stress response genes associated with childhood trauma." *Frontiers in Psychiatry 10*. https://doi.org/10.3389/fpsyt.2019.00808

Johnson, S.B., Blum, R.W., & Giedd, J.N. (2009) "Adolescent maturity and the brain: The promise and pitfalls of neuroscience research in adolescent health policy." *Journal of Adolescent Health 45*, 3, 216–221. doi:10.1016/j.jadohealth.2009.05.016

Kain, K.L. & Terrell, S.J. (2018) *Nurturing Resilience: Helping Clients Move Forward from Developmental Trauma—An Integrative Somatic Approach.* Berkeley, CA: North Atlantic Books.

Khalsa, S.B.S. & Butzer, B. (2016) "Yoga in school settings: A research review." *Annals of the New York Academy of Sciences 1373*, 1, 45–55. doi:10.1111/nyas.13025

Kuhfuß, M., Maldei, T., Hetmanek, A. & Baumann, N. (2012) "Somatic experiencing – effectiveness and key factors of a body-oriented trauma therapy: A scoping literature review." *European Journal of Psychotraumatology 12*(1),1929023. doi:10.1080/20008198.2021.1929023

Landreth, G. (2002) *Play Therapy. The Art of the Relationship.* New York, NY: Routledge.

Lang, R., O'Reilly, M., Healy, O., Rispoli, M. *et al.* (2012) "Sensory integration therapy for autism spectrum disorders: A systematic review." Database of Abstracts of Reviews of Effects (DARE): Quality-assessed Reviews [Internet]. York (UK): Centre for Reviews and Dissemination. Accessed on 12/19/2022 at www.ncbi.nlm.nih.gov/books/NBK100214

Lenzen, M. (2005) "Feeling our emotions (interview with Antonio R. Damasio)." *Scientific American*, April 1. Accessed on 1/26/2023 at www.scientificamerican.com/article/feeling-our-emotions

Levine, E.G. (2015) *Play and Art in Child Psychotherapy: An Expressive Arts Therapy Approach.* London: Jessica Kingsley Publishers.

Levine, P.A. (2008) *Healing Trauma. A Pioneering Program for Restoring the Wisdom of Your Body.* Boulder, CO: Sounds True.

Levine, P.A. (n.d.a) *Somatic Experiencing Training Manual.* Boulder, CO: Foundation for Human Enrichment.

Levine, P.A., PhD. (n.d.b) "About Dr Levine." Ergos Institute of Somatic Education. Accessed on 1/26/2023 at www.somaticexperiencing.com/about-peter

Levine, P.A. & Kline, M. (2007) *Trauma Through a Child's Eyes: Awakening the Ordinary Miracle of Healing.* Berkeley, CA: North Atlantic Books.

Lloyd. S. (2020) *Building Sensorimotor Systems in Children with Developmental Trauma: A Model for Practice.* London: Jessica Kingsley Publishers.

Losinski, M., Sanders, S.A. & Wiseman, N.M. (2016) "Examining the use of deep touch pressure to improve the educational performance of students with disabilities: A meta-analysis." *Research and Practice for Persons with Severe Disabilities 41*, 1, 3–18. doi:10.1177/1540796915624889

McEwen, B.S. & Wingfield, J.C. (2007) "Allostasis and Allostatic Load." In G. Fink (ed.) *Encyclopedia of Stress* (2nd edn). Cambridge, MA: Academic Press. doi:10.1016/B978-012373947-6.00025-8

McLaughlin, K. (2022) "Posttraumatic stress disorder in children and adolescents: Epidemiology, pathogenesis, clinical manifestations, course, assessment, and diagnosis." UpToDate. Accessed on 1/26/2023 at www.uptodate.com/contents/posttraumatic-stress-disorder-in-children-and-adolescents-epidemiology-pathogenesis-clinical-manifestations-course-assessment-and-diagnosis/print

McLeod, S. (2014) "Carl Rogers' humanistic theory of personality development." SimplyPsychology. Accessed on 1/26/2023 at www.simplypsychology.org/carl-rogers.html

McNiff, S. (2011) "Artistic expressions as primary modes of inquiry." *British Journal of Guidance and Counselling 39*(5), 385–396.

Malchiodi, C. (2019) "The Power of Expressive Arts: A Three-Part Process for Engaging the Body in Therapy." Accessed on 1/26/2023 at www.psychotherapynetworker.org/blog/details/1607/the-power-of-expressive-arts

Malchiodi, C. (2020) *Trauma and Expressive Arts Therapy: Brain, Body, and Imagination in the Healing Process.* New York, NY: Guildford Press.

Mallorquí-Bagué, N., Garfinkel, S.N., Engels, M., Eccles, J.A. *et al.* (2014) "Neuroimaging and psychophysiological investigation of the link between anxiety, enhanced affective reactivity and interoception in people with joint hypermobility." *Frontiers in Psychology 5.* doi:10.3389/fpsyg.2014.01162

Massachusetts General Hospital (2019, June 12) "Atlanto-axial instability (AAI): What you need to know." Accessed on 12/19/2022 at www.massgeneral.org/children/down-syndrome/atlantoaxial-instability-aai

Messmer, E.M. (2009) "Emotionale Tränen [Emotional tears]." *Ophthalmologe 106*, 7, 593–602. doi:10.1007/s00347-009-1966-5

Miller, R. (n.d.) "Yoga therapy: Definition, perspective and principles." International Association of Yoga Therapists. Accessed on 12/19/2022 at www.iayt.org/page/YogaTherapyDefinitio

Miller, R. (2012). *The Samkhya Karika.* San Rafael, CA: Integrative Restoration Institute.

Mills, K.L., Goddings, A.L., Herting, M.M., Meuwese, R. *et al.* (2016) "Structural brain development between childhood and adulthood: Convergence across four longitudinal samples." *NeuroImage 141*, 273–281. doi:10.1016/j.neuroimage.2016.07.044

Moszeik, E.N., von Oertzen, T. & Renner, K.H. (2020) "Effectiveness of a short Yoga Nidra meditation on stress, sleep, and well-being in a large and diverse sample." *Current Psychology 41*, 8, 5272–5286. doi:10.1007/s12144-020-01042-2

National Institute of Neurological Disorders and Stroke (n.d.) "Apraxia." Accessed on 12/19/2022 at www.ninds.nih.gov/health-information/disorders/apraxia

National Institute of Neurological Disorders and Stroke (n.d.) "Hypertonia." Accessed on 12/19/2022 at www.ninds.nih.gov/health-information/disorders/hypertonia

National Institute on Deafness and Other Communication Disorders (2022, March 16) "How do we hear?". Accessed on 12/19/2022 at www.nidcd.nih.gov/health/how-do-we-hear

Neurodiversity Hub (n.d.) "What is neurodiversity?" Accessed on 12/19/2022 at www.neurodiversityhub.org/what-is-neurodiversity

Newman, T. (2017, December 8) "What is dyspraxia?" Medical News Today. Accessed on 12/19/2022 at www.medicalnewstoday.com/articles/151951#dyspraxia_symptoms

Page, L.J., Page, L.L., Rezek, S. & Barbosa, C.E. (2013) *Mudras for Healing and Transformation.* Integrative Yoga Therapy.

Patañjali. (1975) *The Yoga Sutras of Patanjali: the book of the spiritual man: an interpretation.* London: Watkins.

Perry, B. (2020) "4. Regulate, Relate, Reason (Sequence of Engagement): Neurosequential Network Stress & Trauma Series" [Video]. Accessed on 1/26/2023 at www.youtube.com/watch?v=LNuxy7FxEVk

Perry, B.D. and Szalavitz, M. (2017) *The Boy Who Was Raised as a Dog: And Other Stories from a Child Psychiatrist's Notebook. What Traumatized Children Can Teach Us About Loss, Love, and Healing.* London: Basic Books.

Perry, B. & Winfrey, O. (2021) *What Happened to You? Conversations on Trauma, Resilience, and Healing.* New York, NY: Flatiron Books.

Porges, S.W. (2017) *The Pocket Guide to the Polyvagal Theory: The Transformative Power of Feeling Safe.* New York, NY: W.W. Norton & Company.

Porges, S.W. (2021a) *Polyvagal Safety: Attachment, Communication, Self-Regulation.* New York, NY: W.W. Norton & Company.

Porges, S.W. (2021b) "Polyvagal theory: A biobehavioral journey to sociality." Comprehensive Psychoneuroendocrinology 7. doi:10.1016/j.cpnec.2021.100069

Porges, S.W. (2022) "Polyvagal theory: A science of safety." *Frontiers in Integrative Neuroscience* 16. doi:10.3389/fnint.2022.871227

Powell, A. (2019, April 27) "The Funga Alafia (Fanga) Song—Part 2 (Lyrics)." Pancocojams. Accessed on 12/19/2022 at https://pancocojams.blogspot.com/2011/11/funga-alafia-fanga-song-part-2-lyrics.html

Rothschild, B. (2000) *The Body Remembers: The Psychophysiology of Trauma and Trauma Treatment.* New York, NY: W.W. Norton & Company.

Schneck, D. & Berger, D. (2006) *The Music Effect: Music Physiology and Clinical Applications.* London: Jessica Kingsley Publishers.

Schneider, A. & Cooper, N.J. (2019) "A brief history of the chakras in human body." Pennsylvania State University. doi:10.13140/RG.2.2.17372.00646

Scoliosis Research Society (n.d.) "Adolescent Idiopathic Scoliosis." Accessed on 12/19/2022 at www.srs.org/patients-and-families/conditions-and-treatments/parents/scoliosis/adolescent-idiopathic-scoliosis

Shah, S. (2020, July 30) "How to make the Yamas and Niyamas work for you in the modern world." The Art of Living. Accessed on 1/26/2023 at www.artofliving.org/us-en/yoga/beginners/yamas-niyamas

Siegel, D.J. (1999). *The Developing Mind: Toward a Neurobiology of Interpersonal Experience.* New York, NY: Guilford Press.

Siegel, D. J. (2014) "Pruning, Mylenation and the Remodeling Adolescent Brain." *Psychology Today*, February 4. Accessed on 12/19/2022 at www.psychologytoday.com/us/blog/inspire-rewire/201402/pruning-myelination-and-the-remodeling-adolescent-brain

Siegel, D.J. (2015) *Brainstorm: The Power and Purpose of the Teenage Brain.* New York, NY: Jeremy P. Tarcher/Penguin.

Siegel, D.J. & Bryson, T.P. (2012) *The Whole-Brain Child: 12 Proven Strategies to Nurture Your Child's Developing Mind.* London: Constable & Robinson.

Siegel, D.J., Siegel, M.W. & Parker, S.C. (2016) "Internal Education and the Roots of Resilience: Relationships and Reflection as the New R's of Education." In K.A. Schonert-Reichl & R.W. Roeser (eds) *Handbook of Mindfulness in Education: Integrating Theory and Research into Practice.* New York, NY: Springer Science+Business Media.

Simon, K.C., McDevitt, E.A., Ragano, R. & Mednick, S.C. (2022) "Progressive muscle relaxation increases slow-wave sleep during a daytime nap." *Journal of Sleep Research 31*, 5. doi:10.1111/jsr.13574

Somatic Experiencing® International (n.d.) "SE 101: What is Somatic Experiencing®?" Accessed on 1/26/2023 at https://traumahealing.org/se-101

Stoler-Miller B. (1998) *Yoga: Discipline of Freedom.* New York, NY: Bantam Books.

Stoler-Miller B. (2004) *The Bhagavad-Gita.* New York, NY: Bantam Classics.

Stoppler, M.C. (2005, May 23) "Progressive muscle relaxation for stress and insomnia." WebMD. Accessed on 12/19/2022 at www.webmd.com/sleep-disorders/muscle-relaxation-for-stress-insomnia

Streeter, C.C., Whitfield, T.H., Owen, L., Rein, T. *et al.* (2010) "Effects of yoga versus walking on mood, anxiety, and brain GABA levels: A randomized controlled MRS study." *Journal of Alternative and Complementary Medicine 16*, 11, 1145–1152. doi:10.1089/acm.2010.0007

Sullivan, M.B., Erb, M., Schmalzl, L., Moonaz, S., Noggle Taylor, J. & Porges, S.W. (2018) "Yoga therapy and Polyvagal Theory: The convergence of traditional wisdom and contemporary neuroscience for self-regulation and resilience." *Frontiers in Human Neuroscience 2018*, 12, 67. https://doi.org/10.3389/fnhum.2018.00067

Sullivan, M.B. & Robertson, L.C.H. (2020). *Understanding Yoga Therapy: Applied Philosophy and Science for Health and Well-Being.* New York, NY: Routledge.

The Philadelphia ACE Project (n.d.) Philadelphia ACE Survey. Accessed on 12/19/2022 at www.philadelphiaaces.org/philadelphia-ace-survey

Tougaw, J. (2020, April 18) "Neurodiversity: The movement." Psychology Today. Accessed on 12/19/2022 at www.psychologytoday.com/us/blog/the-elusive-brain/202004/neurodiversity-the-movement

Toussaint, L., Nguyen, Q.A., Roettger, C., Dixon, K. *et al.* (2021) "Effectiveness of progressive muscle relaxation, deep breathing, and guided imagery in promoting psychological and physiological states of relaxation." *Evidence-Based Complementary and Alternative Medicine 2021*, 5924040. doi:10.1155/2021/5924040

U.S. Department of Veterans Affairs (n.d.) "PTSD for children 6 years and younger." Accessed on 12/19/2022 at www.ptsd.va.gov/professional/treat/specific/ptsd_child_under6.asp#two

Van der Kolk, B.A. (2015) *The Body Keeps the Score: Brain, Mind, and Body in the Healing of Trauma.* New York, NY: Penguin Books.

Van der Kolk, B. (2021) "What is trauma? The author of 'The Body Keeps the Score' explains." Big Think, October 20. https://bigthink.com/series/the-big-think-interview/what-is-trauma

Vinney, C. (2019, October 24) "What is attachment theory? Definition and stages." ThoughtCo. Accessed on 12/19/2022 at www.thoughtco.com/attachment-theory-4771954

Weaver, L.L. & Darragh, A.R. (2015) "Systematic review of yoga interventions for anxiety reduction among children and adolescents." *American Journal of Occupational Therapy 69*, 6, 6906180070p1–6906180070p9. doi:10.5014/ajot.2015.020115

Websters Dictionary 1828. (n.d.). "Discernment." Accessed on 12/19/2022 at https://webstersdictionary1828.com/Dictionary/discernment

Weintraub, A. (2010, December) "Breath of Joy." Yoga International. Accessed on 12/19/2022 at https://yogatherapyalacarte.files.wordpress.com/2019/02/breath-of-joy.pdf

Weir, K. (2020, April 1) "Nurtured by nature." American Psychological Association. Accessed on 12/19/2022 at www.apa.org/monitor/2020/04/nurtured-nature

Whitney, D.G. & Peterson, M.D. (2019) "US national and state-level prevalence of mental health disorders and disparities of mental health care use in children." *JAMA Pediatrics 173*, 4, 389–391. doi:10.1001/jamapediatrics.2018.5399

Wikipedia (2022a) "Allostatic load." Accessed on 12/19/2022 at https://en.wikipedia.org/w/index.php?title=Allostatic_load&oldid=1101824755

Wikipedia (2022b) "Interoception." Accessed on 12/19/2022 at https://en.wikipedia.org/wiki/Interoception

Wood, C. (2017) *Yardsticks: Child and Adolescent Development Ages 4–14* (4th ed.). Turner Falls, MA: Center for Responsible Schools.

# Subject Index

Note: illustrations are referenced by page numbers in *italics*

# Author Index